SECTION 1:

AIRWAY MANAGEMENT

1. a b c d e
2. a b c d e
3. a b c d e
4. a b c d e
5. a b c d e

SECTION 2:

ANESTHESIOLOGY

6. a b c d e
7. a b c d e
8. a b c d e
9. a b c d e

SECTION 3:

CARDIOVASCULAR

10. a b c d e
11. a b c d e
12. a b c d e
13. a b c d e
14. a b c d e
15. a b c d e
16. a b c d e
17. a b c d e
18. a b c d e
19. a b c d e
20. a b c d e
21. a b c d e
22. a b c d e
23. a b c d e
24. a b c d e
25. a b c d e
26. a b c d e
27. a b c d e
28. a b c d e
29. a b c d e
30. a b c d e
31. a b c d e
32. a b c d e
33. a b c d e

SECTION 4:

ENVIRONMENTAL INJURY

34. a b c d e
35. a b c d e
36. a b c d e
37. a b c d e
38. a b c d e

SECTION 5:

GASTROINTESTINAL

39. a b c d e
40. a b c d e
41. a b c d e
42. a b c d e
43. a b c d e
44. a b c d e
45. a b c d e

SECTION 6:

HEMATOLOGIC

46. a b c d e
47. a b c d e
48. a b c d e
49. a b c d e
50. a b c d e
51. a b c d e
52. a b c d e
53. a b c d e

SECTION 7:

HEMODYNAMIC MONITORING

54. a b c d e
55. a b c d e
56. a b c d e
57. a b c d e
58. a b c d e
59. a b c d e
60. a b c d e
61. a b c d e
62. a b c d e
63. a b c d e
64. a b c d e
65. a b c d e
66. a b c d e
67. a b c d e
68. a b c d e
69. a b c d e
70. a b c d e
71. a b c d e
72. a b c d e
73. a b c d e
74. a b c d e
75. a b c d e
76. a b c d e
77. a b c d e
78. a b c d e
79. a b c d e
80. a b c d e
81. a b c d e
82. a b c d e
83. a b c d e
84. a b c d e
85. a b c d e
86. a b c d e
87. a b c d e
88. a b c d e
89. a b c d e
90. a b c d e
91. a b c d e
92. a b c d e
93. a b c d e
94. a b c d e
95. a b c d e
96. a b c d e
97. a b c d e
98. a b c d e
99. a b c d e
100. a b c d e
101. a b c d e
102. a b c d e

ANSWER SHEET (circle correct answer)

103. a b c d e
104. a b c d e
105. a b c d e
106. a b c d e
107. a b c d e
108. a b c d e
109. a b c d e

SECTION 8:

INFECTIOUS DISEASE/ IMMUNOLOGIC

110. a b c d e
111. a b c d e
112. a b c d e
113. a b c d e
114. a b c d e
115. a b c d e
116. a b c d e
117. a b c d e
118. a b c d e
119. a b c d e
120. a b c d e
121. a b c d e
122. a b c d e
123. a b c d e
124. a b c d e
125. a b c d e
126. a b c d e
127. a b c d e
128. a b c d e
129. a b c d e
130. a b c d e
131. a b c d e
132. a b c d e
133. a b c d e
134. a b c d e

SECTION 9:

METABOLIC/ENDOCRINOLOGIC

135. a b c d e
136. a b c d e
137. a b c d e
138. a b c d e
139. a b c d e
140. a b c d e
141. a b c d e
142. a b c d e
143. a b c d e
144. a b c d e
145. a b c d e
146. a b c d e
147. a b c d e
148. a b c d e
149. a b c d e
150. a b c d e
151. a b c d e
152. a b c d e
153. a b c d e
154. a b c d e
155. a b c d e

SECTION 10:

NEUROLOGIC

156. a b c d e
157. a b c d e
158. a b c d e
159. a b c d e
160. a b c d e
161. a b c d e
162. a b c d e
163. a b c d e
164. a b c d e
165. a b c d e
166. a b c d e
167. a b c d e
168. a b c d e
169. a b c d e
170. a b c d e
171. a b c d e
172. a b c d e
173. a b c d e
174. a b c d e
175. a b c d e
176. a b c d e
177. a b c d e
178. a b c d e
179. a b c d e
180. a b c d e
181. a b c d e
182. a b c d e
183. a b c d e
184. a b c d e
185. a b c d e
186. a b c d e

SECTION 11:

OBSTETRIC

187. a b c d e
188. a b c d e
189. a b c d e

SECTION 12:

PEDIATRIC/NEONATOLOGY

190. a b c d e
191. a b c d e
192. a b c d e
193. a b c d e
194. a b c d e

SECTION 13:

PHARMACOLOGY

195. a b c d e
196. a b c d e
197. a b c d e
198. a b c d e
199. a b c d e
200. a b c d e
201. a b c d e
202. a b c d e
203. a b c d e
204. a b c d e
205. a b c d e
206. a b c d e

207. a b c d e
208. a b c d e
209. a b c d e
210. a b c d e
211. a b c d e
212. a b c d e
213. a b c d e
214. a b c d e
215. a b c d e
216. a b c d e
217. a b c d e
218. a b c d e
219. a b c d e
220. a b c d e
221. a b c d e
222. a b c d e
223. a b c d e
224. a b c d e
225. a b c d e
226. a b c d e
227. a b c d e
228. a b c d e
229. a b c d e
230. a b c d e
231. a b c d e
232. a b c d e
233. a b c d e
234. a b c d e
235. a b c d e
236. a b c d e
237. a b c d e
238. a b c d e

SECTION 14:

POISONING/DRUG OVERDOSE

239. a b c d e
240. a b c d e
241. a b c d e
242. a b c d e
243. a b c d e
244. a b c d e
245. a b c d e
246. a b c d e
247. a b c d e
248. a b c d e
249. a b c d e
250. a b c d e
251. a b c d e
252. a b c d e
253. a b c d e
254. a b c d e
255. a b c d e
256. a b c d e
257. a b c d e
258. a b c d e
259. a b c d e
260. a b c d e

SECTION 15:

PULMONARY

261. a b c d e
262. a b c d e
263. a b c d e
264. a b c d e
265. a b c d e
266. a b c d e
267. a b c d e
268. a b c d e
269. a b c d e
270. a b c d e
271. a b c d e
272. a b c d e
273. a b c d e
274. a b c d e
275. a b c d e
276. a b c d e
277. a b c d e
278. a b c d e
279. a b c d e
280. a b c d e
281. a b c d e
282. a b c d e
283. a b c d e
284. a b c d e
285. a b c d e
286. a b c d e
287. a b c d e
288. a b c d e
289. a b c d e
290. a b c d e
291. a b c d e
292. a b c d e
293. a b c d e
294. a b c d e
295. a b c d e
296. a b c d e
297. a b c d e
298. a b c d e
299. a b c d e
300. a b c d e
301. a b c d e
302. a b c d e
303. a b c d e

SECTION 16:

RADIOLOGY/IMAGING

304. a b c d e
305. a b c d e
306. a b c d e
307. a b c d e
308. a b c d e
309. a b c d e
310. a b c d e
311. a b c d e
312. a b c d e
313. a b c d e
314. a b c d e
315. a b c d e
316. a b c d e
317. a b c d e

ANSWER SHEET (circle correct answer)

SECTION 17:

RENAL/FLUIDS/ELECTROLYTES

318. a b c d e
319. a b c d e
320. a b c d e
321. a b c d e
322. a b c d e
323. a b c d e
324. a b c d e
325. a b c d e
326. a b c d e
327. a b c d e
328. a b c d e
329. a b c d e
330. a b c d e
331. a b c d e
332. a b c d e
333. a b c d e
334. a b c d e
335. a b c d e
336. a b c d e
337. a b c d e
338. a b c d e

SECTION 18:

RESUSCITATION

339. a b c d e
340. a b c d e
341. a b c d e
342. a b c d e
343. a b c d e
344. a b c d e

SECTION 19:

SURGERY

345. a b c d e
346. a b c d e
347. a b c d e
348. a b c d e
349. a b c d e
350. a b c d e
351. a b c d e
352. a b c d e
353. a b c d e
354. a b c d e
355. a b c d e
356. a b c d e

SECTION 20:

TRAUMA

357. a b c d e
358. a b c d e
359. a b c d e
360. a b c d e
361. a b c d e
362. a b c d e
363. a b c d e
364. a b c d e
365. a b c d e
366. a b c d e
367. a b c d e
368. a b c d e
369. a b c d e
370. a b c d e
371. a b c d e
372. a b c d e
373. a b c d e
374. a b c d e
375. a b c d e
376. a b c d e
377. a b c d e
378. a b c d e
379. a b c d e
380. a b c d e

SOCIETY OF CRITICAL CARE MEDICINE

SELF-ASSESSMENT IN MULTIDISCIPLINARY CRITICAL CARE: A COMPREHENSIVE REVIEW

Edited By:
R. Phillip Dellinger, MD
Robert W. Taylor, MD

The Society of Critical Care Medicine Comprehensive Review has resulted from the efforts of many contributors. It is intended to represent the body of knowledge which is necessary in the care of the critically ill patient.

SCCM has no knowledge of the content of any certifying examination and makes no claims as to the relevance of the enclosed material for preparations for such examination.

The opinions expressed herein are those of the authors and editors and are not to be construed as reflecting the views of the United States Air Force or of the Department of Defense.

Printed in the United States of America

The Society of Critical Care Medicine
251 East Imperial Highway, Suite 480
Fullerton, California 92635

Library of Congress Catalog Card Number: 86-60806
International Standard Book Number: 0-936145-25-0

Fourth Printing: May 1987

EDITORS:

R. Phillip Dellinger, MD

Associate Professor of Medicine
Baylor College of Medicine
Section of Pulmonary/Critical Care
Director, Medicine Service, Emergency Center
Ben Taub General Hospital
Houston, Texas

Robert W. Taylor, MD

Major, USAF, MC
Assistant Professor of Medicine
Uniformed Services University of the Health Sciences
Bethesda, Maryland
Director, Special Care Units
USAF Medical Center, Scott
Scott Air Force Base, Illinois

CONTRIBUTORS

Arnold Aberman
Jack J. Applefeld
Donald Armstrong
Ralph A. Babcock
Robert F. Bedford
Roger C. Bone
Michael J. Brischetto
Howard R. Bromley
David L. Brown
Charles Bryan
Christopher W. Bryan-Brown
John F. Burke
Graziano C. Carlon
Richard W. Carlson
Frank B. Cerra
Bart Chernow
Joseph D. Cohn
Alan W. Conn
Robert K. Crone
David J. Cullen
William R. Davis
R. Phillip Dellinger
Scott A. Deppe
William P. Dole
James F. Dorethy
John B. Downs
Joseph P. Ducey
Charles A. Duncan
J. Christopher Farmer
Alan Fields
H. Stephen Fletcher
Joseph G. Gabel
Franklin H. Gafford IV
Gary Gammage
Leland Garrett
Michael G. Gesenovesi
Dennis M. Greenbaum
A. Gerson Greenburg
George A. Gregory
Ake Grenvik
Betty L. Grundy
Thomas P. Hackett
Robert J. Henning
Peter R. Holbrook
Alan J. Hyman
David L. Jackson
Michael S. Jastremski
Charles C. Jeffrey
Robert Joyner
Barbara Kemper
Satish C. Khaneja
Kathryn A. Koch
Dan F. Kopen
James M. Lamiell
A. Martin Lerner
Frank R. Lewis, Jr.
Carolyn Lynch
Douglas L. Mallory
Joao A. Mattar
John Mayer
Thomas L. McKiernan
Gerald Moss
Hiltrud Mueller
Dennis L. Myers
Loren D. Nelson
Nicholas P. Ninos
Scott H. Norwood
Heida Olin
Hope Olivo
Rosanne O'Toole
Alan R. Patterson
E. Converse Peirce II
Marvin D. Peyton
William C. Pinkston
Henning Pontoppidan
Stephen H. Powell
C. Daniel Procter
Vinod K. Puri
Ron Quinton
Gladys Ranck
Robert Rangno
S. David Register III
M. Frances Rhoton
Charles L. Rice
Mark C. Rogers
Greg Ruhland
Peter Safar
Brenda Sanders
Robert Schlichtig
Robert Shepperd
William C. Shoemaker
Christopher M. Sholer
James V. Snyder
Thomas H. Spence
Robert W. Taylor
Daniel Teres
W. Leigh Thompson
Alan S. Tonnesen
William Van de Graaff
Anton F. Van Eeden
Richard M. Vazquez
Bahman Venus
Christopher Veremakis
James Vevaina
Dharmapuri Vidyasagar
Alberto Villazon-Sahagun
Thomas Vitale
Burton A. Waisbren
Max Harry Weil
Fredrick Weiland
Andrew Wilkerson
Robert F. Wilson
Mihae Yu
Susan D. Zemljic

ACKNOWLEDGMENTS

The editors are indebted to the many contributors to the SCCM Critical Care Self-Assessment Programs who provided the inspiration for this project. We have been fortunate indeed to have the support of the entire SCCM staff. Most importantly, we would like to thank our wives and families who waited patiently once again as another project required much more time than initially anticipated.

R.P.D.
R.W.T.

PREFACE

Selected questions submitted to the Society of Critical Care Medicine over the past six years have been divided into 20 sections. Each question and rationale has been updated. Related editorial comments supplement the core material. Relevant new references have been added throughout.

The questions in each section are grouped without answers. After reviewing the questions the reader simply needs to turn the page to find correct answers, rationales, up-to-date references and pertinent editorial comments.

This program serves not only as self-assessment but also as a comprehensive review of many of the most important topics in critical care and as a guide for the participant to the "classic" and the "latest" articles in the critical care literature.

CONTENTS

CONTENTS

CONTENTS

CONTENTS

Section 1

AIRWAY MANAGEMENT

1. In adults, tracheal damage during endotracheal intubation with continuous positive pressure breathing is MOST closely related to:

   a. Diameter of the endotracheal tube
   b. Shape of the pneumatic cuff
   c. Compliance of the pneumatic cuff
   d. Length of the endotracheal tube
   e. Sex of the patient

2. When considering prolonged endotracheal intubation, which ONE of the following statements is TRUE?

   a. Tracheotomy should be performed if the patient cannot be extubated within 7 days.
   b. Cuff pressure should ideally be maintained at a level less than 20-25 mm Hg to decrease the incidence of pressure necrosis of the trachea.
   c. Replacement of an endotracheal tube with a tracheostomy tube increases anatomic dead space.
   d. Tracheal stenosis is more likely to result after prolonged oro-tracheal intubation with high volume, low pressure cuffs than after tracheotomy.

3. A 35-year-old patient developed acute respiratory failure secondary to pneumonia. The patient was tracheally intubated and mechanically ventilated. A left pneumothorax occurred during insertion of a left subclavian catheter. Figure 1 demonstrates an AP portable chest radio-graph obtained following left thoracostomy tube insertion.

   The appropriate NEXT step in patient management is:

   a. The patient has developed a large left parapneumonic effusion which should be drained by needle or catheter thoracentesis.
   b. The chest tube should be withdrawn and another placed.
   c. A second chest tube should be inserted through the left second intercostal space in the mid-clavicular line.
   d. The chest tube should be removed from water seal and placed directly on 60 cm H_2O suction.
   e. None of the above

4. A neonate with Infant Respiratory Distress Syndrome (IRDS) is intubated with considerable difficulty. Following intubation, the infant becomes more hypoxic and hypercapnic. A chest radiograph is obtained and is shown in Figure 2.

   The MOST likely cause of the worsening respiratory status in this patient is:

   a. Pneumothorax
   b. Increased abdominal distention
   c. Rapid worsening of IRDS
   d. None of the above

5. An adult is orotracheally intubated and is receiving positive pressure ventilation and positive end-expiratory pressure. A significant leak acutely develops around the endotracheal (ET) tube and the patient's respiratory status rapidly deteriorates. The ICU nurse reports that the cuff inflation pressure is 25 cm H_2O and is unchanged from four hours previously.

Which ONE of the following is most appropriate in initial management of this patient?

a. Replace the ET tube.
b. Withdraw the ET tube 4-5 cm and recheck for leaking.
c. Perform direct laryngoscopy.
d. Perform emergent tracheostomy.
e. Further inflation of the ET tube cuff

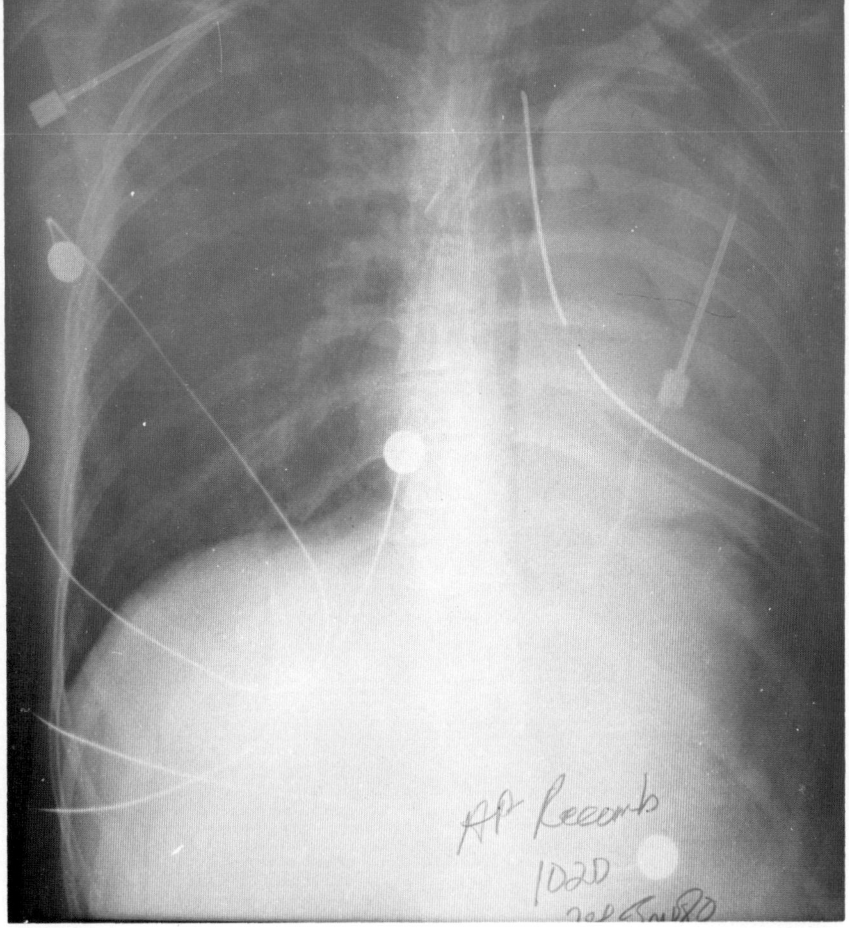

Figure 1

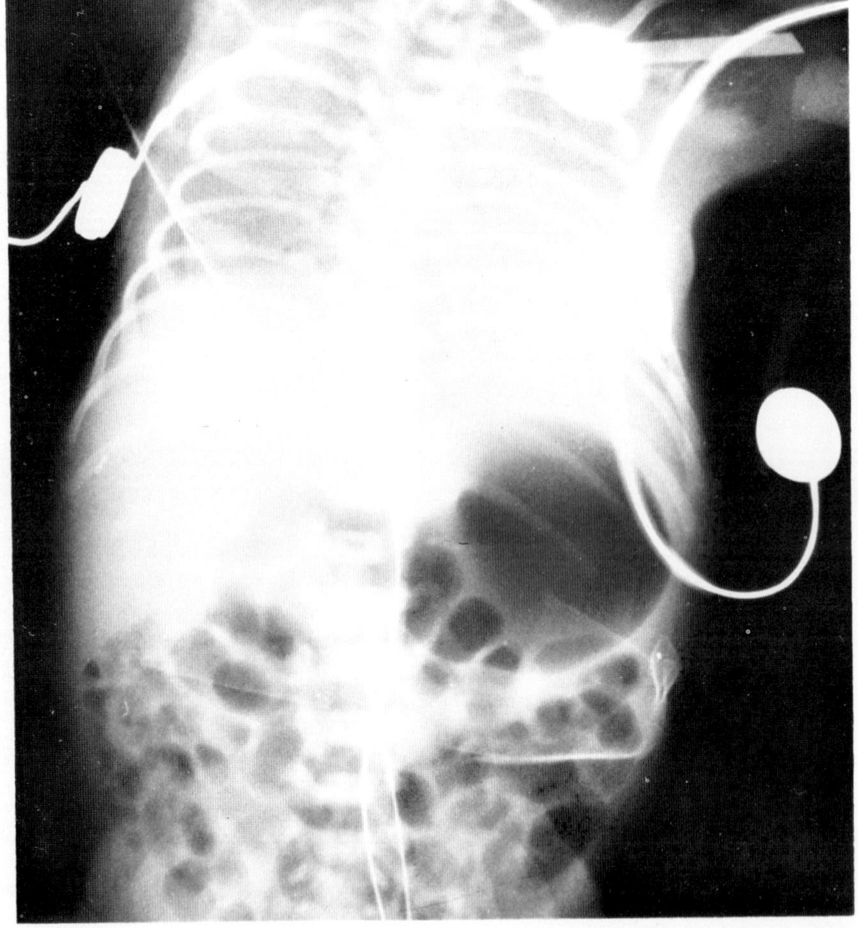

Figure 2

AIRWAY MANAGEMENT

ANSWERS

1-c 2-b 3-e 4-d 5-c

RATIONALE 1-c

Endotracheal tubes cause damage at three points. The nasopharynx or oropharynx may be eroded or inflamed causing bleeding, ulcers, and blocked drainage of the ears and sinuses. The larynx may be damaged, especially if a large tube is used in a small larynx. Swallowing causes laryngeal motion against the tube and may increase laryngeal injury. Tracheal damage is most closely related to the pressure within the balloon. Cuffs that maintain tracheal contact throughout the breathing cycle are needed for continuous positive pressure breathing. A high-compliance cuff allows safe apposition of the cuff with the tracheal mucosa at low cuff pressures thereby reducing pressure injury of the trachea.

REFERENCES

Blanc VF, Tremblay HA: The complications of tracheal intubation: A new classification and review of the literature. Anesth Analg 1974; 53:202

Bryant CR, Trinkle JK, Dubilier L: Reappraisal of tracheal injury from cuffed tracheostomy tubes: Experiments in dogs. JAMA 1971; 215:625

De Angelis J: Endotracheal intubation vs. tracheostomy. In: Critical Care Medicine Handbook. Weil MH, Shubin H (Eds). New York, John N Kolen, 1974, pp 15-20

Sykes MK, McNicol MW, Campbell EJM: Respiratory Failure. Second Edition. Philadelphia, JB Lippincott Co., 1976, p 173

RATIONALE 2-b

Complications including tracheoesophageal fistula, tracheal stenosis, tracheo-arterial fistula, and cuff trachiectasis can follow prolonged intubation. Most major acute complications from both tracheotomy and from endotracheal intubation result from excessive pressure by the endotracheal tube or tracheostomy tube cuff. These may produce mucosal ulceration, cartilaginous destruction, tracheomalacia, and tracheal wall necrosis. When capillary perfusion pressure (approximately 30 mm Hg) is exceeded, the risk of ischemia is markedly increased. Maintenance of pressure greater than 30 mm Hg for prolonged periods of time may lead to progressive tracheal wall necrosis, resulting in erosion into adjacent structures. Therefore, cuff pressure should be monitored and maintained at less than 30 mm Hg.

Current literature does not support the need for early tracheotomy. Patients tolerate low pressure, high compliance endotracheal tubes up to 3 weeks and possibly longer without significant problems. Recent data suggests that tracheal stenosis is more likely to occur after tracheotomy than after prolonged endotracheal intubation with low pressure cuffs. Trauma to the vocal cords at the time of endotracheal tube intubation is common and is usually self-limited. Small ulcerations have been noted posteriorly on the vocal cords at the time of extubation, however, they rarely cause problems.

Tracheotomy may, however, improve the patient's ability to communicate and facilitate removal of airway secretions.

REFERENCES

Lewis FR, Schlobohm RM, Thomas AN: Prevention of complications from prolonged tracheal intubation. Am J Surg 1978; 135:452

Stauffer JL, Olson DE, Petty TL: Complications and consequences of endotracheal intubation and tracheotomy: A prospective study of 150 critically ill adult patients. Am J Med 1981; 70:65

Via-Reque E, Rattenborg CC: Prolonged oro- or nasotracheal intubation. Crit Care Med 1981; 9:637

RATIONALE 3-e

The opacified left lung in Figure 1 vividly demonstrates lack of total re-expansion following the antecedent chest tube insertion. This is an excellent example of right mainstem bronchus intubation. The resultant obstruction of the left mainstem bronchus is due to endotracheal tube displacement into the right mainstem bronchus. Withdrawal of the endotracheal tube to mid-trachea in this patient resulted in marked reaeration of the left lung.

REFERENCES

Caldwell SL, Sullivan KN: Artificial airways. In: Respiratory Care: A Guide to Clinical Practice. Second Edition. Burton GG, Hodgkin JE (Eds). Philadelphia, JB Lippincott Co., 1984, pp 493-521

Fraser RG, Pare JAP: Diagnosis of Diseases of the Chest. Philadelphia, WB Saunders Co., 1977, p 361

Goodman LR, Putman CE: Intensive Care Radiology: Imaging of the Critically Ill. St. Louis, CV Mosby Co., 1978, pp 29-63

Stauffer JL, Olson DE, Petty TL: Complications and consequences of endotracheal intubation and tracheotomy. A prospective study of 150 critically ill adult patients. Am J Med 1981; 70:65

Zwillich CW, Pierson DJ, Creagh CE, et al: Complications of assisted ventilation: A prospective study of 354 consecutive episodes. Am J Med 1974; 57:161

RATIONALE 4-d

Abdominal distention, hypoxia and hypercapnia following endotracheal intubation suggest a malpositioned tube. Although a radiograph should never be waited upon to confirm this diagnosis, Figure 2 demonstrates the tracheal air column anterior to an endotracheal tube that is in the esophagus.

This complication is best prevented by visually assuring that the endotracheal tube tip has passed through the vocal cords at the time of laryngoscopy. Observation of the thorax for symmetrical expansion and auscultation of the chest for symmetrical breath sounds are also important, but may be difficult. Auscultation over the left upper quadrant of the abdomen may reveal a "gurgling" sound during inspiration, further suggesting an esophageal position of the tube. The abdomen usually becomes rapidly distended with gas in this setting.

Bilateral chest movement during inspiration has been reported with esophageal intubation. This may be secondary to esophageal distention and a subsequent "lifting" of the heart and mediastinal structures.

REFERENCES

Cundy J: Accidental intubation of the esophagus. Anaesth Intensive Care 1981; 9:76

Ogden PN: Endotracheal tube misplacement. Anaesth Intensive Care 1983; 11:273

Salem MR, Mathrubhutham M, Bennett EJ: Difficult intubation. N Engl J Med 1976; 295:879

Stirt JA: Endotracheal tube misplacement. Anaesth Intensive Care 1982; 10:274

RATIONALE 5-c

Endotracheal tube cuff leaks and tracheomalacia are potential causes for gas leakage around the tube during mechanical ventilation. Another common cause, however, is proximal endotracheal tube cuff herniation through the vocal cords. Direct laryngoscopy allows documentation of tube and cuff position. If herniation has occurred, the cuff is deflated, the tube is advanced to the mid-tracheal position, after which the cuff is reinflated. An AP chest radiograph may also help in documenting tube position.

Replacing the endotracheal tube in this setting may be unnecessary. "Blind" withdrawal of the tube may cause loss of airway control. Emergent tracheostomy is NOT indicated.

REFERENCES

Ching N, Nealon TF: Cuff pressure measurements. Chest 1974; 66:604

Leigh JM, Maynard JP: Pressure on the tracheal mucosa from cuffed tubes. Br Med J 1979; 1:1173

Lewis FR, Schlobohm RM, Thomas AN: Prevention of complications from prolonged tracheal intubation. Am J Surg 1978; 135:452

Mathias DB, Wedley JR: The effects of cuffed endotracheal tubes on the tracheal wall. Br J Anaesth 1974; 46:849

Off D, Braun SR, Tompkins B, et al: Efficacy of the minimal leak technique of cuff inflation in maintaining proper intracuff pressures for patients with cuffed artificial airways. Resp Care 1983; 28:1115

Via-Reque E, Rattenborg CC: Prolonged oro- or nasotracheal intubation. Crit Care Med 1981; 9:637

EDITORIAL COMMENT

Endotracheal intubation with the currently used low-pressure, high-volume cuffed tubes is generally well tolerated. Tube related complications, however, even in the best of circumstances are legion and in an an occasional patient may be devastating. Many of these complications are listed below.

- Abrasion, laceration or perforation of nasal cavity, nasopharynx, oropharynx, hypopharynx, larynx, trachea, esophagus
- Nasal septum perforation, fracture or dislocation
- Epistaxis
- Mandibular fracture or dislocation
- Dental injury
- Tooth aspiration
- Vocal cord paralysis
- Mainstem bronchus intubation
- Tube herniation or dislodgement
- Esophageal intubation
- Equipment failure, tube obstruction, cuff leak
- Hypoxemia and hypercapnia associated with difficult intubation
- Adverse cardiovascular response to laryngoscopy and tracheal intubation
- Altered airway immune defense mechanisms
- Infection
- Altered eustachian tube function
- Sinusitis
- Stenosis - larynx, trachea
- Tracheoesophageal fistulae

ADDITIONAL REFERENCES

Bernhard WN, Yost L, Joynes D, et al: Intracuff pressures in endotracheal and tracheostomy tubes: Related cuff physical characteristics. Chest 1985; 87:720

Cavo JW: True vocal cord paralysis following intubation. Laryngoscope 1985; 95:1352

Kastanos N, Estopa-Miro R, Marin PA, et al: Laryngotracheal injury due to endotracheal intubation: Incidence, evolution and predisposing factors. A prospective long-term study. Crit Care Med 1983; 11:362

Keane WM, Denneny JC, Rowe LD, et al: Complications of intubation. Ann Otol Rhinol Laryngol 1982; 91:584

Lund T, Goodwin CW, McManus WF, et al: Upper airway sequelae in burn patients requiring endotracheal intubation or tracheostomy. Ann Surg 1985; 201:374

Mehta S, Mickiewicz M: Pressure in large volume, low pressure cuffs: Its significance, measurement and regulation. Intensive Care Med 1985; 11:267

O'Neill JE, Giffin JP, Cottrell JE: Pharyngeal and esophageal perforation following endotracheal intubation. Anesthesiology 1984; 60:487

Saunders CE, Sedman AJ: Left mainstem bronchus intubation. Am J Emerg Med 1984; 2:406

Whited RE: Posterior commissure stenosis post long-term intubation. Laryngoscope 1983; 93:1314

Section 2

6. Which ONE of the following statements is TRUE about the postoperative administration of 10 mg of morphine into the lumbar epidural space?

   a. Postoperative analgesia will be provided but will be limited to the lumbosacral distribution.
   b. Lower extremity motor strength is usually not affected.
   c. Respiratory depression should resolve within 4-6 hours.
   d. Orthostatic hypotension commonly occurs as a result of sympathectomy following epidural morphine injection.
   e. Only mechanically ventilated patients should receive epidural morphine, regardless of dosage, in order to prevent respiratory acidemia.

7. A 35-year-old female is admitted to the ICU after an attempted elective cholecystectomy. The operation was terminated prematurely when the patient developed a superventricular tachycardia, PVCs, cyanosis and muscular rigidity. The patient has no prior history of cardiac or pulmonary disease. On initial evaluation the patient is cyanotic, diaphoretic, tachypneic and tachycardiac.

   Temperature - 38.5°C (101.3°F) Pulse - 150/min
   Respiratory rate - 15/min BP - 100/60

   Arterial blood gases (FIO_2 0.4, Tidal volume 800 cc) are as follows:

   pH 7.01 $PaCO_2$ 65 mm Hg PaO_2 55 mm Hg

   Which ONE of the following statements about the patient's condition and its therapy is FALSE?

   a. There is a hereditary predisposition for this disorder.
   b. Anesthetic agents or muscle relaxants likely precipitated this patient's illness.
   c. Proper preoperative therapy may have prevented this disorder.
   d. Intravenous procainamide is the treatment of choice.

8. When managing tetanus or strychnine poisoning, it is often necessary to paralyze neuromuscular transmission for prolonged periods. Which ONE of the following drugs is MOST likely to have the shortest duration of muscle relaxing effect?

   a. D-tubocurarine chloride
   b. Gallamine triethiodide
   c. Pancuronium bromide
   d. Succinylcholine chloride

9. Which nondepolarizing neuromuscular blocking agent is MOST likely to cause prolonged blockade in a 68-year-old male with the adult respiratory distress syndrome and oliguric acute tubular necrosis?

   a. Vecuronium
   b. Pancuronium bromide
   c. D-tubocurarine
   d. Metocurine
   e. Atracurium

ANSWERS

6-b 7-d 8-d 9-d

RATIONALE 6-b

Administration of morphine into the lumbar epidural space can provide analgesia, not only in the lumbosacral regions, but in the thoracic region as well. This probably occurs because of cephalad diffusion of the relatively lipid-insoluble morphine within the CSF. Lower extremity strength should not be affected nor should sympathectomy occur if only morphine and not a local anesthetic are injected in the epidural space. Early respiratory depression secondary to rapid uptake of morphine into the epidural venous plexus peaks at about 15-20 minutes. Recent studies show that measurable respiratory depression persists for up to 17 hours after epidural administration of 10 mg morphine. Lower doses result in less profound and less significant respiratory depression and are frequently given to patients not receiving mechanical ventilation.

REFERENCES

Christensen P, Larsen VH, Iversen AD, et al: Thoracic and lumbar epidural morphine after upper laparotomy. Abstract 89, Scandinavian Society of Anesthesiologists, 17th Congress, 1983

Nordberg G, Hedner T, Melstrand T, Dahlstrom B: Pharmacokinetic aspects of epidural morphine analgesia. Anesthesiology 1983; 58:545

Rawal N, Wattwil M: Respiratory depression after epidural morphine - An experimental and clinical study. Anesth Analg 1984; 63:8

Yaksh TL: Spinal opiate analgesia: Characteristics and principles of action. Pain 1981; 11:293

EDITORIAL COMMENT

The use of epidural narcotics has revolutionized postoperative analgesia and is finding increased application in the intensive care unit. Postoperative pulmonary function is often less compromised when this technique is used rather than other forms of analgesia.

Epidural narcotics have been successfully used in thoracic, abdominal, orthopedic, urologic, gynecologic and other surgeries. This technique has also been useful in the management of patients with intractable pain secondary to malignancy or other conditions.

Side effects are usually mild or easily treated. These include urinary retention, pruritus, nausea/vomiting, and respiratory depression. Respiratory depression appears to be a rare occurrence. Sellevold reported its occurrence in less than 1% of 1085 patients who had received epidural morphine.

ADDITIONAL REFERENCES

Bromage PR: Epidural and spinal narcotics. Seminars in Anesthesia 1983; 2:75

Bromage PR, Camporesi E, Chestnut D: Epidural narcotics for postoperative analgesia. Anesth Analg 1980; 59:473

Fromme GA, Steidl LJ, Danielson DR: Comparison of lumbar and thoracic epidural morphine for relief of post-thoracotomy pain. Anesth Analg 1985; 64:454

Nordberg G: Pharmacokinetic aspects of spinal morphine analgesia. Acta Anaesthesiol Scand [Suppl] 1984; 28:7

Pflug AE, Bonica JJ: Physiopathology and control of postoperative pain. Arch Surg 1977; 112:773

Stenseth R, Sellevold O, Breivik H: Epidural morphine for postoperative pain: Experience with 1085 patients. Acta Anaesthesiol Scand 1985; 29:148

Yablonski-Perety T, Klin B, Beilin Y, et al: Continuous epidural narcotic analgesia for intractable pain due to malignancy. J Surg Oncol 1985; 29:8

RATIONALE 7-d

Malignant hyperthermia (MH) is a syndrome usually precipitated in genetically susceptible individuals by volatile anesthetic agents or succinylcholine. During episodes of MH, skeletal muscle increases its oxygen consumption, CO_2 production, and lactate production, resulting in the development of a metabolic and respiratory acidosis, tremendous heat production and prolonged muscle contraction. The pathophysiology is not definitely known but probably involves abnormal membrane permeability and calcium flux within the muscle fiber. Mild cases may be terminated simply by stopping the inciting agents. Severe cases may result in temperatures as high as 43°C, massive muscle necrosis, irreversible metabolic acidosis, cardiovascular collapse and death. The treatment of choice is intravenous dantrolene, and supportive therapy directed at the hyperthermia and mixed acidosis. Pretreatment with oral dantrolene for 24 hours prior to anticipated surgery is beneficial. Anesthetic agents less likely to cause MH include opiates, thiopental, droperidol, nitrous oxide and pancuronium.

REFERENCES

Ellis FR: Malignant hyperpyrexia. Arch Dis Child 1984; 59:1013

Flewellen TE, Nelson TE, Jones WP, et al: Dantrolene dose response in awake man: Implications for management of malignant hyperthermia. Anesthesiology 1983; 59:275

Gronert G: Malignant hyperthermia. Anesthesiology 1980; 53:395

EDITORIAL COMMENT

Several investigators have recently suggested that end-tidal CO_2 measurement and/or measurement of O_2 consumption are effective in the early diagnosis and management of malignant hyperthermia.

ADDITIONAL REFERENCES

Bandendistel L, Goudsouzian N, Cote C, et al: End-tidal CO_2 monitoring: Its use in the diagnosis and management of malignant hyperthermia. Anaesthesia 1984; 39:1000

Baumgarten RK, Reynolds WI: Early detection of malignant hyperthermia (Letter). Anesthesiology 1985; 63:123

Neubauer KR, Kaufman RD: Another use for mass spectrometry: Detection and monitoring of malignant hyperthermia. Anesth Analg 1985; 64:837

Triner L, Sherman J: Potential value of expiratory carbon dioxide measurement in patients considered to be susceptible to malignant hyperthermia (Letter). Anesthesiology 1981; 55:482

RATIONALE 8-d

Succinylcholine chloride has the shortest duration of action. Gallamine triethiodide has the shortest duration of action among the remaining choices. With large doses, however, gallamine's duration of action can be prolonged. Pancuronium bromide in small doses has a shorter duration of action than D-tubocurarine chloride. When very large doses are used, as might be employed in treating tetanus or strychnine poisoning, the duration of actions of gallamine triethiodide, D-tubocurarine chloride, and pancuronium bromide are relatively equivalent. Most published studies have employed the older D-tubocurarine in treatment of tetanus. Pancuronium bromide may, however, be a better option because of its relative lack of cardiovascular effects.

REFERENCES

Ablett JJ: Tetanus and the anaesthetist: A review of the symptomatology and the recent advances in treatment. Br J Anaesth 1956; 28:258

American Medical Association, Department of Drugs: Nondepolarizing (competitive) blocking agents. AMA Drug Evaluations. Third Edition. Littleton, MA, PSG Publishing Co., 1977, pp 311-314

Churchill-Davidson HC: A Practice of Anaesthesia. Fourth Edition. Philadelphia, WB Saunders Co., 1978, pp 897-899

Collins VJ: Relaxants--pharmacology and use. In: Principles of Anesthesiology. Second Edition. Philadelphia, Lea & Febiger, 1976, pp 594-626

Dripps R, Eckenhoff JE, Vandam LD: Introduction to Anesthesia - The Principles of Safe Practice. Fifth Edition. Philadelphia, WB Saunders Co., 1982, pp 160-179

Shackleton RP: The treatment of tetanus: Role of the anaesthetist. Lancet 1954; 2:155

Wright R, Sykes MK, Jackson BG, et al: Intermittent positive pressure respiration in tetanus neonatorium. Lancet 1961; 2:678

RATIONALE 9-d

Metocurine (Metubine), like gallamine, another nondepolarizing neuromuscular blocking agent, is entirely dependent on renal excretion for elimination. Pancuronium is more dependent on renal excretion than is d-tubocurarine but both have significant hepatobiliary excretion and can therefore be used in reduced doses in patients with renal failure. Atracurium and vecuronium are new intermediate-duration, nondepolarizing neuromuscular blockers which are chemically and enzymatically cleared and can be safely used in patients with both renal and hepatobiliary disease.

Succinylcholine is a depolarizing neuromuscular blocker whose half-life is prolonged slightly in patients with chronic renal failure but not in acute renal failure.

REFERENCES

Dripps R, Eckenhoff JE, Vandam LD: Introduction to Anesthesia - The Principles of Safe Practice. Fifth Edition. Philadelphia, WB Saunders Co., 1982, pp 160-179

Hughes R: Experimental and clinical evaluation of neuromuscular blocking agents. J Pharmacol Methods 1984; 12:1

Lebrault C, Berger JL, D'Hollander AA, et al: Pharmacokinetics and pharmacodynamics of vecuronium (ORG NC 45) in patients with cirrhosis. Anesthesiology 1985; 62:601

Miller RD (Ed): Anesthesia. Vol 1. New York, Churchill Livingstone Inc., 1981, pp 487-538

Nigrovic V, Auen M, Wajskol A: Enzymatic hydrolysis of atracurium in vivo. Anesthesiology 1985; 62:606

Orko R, Heino A, Rosenberg PH: Vecuronium in patients with and without renal failure. Acta Anaesthesiol Scand 1985; 29:326

Section 3

10. Which of the following is LEAST likely to decrease dP/dt in a dissecting aortic aneurysm associated with central arterial pressures of 160/100 mm Hg:

a. Trimethaphan camsylate
b. Reserpine
c. Propranolol
d. Hydralazine
e. Guanethidine

Questions 11-12 refer to the following patient: A 55-year-old male with a strong family history of myocardial infarction was admitted to the ICU with the sudden onset of excruciating persistent chest pain. The pain was retrosternal in location and radiated to the back between the scapulae. The patient was observed to have a syncopal episode shortly after the pain began. There was a history of untreated hypertension and a 35 pack-year history of smoking. There was no previous history of heart disease.

Vital signs:

Temperature - 37°C	Pulse - 110
Respiratory rate - 24	BP - 210/125

Cardiovascular Exam:

- loud A2
- grade II diastolic decrescendo murmur at the left sternal border in the 2nd interspace
- decreased R carotid pulse with an associated bruit
- normal pulses elsewhere

An AP portable chest film revealed borderline cardiomegaly and a prominent ascending aorta and arch.

11. Which ONE of the following statements describes the MOST appropriate initial management?

a. Observation in a quiet environment with nasal oxygen and prophylactic lidocaine infusion
b. Immediate institution of intra-arterial pressure monitoring and treatment with intravenous diazoxide or nitroprusside
c. Institution of intra-arterial pressure monitoring and treatment with iv propranolol and iv nitroprusside
d. Immediate transfer to the cardiac catheterization laboratory for coronary angiography and intra-coronary streptokinase therapy

12. Which ONE of the following is the MOST important diagnostic measure?

a. Serial determinations of the MB dimer of CPK
b. Echocardiography
c. Technetium pyrophosphate myocardial scan
d. Serial electrocardiography
e. Emergency angiography after the patient is stabilized

13. On a warm summer day, a 40-year-old female complained of being very hot, fatigued, lightheaded and of a retrosternal chest pressure. Several minutes later she momentarily lost consciousness. She was driven to the hospital by her daughter and subsequently admitted to the ICU. She denied a history of similar episodes, hypertension, diabetes mellitus or tobacco use. She stated that both her father and a paternal uncle died suddenly in their early forties.

Physical examination revealed:

Temperature - 37°C (98.6°F)	Pulse - 108
Respiratory rate - 16	BP - 100/60

The patient was alert and was resting comfortably in bed. There was no jugular venous distention. A bifid carotid pulse was noted without associated carotid bruits. The lung fields were clear. There was a double precordial impulse. A systolic ejection murmur was heard along the left sternal border and was accentuated during a valsalva maneuver. There was, in addition, a paradoxical splitting of S2, a soft S3 and a loud S4. The remainder of the physical examination was normal.

A chest roentgenogram revealed a prominent left ventricle but was otherwise normal. An EKG revealed broad Q waves in leads II, III, aVF and V_1 - V_3. There was no ST segment elevation.

Which ONE of the following statements about this condition is TRUE?

a. Nitroglycerin will probably improve symptoms.
b. Mitral regurgitation is rarely present.
c. Digoxin will probably improve symptoms.
d. Up to 50% of first degree relatives may have evidence of a similar condition.

14. Which ONE of the following maneuvers is NOT expected to increase the intensity of the systolic outflow murmur heard in hypertrophic obstructive cardiomyopathy (idiopathic hypertrophic subaortic stenosis)?

a. Squatting
b. Amyl nitrate
c. Isoproterenol
d. Upright posture

15. Which ONE of the following statements about verapamil is TRUE?

a. Positive inotropic action
b. Negative chronotropic action
c. Positive dromotropic action
d. Vasoconstrictor action

16. In atrial fibrillation both aberrant conduction and ventricular ectopic beats may cause alteration in QRS and T morphology. Which ONE of the following findings MOST favors such beats being caused by a ventricular ectopic focus rather than aberrant conduction?

a. Abnormal beats have a right bundle branch block configuration in lead V_1.
b. Abnormal beats appear only at the end of a long RR interval.
c. Abnormal beats occur sometimes in runs of 2 or 3.
d. Initial vector of abnormal beats is same as the normal beats.

17. In which ONE of the following conditions is electrocardioversion of atrial fibrillation MOST likely to be successful in establishing a stable (long-term) sinus rhythm?

a. Severe mitral valve disease
b. Paroxysmal history of atrial fibrillation
c. Digitalis intoxication
d. New onset of atrial fibrillation

18. A 40-year-old male is noted to have recurrent episodes of ventricular tachycardia in the immediate postoperative period, following a cholecystectomy. The episodes have terminated spontaneously after 20-30 seconds. The patient has no previous history of heart disease. His preoperative 12-lead electrocardiogram is normal with the exception of a prolonged QT interval. His serum K^+ is 2.5 mEq/L. An electrocardiographic recording of one of these episodes is shown below.

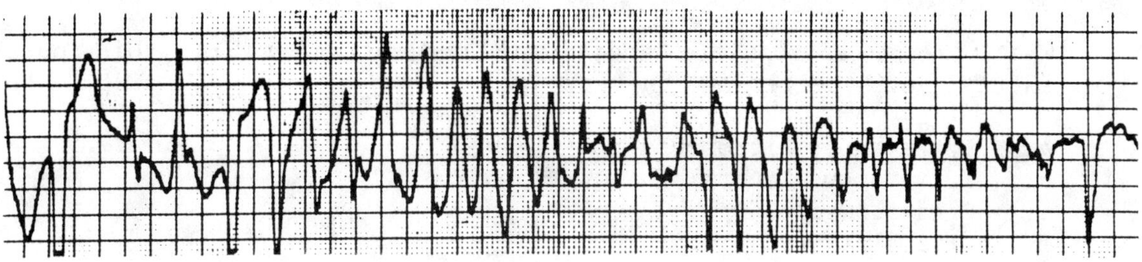

Which ONE of the following is LEAST appropriate in the treatment of this disorder?

a. KCl administration
b. Procainamide
c. Isoproterenol
d. Overdrive pacing

19. Multifocal atrial tachycardia (MAT) is a common dysrhythmia in critically ill patients, especially in those with which ONE of the following?

a. Mitral valve disease
b. Renal failure
c. Hepatic failure
d. Chronic obstructive pulmonary disease

20. Paroxysmal supraventricular tachycardia is MOST effectively treated with which ONE of the following?

a. Verapamil
b. Digoxin
c. Propranolol
d. Edrophonium (Tensilon)
e. Norepinephrine (overdrive suppression)

21. Which ONE of the following statements concerning hypertensive encephalopathy is TRUE?

a. Theoretically autoregulation is lost and vasospasm leads to cerebral ischemia.
b. After lowering the blood pressure, symptoms are generally slow to resolve.
c. Theoretically autoregulation is maintained but overperfusion and cerebral edema occur.
d. Nitroprusside is contraindicated because it is a cerebral vasodilator and increases cerebral blood flow.

22. A 37-year-old male is admitted to the ICU from the ER with a blood pressure of 240/150 and mental confusion for the last 6 hours. The patient has papilledema, mental confusion and a left ventricular heave. The physical exam is otherwise unremarkable. The EKG shows left ventricular strain, his chest radiograph shows cephalization of flow without infiltrates and a large cardiac shadow. The patient was given a 40 mg iv bolus of furosemide in the emergency room.

What is/are appropriate additional medication(s) for this patient's initial antihypertensive therapy?

a. Intravenous nitroprusside
b. Intravenous labetalol
c. Oral clonidine
d. Oral alpha methyldopa
e. Either a or b

23. The hemodynamic changes in response to intra-aortic balloon counterpulsation include all of the following EXCEPT:

a. A rise in diastolic aortic pressure
b. An increase in coronary blood flow
c. A fall in left atrial pressure
d. A rise in systolic aortic pressure
e. A decrease in systemic vascular resistance

Questions 24-27: For EACH numbered statement, select the ONE lettered heading that is most closely associated with it. Each lettered heading may be selected once, more than once, or not at all.

a. ST segment depression and T wave inversion in leads V_1 - V_5
b. Tall R waves and ST segment depression in leads V_1 and V_2
c. Q waves in leads V_1, V_2 and V_3
d. A frontal plane QRS axis of +90° to +180° and an S_1 Q_3 pattern
e. Deep broad Q waves in leads II, III and aVF

24. Anteroseptal myocardial infarction

25. Inferior myocardial infarction

26. Subendocardial myocardial infarction

27. Posterior myocardial infarction

28. Which ONE of the following statements about postoperative myocardial infarction is FALSE?

a. Is associated with an overall mortality of about 50%
b. Is more likely to present as a rate or rhythm disturbance than as chest pain
c. Is more likely to occur in a patient with a prior history of infarction
d. Is associated with a mortality rate very similar to that of non-surgical hospitalized patients with myocardial infarction

29. Which ONE of the following statements about cardiogenic shock due to right ventricular (RV) infarction is FALSE?

a. RV infarction causing shock is usually more amenable to medical therapy than left ventricular infarction and shock.
b. A low pulmonary artery occlusion pressure found in RV cardiogenic shock usually implies minimal left ventricular damage.
c. Right ventricular function can be assessed accurately by two-dimensional echocardiography.
d. Distended neck veins and hypotension are predominant clinical findings in right ventricular cardiogenic shock.

30. Which ONE of the following is NOT an indication for emergency temporary cardiac pacing?

a. Ventricular asystole unresponsive to drug therapy
b. Third degree heart block with hypotension
c. New right bundle branch block and left anterior hemiblock with Mobitz II AV block in the setting of an acute anterior wall myocardial infarction
d. Electromechanical dissociation during cardiac resuscitation

31. Abnormal pulsus paradoxus is LEAST commonly observed in association with which ONE of the following?

a. Hypovolemia with hypotension
b. Acute asthma
c. Pericardial tamponade
d. Pulmonary emphysema
e. Pneumonia

32. Which ONE of the following mechanisms best explains pulsus paradoxus?

a. A negative pleural pressure
b. An increase in left ventricular afterload
c. An increase in venous return
d. An increase in left ventricular compliance

33. A 47-year-old male is admitted to your ICU for observation. He was the victim of vehicular trauma 6 hours earlier, had multiple long bone fractures and several deep lacerations. He has a past history of excessive alcohol ingestion, cigarette smoking and an allergy to penicillin. His medications include meperidine, cefotaxime sodium, thiamine and multivitamins. During the second infusion of cefotaxime he is noticed to develop a generalized maculopapular rash, inspiratory stridor, diffuse bronchospasm and hypotension.

Which of the following statements about this condition is true?

a. The patient has suffered pulmonary fat embolization.
b. This condition represents a Type II-antibody-dependent cytotoxic hypersensitivity reaction.
c. Endotracheal intubation, supplemental oxygen, rapid fluid infusion and dopamine hydrochloride (2-10 mcg/kg•min titrated to response) represent the optimum initial form of therapy.
d. This condition is identical pathophysiologically to that caused by radiographic contrast media.
e. None of the above

CARDIOVASCULAR

ANSWERS

10-d	11-c	12-e	13-d	14-a	15-b	16-c	17-d	18-b
19-d	20-a	21-a	22-e	23-d	24-c	25-e	26-a	27-b
28-d	29-b	30-d	31-e	32-a	33-e			

===

AORTIC DISSECTION

===

RATIONALE 10-d

The critical factor causing dissecting aneurysms of the aorta is not the mean arterial pressure, but the rate of rise of the aortic pressure during systole (dP/dt). This can be reduced quickly by intravenous administration of trimethaphan camsylate (inhibits ganglionic transmission) or propranolol (inhibits beta-adrenergic receptors), both of which reduce contractility. Reserpine (depletes norepinephrine from postganglionic sympathetic nerves) acts more slowly and oral guanethidine (reduces norepinephrine release) takes several days for maximum effect. All of these treatments, however, decrease contractility, slow ejection, and reduce dP/dt by inhibiting the influences of the sympathetic nervous system on the heart. Hydralazine, a direct dilator of arterial smooth muscle, lowers arterial pressure but allows the reflex increase in sympathetic nervous system activity that generally increases heart rate and contractility, thereby increasing dP/dt. Hydralazine thus is contraindicated in a patient with a dissecting aortic aneurysm. Nitroprusside sodium, a direct vasodilator similar to hydralazine, may also lead to increased heart rate and contractility and should be used with caution. Of course, either hydralazine or nitroprusside sodium may be used safely if the reflex increase in sympathetic nervous system activity is inhibited, preferably with propranolol or another beta-adrenergic blocker.

REFERENCES

Anagnostopoulos CE: Acute Aortic Dissectons. Baltimore, University Park Press, 1975

Lindsay J Jr, Hurst JW: Dissecting aneurysm of the aorta. In: Critical Care Medicine. Weil MH, Shubin H (Eds). Maryland, Harper and Row, 1976, pp 130-134

Schlatmann TJM, Becker AF: Pathogenesis of dissecting aneurysm of the aorta. Am J Cardiol 1977; 39:21

Wheat MW Jr: Intensive drug therapy. In: Aortic Dissection. Doroghazi RM, Slater EE (Eds). New York, McGraw-Hill Book Company, 1983, p 165

Wheat MW Jr, Palmer RF: Dissecting aneurysms of the aorta: Present status of drug versus surgical therapy. Prog Cardiovasc Dis 1968; 11:198

RATIONALE 11-c 12-e

The patient's presentation is consistent with an acute myocardial infarction but certain data strongly suggest aortic dissection. The acute severity of the pain, its persistent quality, and its radiation are atypical of myocardial infarction. Patients with aortic dissection are usually free of pain prior to the event. Hypertension is common in coronary disease but is almost universal in dissection. Syncope is unusual in myocardial infarction and should always prompt an investigation for another problem. The murmur of aortic insufficiency and asymmetric carotid pulses demand further explanation. These findings are not unusual with dissection of the ascending aorta.

Appropriate therapy for acute aortic dissection of the ascending aorta includes rapid correction of hypertension with agents that do not increase the velocity of ejection (dP/dt). Agents thus contraindicated include nitroprusside (used as a single agent), diazoxide and hydralazine. The agents of choice are trimethaphan or intravenous propranolol followed by intravenous nitroprusside.

Once the diagnosis of acute aortic dissection is suspected and the patient is stabilized, emergency diagnostic procedures are in order. Serial cardiac enzyme determinations and EKGs are reasonable to evaluate for myocardial infarction from associated coronary artery dissection. Echocardiography is useful in the evaluation of associated acute aortic insufficiency and hemopericardium and occasionally demonstrates the dissection. However, emergency angiography is the most important study and is required to make the definitive diagnosis. The extent of the dissection, the site of origin of the dissection and the origins of the great vessels may be visualized in anticipation of urgent surgical repair.

REFERENCES

Moothart RW, et al: Echocardiography in aortic root dissections and dilation. Am J Cardiol 1975; 36:11

Ram CV: Hypertensive emergencies: Recognition and management. Curr Probl Cardiol 1982; 7:7

Ram CV, Kaplan NM: Hypertensive emergencies. In: Textbook of Critical Care. Shoemaker WC, Thompson WL, Holbrook PR (Eds). Philadelphia, WB Saunders Co., 1984, pp 464-465

Slater E, DeSanctis R: Dissection of the aorta. Med Clin North Am 1979; 63:141

Wheat MW Jr: Treatment of dissection aneurysms of the aorta: Current status. Prog Cardiovasc Dis 1973; 16:87

EDITORIAL COMMENT

Presently aortography remains the single most important study in the diagnosis of dissecting aortic aneurysm, however, several noninvasive studies deserve mention.

Contrast-enhanced computerized tomography appears to be highly accurate in the diagnosis of acute aortic dissection.

Improved results utilizing transthoracic two-dimensional echocardiography for detection of ascending aortic dissection have recently been reported. Granato found the test to be 100% sensitive and 88% specific for diagnosis of ascending aortic dissection. Its role in diagnosing distal aortic dissection, however, is limited.

Borner reported successful use of transesophageal echocardiography in a single case of distal aortic dissection. Because of the close anatomic relationship of the esophagus and the descending aorta this technique may prove to be valuable.

Early experience with magnetic resonance imaging suggests that it may also be useful in the diagnosis of aortic dissection.

ADDITIONAL REFERENCES

Amparo EC, Higgins CB, Hricak H, et al: Aortic dissection: Magnetic resonance imaging. Radiology 1985; 155:399

Borner N, Erbel R, Braun B, et al: Diagnosis of aortic dissection by transesophageal echocardiography. Am J Cardiol 1984; 54:1157

Diehl JT, Kaiser LR, Howard RJ: Two-dimensional echocardiography for diagnosing acute ascending aortic dissection. Can J Surg 1985; 28:345

Geisinger MA, Risius B, O'Donnell JA, et al: Thoracic aortic dissections: Magnetic resonance imaging. Radiology 1985; 155:407

Granato JE, Dee P, Gibson RS: Utility of two-dimensional echocardiography in suspected ascending aortic dissection. Am J Cardiol 1985; 56:123

Heiberg E, Wolverson M, Sundaram M, et al: CT findings in thoracic aortic dissection. AJR 1981; 136:13

Larde D, Belloir C, Vasile N, et al: Computerized tomography in dissection of the thoracic aorta. Radiology 1980; 136:147

Moncada R, Churchill R, Reynes C, et al: Diagnosis of dissecting aortic aneurysm by computerized tomography. Lancet 1981; 1:238

ASYMMETRIC SEPTAL HYPERTROPHY

RATIONALE 13-d

Idiopathic hypertrophic subaortic stenosis (IHSS) is also referred to as asymmetric septal hypertrophy (ASH). It is associated with distorted myocardial architecture and a hypertrophied interventricular septum. During systole, the anterior mitral valve leaflet may abut upon the hypertrophied septum and cause obstruction to ventricular outflow. The disorder is familial and up to 50% of first degree relatives may have evidence of septal abnormality. In any given individual the severity of the obstruction seems to be related to the left ventricular end-diastolic volume, the contractile state of the myocardium and the pressure that distends the outflow tract during systole.

When left ventricular volume is decreased (dehydration, valsalva, nitroglycerin, etc.), obstruction is intensified. When the force of contraction is increased (digoxin, isoproterenol, etc.), the size of the ventricular cavity is also decreased and obstruction increased. Elevation of arterial pressure (phenylephrine, isometric hand-grip, etc.) increases the distending pressure of the left ventricular outflow tract during systole and therefore decreases obstruction. Classic historical and physical findings in this disorder include: dyspnea, chest pain, lightheadedness, syncope, a bifid carotid pulse, a double or triple apical impulse, a paradoxically split S2, third and fourth heart sounds and a systolic ejection murmur heard at the left sternal border. The murmur is usually intensified by maneuvers that increase obstruction such as valsalva. Some degree of mitral regurgitation is present in most patients with this disorder. This occurs presumably as a result of displacement of the mitral valve by the left ventricular hypertrophy. Chest radiographs may demonstrate left ventricular enlargement. Because of gross septal hypertrophy the EKG usually displays diffuse broad Q waves.

REFERENCES

Epstein SE, et al: Asymmetric septal hypertrophy. Ann Intern Med 1974; 81:650

Wigle ED, Sasson Z, Henderson MA, et al: Hypertrophic cardiomyopathy. The importance of the site and extent of hypertrophy. Prog Cardiovasc Dis 1985; 28:1

Wynne J, Braunwald E (Eds): The cardiomyopathies and myocarditis. In: Heart Disease. Philadelphia, WB Saunders Co., 1984, pp 1399-1456

RATIONALE 14-a

Hypertrophic obstructive cardiomyopathy is often diagnosed by performing auscultatory maneuvers. The murmur caused by outflow obstruction is made louder by any maneuver that increases the severity of the obstruction. In general, a decrease in ventricular intracavity volume will increase outflow obstruction and enhance the murmur. Amyl nitrate produces vasodilatations and hypotension. The resultant reflex tachycardia shortens diastolic filling time which, in turn, decreases intracavity volume and increases obstruction. Isoproterenol augments the contractile state of the myocardium and produces tachycardia. Diastolic filling time and ventricular compliance are therefore decreased and outflow obstruction subsequently increased. Squatting increases venous return by compression of abdominal veins and increases afterload by aortic compression. This results in an increase in the volume of the ventricular cavity with reduction in outflow obstruction and subsequent decrease in the intensity of the murmur. If an upright posture is resumed, the opposite effect will occur.

REFERENCE

Wynne J, Braunwald E (Eds): The cardiomyopathies and myocarditis. In: Heart Disease. Philadelphia, WB Saunders Co., 1984, pp 1399-1456

EDITORIAL COMMENT

The mainstay of medical therapy in this disorder has been beta-adrenergic blocking drugs such as propranolol. Calcium-channel blocking agents are becoming increasingly utilized in hypertrophic cardiomyopathy. Clinical trials with verapamil and nifedipine suggest improvement in symptomatic status and exercise tolerance in many patients. The exact mechanisms are not understood but may relate to improved diastolic relaxation and filling. McKenna reported improved survival with amiodarone in patients with hypertrophic cardiomyopathy and ventricular tachycardia.

ADDITIONAL REFERENCES

Bonow RO: Effects of calcium-channel blocking agents on left ventricular diastolic function in hypertrophic cardiomyopathy and in coronary artery disease. Am J Cardiol 1985; 55:172B

Lorell BH: Use of calcium-channel blockers in hypertrophic cardiomyopathy. Am J Med 1985; 78(Suppl 2B):43

McKenna WJ: Does treatment influence the natural history of patients with hypertrophic cardiomyopathy? Drugs 1985; 29:53

McKenna WJ, Oakley CM, Krikler DM, et al: Improved survival with amiodarone in patients with hypertrophic cardiomyopathy and ventricular tachycardia. Br Heart J 1985; 53:412

DYSRHYTHMIAS

RATIONALE 15-b

Verapamil exerts its primary effect during phase 2 of the action potential. Like the other calcium-channel blocking agents, verapamil interferes with the inward transmembrane flux of calcium through so-called "slow channels." These agents have a vasodilation action which accounts in part for their usefulness in atherosclerotic and vasospastic coronary artery disease. They possess negative chronotropic, inotropic and dromotropic action.

REFERENCES

Antman EM, Stone PH, et al: Calcium channel blocking agents in the treatment of cardiovascular disorders. Part I. Basic and clinical electrophysiologic effects. Ann Intern Med 1980; 93:875

Eichelbaum M, Echizen H: Clinical pharmacology of calcium antagonists: A critical review. J Cardiovasc Pharmacol 1984; 6:S963

Singh BN: Calcium antagonists: Part I. Pharmacologic basis for therapeutic applications. Hosp Forum 1984; 19:318

Stone PH, Antman EM, et al: Calcium channel blocking agents in the treatment of cardiovascular disorders. Part II. Hemodynamic effects and clinical applications. Ann Intern Med 1980; 93:886

RATIONALE 16-c

An abnormal beat found only at the end of a long RR interval is most likely ectopic. The longer the RR interval, the more likely there will be an ectopic escape beat and the less likely that the bundle branches are still refractory. Therefore, an aberrantly conducted beat would not be expected. After a ventricular beat, the ventricular conduction system remains refractory to any impulse conduction for a short time. If a supraventricular impulse arrives at the conduction system during this time, the beat will not be conducted to the ventricles. If the impulse arrives after the entire conducting system has recovered, the beat will be normally conducted to both ventricles. When an impulse arrives sometime between these two extremes, when part of the conduction system is still refractory, the beat will be conducted abnormally. The right bundle-branch system is usually the last to recover, therefore, most aberrant beats have a right bundle-branch block pattern.

The refractory period of the conduction system is proportional to the length of the preceding RR interval. Therefore, if an abnormal beat is found after a long preceding RR interval, the beat is more likely to be an aberrantly conducted rather than ectopic beat. If beats are conducted in rapid succession, the conduction system may still be partially refractory resulting in aberrantly conducted beats.

Ectopic beats may occur in runs, and the morphology of the beat must be examined. The initial vector of a normally conducted beat is due to septal depolarization via the left bundle branch. During an aberrantly conducted beat due to refractory right bundle, the initial vector should remain normal as the septum is being depolarized by the left bundle. The initial vector during a ventricular ectopic beat is often abnormal.

REFERENCES

Chung EK: Electrocardiography. Third Edition. Norwalk, CT, Appleton-Century-Crofts, 1985, p 352

Marriott HJL: Practical Electrocardiography. Sixth Edition. Baltimore, Williams & Wilkins Co., 1977, p 172

Marriott HJL, Myerburg RJ: Recognition and treatment of cardiac arrhythmias and conduction disturbances. In: The Heart. Fourth Edition. Hurst JW, Logue RB, Schlant RC, et al (Eds). New York, McGraw-Hill Book Company, 1978, p 664

RATIONALE 17-d

In severe mitral valve disease, electrocardioversion is unlikely to be successful even at high energy settings. There is usually significant left atrial enlargement and an unacceptably high probability of clot embolization. Patients with histories of paroxysmal arrhythmias including atrial fibrillation generally should not undergo electrocardioversion as they have already demonstrated their propensity to return to atrial fibrillation on a sporadic basis. In the presence of digitalis toxicity, electrocardioversion may induce a lethal ventricular dysrhythmia such as ventricular fibrillation which usually cannot be ablated. Sinus rhythm is difficult to maintain following electro-cardioversion in the thyrotoxic patient with atrial fibrillation. Because of the tendency to revert back to atrial fibrillation in this setting the hyperthyroidism should be brought under control before electrocardioversion is attempted. The documented onset of atrial fibrillation as a new dysrhythmia provides an excellent opportunity for electrocardioversion if the patient does not have a contraindication. In addition to the ones previously mentioned, relative contraindications include acute carditis, bradycardia-tachycardia syndrome, severe left ventricular failure and idiopathic atrial fibrillation ("lone fibrillator").

REFERENCES

Resnekov L: Theory and practice of electrocardioversion of cardiac dysrhythmias. Med Clin North Am 1976; 60:325

Zipes DP: Management of Cardiac Dysrhythmias. In: Heart Disease. Second Edition. Braunwald E (Ed). Philadelphia, WB Saunders Co., 1984, pp 648-682

RATIONALE 18-b

"Torsade de pointes" is an interesting form of ventricular tachycardia. As the name implies, the QRS complexes appear to twist around the isoelectric line. A good example of this serious dysrhythmia is shown in the electrocardiographic recording. It has been reported in all age groups, often without evidence of coexistent heart disease. It often occurs in the setting of a prolonged QT interval, either congenital or acquired. The dysrhythmia usually terminates spontaneously, however, it may lead to ventricular fibrillation and death. General treatment involves rapid recognition, discontinuation of any offending drugs, and correction of electrolyte disturbances. Drugs that further prolong the QT interval such as procainamide and quinidine are contraindicated. Treatment successes and failures have been reported with lidocaine and propranolol. Bretylium antagonizes many of the effects of quinidine and has been used successfully in this setting. Isoproterenol infusion has been recommended in the emergency treatment of this dysrhythmia. It reduces the dispersion of myocardial recovery times directly and by inducing a sinus tachycardia. Over-drive pacing is also useful in the emergency treatment of "torsade de pointes." Some cases of this disorder are thought to be secondary to excessive left-sided sympathetic activity, and temporary ablation of the left stellate ganglion has been effective.

Magnesium deficiency has been reported as a cause of "torsade de pointes." This diagnosis should be considered in all patients with "torsade de pointes" since magnesium therapy can correct and possibly prevent this dysrhythmia.

REFERENCES

Fontaine G, et al: Torsades de pointes: Definition and management. Mod Concepts Cardiovasc Dis 1982; 51:103

Levine SR, Crowley TJ, Hai HA: Hypomagnesemia and ventricular tachycardia. A complication of ulcerative colitis and parenteral hyperalimentation in a non-digitalized patient. Chest 1982; 81:244

Loeb HS, Pietras RJ, Gunnar RM, et al: Paroxysmal ventricular fibrillation in two patients with hypomagnesemia: Treated by transvenous pacing. Circulation 1968; 37:210

Moss AJ, Schwartz PJ: Delayed repolarization (QT or QTU prolongation) and malignant ventricular arrhythmias. Mod Concepts Cardiovasc Dis 1982; 51:85

Ramee SR, White CJ, Svinaridi JT: Torsade de pointes and magnesium deficiency. Am J Cardiol 1985; 109:164

Smith W, Gallagher TJ: "Les torsade de pointes": An unusual ventricular arrhythmia. Ann Intern Med 1980; 93:578

RATIONALE 19-d

Multifocal atrial tachycardia is a specific electrocardiographic entity characterized by an atrial rate of greater than 100 beats per minute, the presence of at least three different P-wave forms, and variation in PR and PP intervals.

Mitral valve disease and hepatic failure (associated with alcoholism) are most often associated with atrial fibrillation. Renal failure is not particularly associated with a specific dysrhythmia whereas MAT is most often seen in COPD. The most effective form of therapy for MAT is treatment of the lung condition. MAT is usually not responsive to digoxin therapy.

Verapamil has been found by Levine and others to consistently reduce the atrial and ventricular rate and occasionally convert multifocal atrial tachycardia to sinus rhythm.

REFERENCES

Clark ANG: Multifocal atrial tachycardia. Internal Medicine for the Specialist 1981; 2:10

Chung EK: Electrocardiography. Third Edition. Norwalk, CT, Appleton-Century-Crofts, 1985, p 186

DiMarco JP: Antiarrhythmics. In: The Pharmacologic Approach to the Critically Ill Patient. Chernow B (Ed). Baltimore, Williams & Wilkins Co., 1983, pp 331-369

Levine JH, Michael JR, Guarmieri T: Treatment of multifocal atrial tachycardia with verapamil. N Engl J Med 1985; 312:21

Shine KI, Kastor JA, Yurchak PM: Multifocal atrial tachycardia: Clinical and electrocardiographic features in 32 patients. N Engl J Med 1968; 279:344

RATIONALE 20-a

Although digoxin may be efficacious in this setting, its effect is slow in the non-digitalized patient and it has a narrow toxic-therapeutic ratio. Propranolol can be effective, but it can exacerbate asthma and heart failure and may be contraindicated in a patient requiring beta-adrenergic agonist therapy.

REFERENCES

DiMarco JP: Antiarrhythmics. In: The Pharmacologic Approach to the Critically Ill Patient. Chernow B (Ed). Baltimore, Williams & Wilkins Co., 1983, pp 331-369

Rosen KM, Bauernfeind RA: The tachyarrhythmias. In: Harrison's: Principles of Internal Medicine. Tenth Edition. Petersdorf HG, et al (Eds). New York, McGraw-Hill Book Company, 1983, 1372-1383

EDITORIAL COMMENT

Multiple new antidysrhythmic agents are under investigation and will be available for clinical use in the next few years. Each drug is unique with respect to chemical structure, indications, metabolism and complications. Podrid has recently succinctly reviewed the old and new antidysrhythmic agents. (See Section 13, page 229.)

ADDITIONAL REFERENCE

Podrid PI: Antiarrhythmic drug therapy (Parts I and II). Chest 1985; 88:452,618

HYPERTENSION

RATIONALE 21-a

Hypertensive encephalopathy is a syndrome characterized by high blood pressure, headache, visual disturbance, altered mental status and convulsions. Byroms' classical work supported the theory that loss of autoregulation with subsequent vasospasm was responsible for the symptoms. Recently, another theory, the "break through" theory, has suggested that the elevated blood pressure leads to break through hyperperfusion which results in cerebral edema.

The differential diagnosis includes cerebral infarction or hemorrhage. The best criteria for confirming the diagnosis is the rapid response of the patient's condition to antihypertensive therapy. Many authorities feel that nitroprusside is the therapeutic agent of choice. Nitroprusside increases cerebral blood flow and may raise ICP in a patient with decreased intracranial compliance, but this has never been shown to be an important consideration in hypertensive encephalopathy.

REFERENCES

Chester EM, et al: Hypertensive encephalopathy: A clinicopathologic study of 20 cases. Neurology 1978; 28:928

Palmer RF, Lasseter KC: Sodium nitroprusside. N Engl J Med 1975; 292:294

Ram CVS: Hypertensive encephalopathy - Recognition and management. Arch Intern Med 1978; 138:1851

RATIONALE 22-e

This patient has presented in a hypertensive crisis; the presence of mental confusion, papilledema, and severe elevation of his blood pressure necessitate rapid and effective pressure lowering to prevent death. Nitroprusside in the dosage given has become the most reliable medication for this situation and is probably the most commonly used. Several studies have also indicated the effectiveness of diazoxide infusions under similar circumstances.

Although oral clonidine (also prazosin, hydralazine, and minoxidil) is frequently used in the patient with severe elevation of blood pressure without evidence of hypertensive encephalopathy, its use in patients with encephalopathy is inappropriate. Oral aldomet should not be used in this setting.

Although rapid lowering of arterial pressure is desired, it should not be lowered too drastically. A diastolic level of 100 to 110 mm Hg is reasonable in a patient presenting in this manner.

REFERENCES

Kaplan NM: Management strategies in hypertension. In: Contemporary Issues in Nephrology. Vol 8, Hypertension. Brenner BM, Stein JH (Eds). New York, Churchill Livingstone Inc., 1981, pp 339-366

Wilson DJ, Wallin JD, Vlachakis ND, et al: Intravenous labetalol in the treatment of severe hypertension and hypotensive emergencies. Am J Med 1983; 75:595

EDITORIAL COMMENT

Hypertensive emergencies require rapid and aggressive treatment to prevent end-organ damage and death. Multiple drugs (some old, some new) are highly effective in management.

Drug	Dose	Comment
Sodium Nitroprusside	0.05-10 μg/kg•min continuous iv infusion	immediate onset, requires constant monitoring
Diazoxide	5 mg/kg rapid iv bolus	may produce reflex tachycardia, hypotension
Labetalol	20 mg iv bolus, bolus of 40-80 mg repeated as necessary q 10-15 min	avoid in patients with decompensated CHF, heart block, bronchospasm, and pregnancy
Captopril	0.5-1.0 mg/kg iv bolus	limited experience
Nifedipine	5-10 mg sublingually; repeat in 30 minutes if needed	puncture capsule before use

ADDITIONAL REFERENCES

AMA Committee on Hypertension: The treatment of malignant hypertension on hypertensive emergencies. JAMA 1974; 228:1673

Beer N, Gallegor I, Cohen A, et al: Efficacy of sublingual nifedipine in the acute treatment of systemic hypertension. Chest 1981; 79:571

Burris JF: Hypertensive emergencies. Am Fam Physician 1985; 32:97

Papademetrian V, Notargiacomo AV, Khatri IM, et al: Treatment of severe hypertension with intravenous labetalol. Clin Pharmacol Ther 1982; 32:431

Redgrave JE, Swartz SL: Diagnosis and management of malignant hypertension. Compr Ther 1985; 11:6

Tifft CP, Gavras H, Kershaw GR, et al: Converting enzyme inhibition in hypertensive emergencies. Ann Intern Med 1979; 90:43

INTRA-AORTIC BALLOON COUNTERPULSATION

RATIONALE 23-d

The intra-aortic balloon inflates during diastole and deflates during systole. During diastole the aortic valve is closed, and as the balloon inflates, coronary perfusion is increased as is pressure throughout the arterial circuit. The balloon's deflation during systole decreases systolic arterial pressure and left ventricular afterload. Left ventricular performance is improved because of diminished afterload and improved coronary perfusion. The improved left ventricular performance coupled with diastolic circulatory augmentation increases cardiac output and enhances tissue perfusion.

REFERENCES

Berger RL, Merin G: Mechanical support of the failing left ventricle. In: Handbook of Critical Care. Second Edition. Berle JC, Sampliner JE (Eds). Boston, Little, Brown and Co., 1982

Buckley MJ, Leinbach RC: Hemodynamic evaluation of intra-aortic balloon pumping in man. Circulation 1970; 41(Suppl II):130

McEvary MT, Kay HR, et al: Clinical experience with intra-aortic balloon pump support in 728 patients. Circulation 1977; 58(Suppl I):124

Mueller HS: Treatment of acute myocardial infarction. In: Critical Care: State of the Art. Vol 3. Shoemaker WC, Thompson WL (Eds). Fullerton, CA, Society of Critical Care Medicine, 1982, pp III(G):1-34

Rosenzweig J, Chatterjee S: Restoration of normal cardiac metabolism and hemodynamics after acute coronary occlusion. Ann Thorac Surg 1968; 6:146

Vigneswaran WT, Reece IJ, Davidson KG: Intra-aortic balloon pumping: Seven years' experience. Thorax 1985; 40:858

MYOCARDIAL INFARCTION

RATIONALE 24-c 25-e 26-a 27-b

The QRS complex represents the summation of the electrical forces generated from the various portions of the myocardium during ventricular depolarization. Infarcted tissue becomes electrically silent. The balance of the electrical forces point away from the infarcted area. During depolarization, an abnormal negative deflection will therefore be recorded in the electrode facing the infarcted myocardium. If the infarcted portion of the myocardium normally depolarizes early in the sequence of activation, an initial negative wave (Q wave) will be observed.

Anterior myocardial infarction is associated with Q waves in the precordial leads. Q waves in leads II, III and aVF are typical of inferior myocardial infarction.

Because posterior chest leads are not taken in the routine electrocardiogram, reciprocal changes in the anterior precordial leads are utilized to distinguish posterior infarction. Tall R waves in leads V_1 and V_2 with ST segment depression often signify acute posterior infarction.

The subendocardium contributes little voltage to the surface electrocardiogram. The most consistent electrocardiographic finding in subendocardial infarction is ST segment depression and Q wave inversion in the leads that face the epicardial surface overlying the infarcted area.

REFERENCES

Chou T: Electrocardiography in Clinical Practice. New York, Grune & Stratton, 1979

Marriott HJL: Practical Electrocardiography. Sixth Edition. Baltimore, Williams & Wilkins Co., 1977

RATIONALE 28-d

Postoperative myocardial infarction causes a mortality that is nearly double that of the nonsurgical myocardial infarction. Mortality rates of 50% are not uncommon in this group of patients. The likelihood of a postoperative MI is at least 10 times greater for those patients who have had a previous MI, as compared to those with no history of previous infarction. Due to the effects of narcotics and the surgery itself, chest pain is not the most common presentation of MI in these patients. Rather, the appearance of dysrhythmias, hypertension, CHF or tachypnea more commonly suggests the possibility of infarction. Portable nuclear imaging techniques have increased the accuracy of diagnosis for the postsurgical patient, in whom both EKG and enzyme determinators can be clouded by the effects of surgery.

REFERENCES

Goldman DR, Brown FH, Levy WK, et al: Medical Care of the Surgical Patient. Philadelphia, JB Lippincott Co., 1982, p 96

Manual of Surgical Intensive Care by the Committee on Pre and Postoperative Care of the American College of Surgeons. Philadelphia, WB Saunders Co., 1977, pp 264-265

Steen PA: Myocardial reinfarction after anesthesia and surgery. An update: Incidence, mortality and predisposing factors. JAMA 1978; 239:2566

Tarhan S, et al: Myocardial infarction after general anesthesia. JAMA 1972; 220:1451

RATIONALE 29-b

Early treatment and recognition of right ventricular infarction causing cardiogenic shock is essential because the mortality of patients in shock caused by RV infarction approaches 50%-75% as contrasted to 90%-95% in shock secondary to left ventricular (LV) infarction. Fourteen percent of patients dying of transmural LV infarction have some involvement of the right ventricular wall as well. RV infarction is rare as an isolated event. A low pulmonary artery wedge pressure found in RV infarction and shock does not necessarily imply that LV damage is slight; more often it implies that the injured RV is unable to pump enough blood to fill the left ventricular cavity effectively during diastole. In myocardial infarction, an elevated jugular venous pressure is not necessarily an indication for diuretic therapy; in particular, if RV infarction and shock has occurred, RV cardiac output which is dependent upon a high right-sided filling pressure markedly deteriorates after administration of an effective diuretic agent. The initial treatment for hypotension with RV infarct is vigorous volume therapy even in the presence of distended neck veins.

REFERENCES

Cohn JN, Guiha NH, Broder ML, et al: Right ventricular infarction. Clinical and hemodynamic features. Am J Cardiol 1974; 33:209

Elkayam U, Halprin SL, Frishman W, et al: Echocardiographic findings in cardiogenic shock due to right ventricular myocardial infarction. Cathet Cardiovasc Diagn 1979; 5:289

Fehir KM: Right ventricular infarction. Johns Hopkins Med J 1980; 147:117

Furey SA, Zieska HA, Levy MN: The essential function of the right ventricle. Am Heart J 1984; 107:404

Gewirtz H, Gold HK, Fallon JT, et al: Role of right ventricular infarction in cardiogenic shock associated with inferior myocardial infarction. Br Heart J 1979; 42:719

Jugdutt BL, Sussex BA, Sivaram CA, et al: Right ventricular infarction: Two-dimensional echocardiographic evaluation. Am Heart J 1984; 107:505

Kaul S, Tei C, Hopkins JM, et al: Assessment of right ventricular function using two-dimensional echocardiography. Am Heart J 1984; 107:526

EDITORIAL COMMENT

The treatment of acute myocardial infarction continues to undergo intense investigation. Recanalization of coronary arteries utilizing intracoronary or intravenous streptokinase is promising. Whether this reverses or limits the acute infarction has not yet been established.

Intracoronary streptokinase, if given within the first four hours after the onset of symptoms, can reduce myocardial damage. Intravenous streptokinase can also produce recanalization but probably less often than intraarterial.

Tissue-type plasminogen activator is almost twice as effective as intravenous streptokinase in recanalizing coronary arteries.

Emergency coronary artery bypass surgery is promising yet requires further study. It has been performed safely in the setting of acute myocardial infarction, however, definite patient benefit remains to be established.

ADDITIONAL REFERENCES

DeWood MA, Spores J, Notske RN, et al: Medical and surgical management of myocardial infarction. Am J Cardiol 1979; 44:1356

Gang W, Buchbinder N, Marcus H, et al: Intracoronary thrombolysis in evolving myocardial infarction. Am Heart J 1981; 101:4

Koren G, Weiss AT, Hasin Y: Prevention of myocardial damage in acute myocardial ischemia by early treatment with intravenous streptokinase. N Engl J Med 1985; 313:1384

Mathey DG, Kuck KH, Tilsner V, et al: Nonsurgical coronary artery recanalization in acute transmural myocardial infarction. Circulation 1981; 63:489

Mayer G, Story WE, Seco JE: Intravenous streptokinase in acute myocardial infarction. Ann Emerg Med 1985; 14:410

Phillips SJ, Kongtahworn C, Zeff RH, et al: Emergency coronary artery revascularization: A possible role for acute infarction. Circulation 1979; 60:241

Relman AS: Intravenous thrombolysis in acute myocardial infarction: A progress report (Editorial). N Engl J Med 1985; 312:915

Swan HJC: Thrombolysis in acute evolving myocardial infarction: A new potential for myocardial salvage (Editorial). N Engl J Med 1983; 308:1354

The TIMI Study Group: The thrombolysis in myocardial infarction (TIMI) trial: Phase I findings. N Engl J Med 1985; 312:932

PACEMAKERS

RATIONALE 30-d

Ventricular asystole and heart block associated with hypotension represent life-threatening situations due to malfunction of the electrical conduction system within the heart. The presence of new trifascicular block in the setting of acute anterior wall ischemia is associated with development of complete AV block in approximately 35% of patients. Temporary cardiac pacing is indicated in each of these situations.

Electromechanical disassociation represents failed myocardial function and not failure of impulse generation or conduction. Cardiac pacing, therefore, is unlikely to be of benefit in this setting.

REFERENCES

Escher DJW: Temporary cardiac pacing. In: Textbook of Critical Care. Shoemaker WC, Thompson WL, Holbrook PR (Eds). Philadelphia, WB Saunders Co., 1984, pp 439-445

Hindman MC, Wagner GS, Jaro M, et al: The clinical significance of bundle branch block complicating acute myocardial infarction: II. Indications for temporary and permanent pacemaker insertion. Circulation 1978; 58:689

McAnulty JH, Rahintoola SH, Murphy E, et al: Natural history of "high-risk" bundle-branch block: Final report of a prospective study. N Engl J Med 1982; 307:137

Rosen KM, Dhingra RC, Loeb HS, et al: Chronic heart block in adults: Clinical and electrophysiologic observation. Arch Intern Med 1973; 131:663

EDITORIAL COMMENT

Cardiac pacing techniques have changed rapidly over the past several years. Bradycardias and tachycardias may be effectively managed by artificial pacing. Temporary emergency cardiac pacing is indicated for sustained symptomatic bradycardia. Prophylactic pacing in the setting of acute myocardial infarction remains controversial. Indications for temporary cardiac pacing in acute myocardial infarction are given below. Rapid atrial or ventricular pacing is an alternative to cardioversion in atrial flutter and ventricular tachycardia.

Indications for prophylactic temporary cardiac pacing in acute myocardial infarction:

- Generally Accepted -

1. Newly acquired bifascicular block
2. Second degree AV block, type II
3. Complete AV block

- Controversial -

1. Acute anterior MI with a new right bundle branch block and a normal axis.
2. Acute anterior MI with a new left bundle branch block and a normal PR interval.

ADDITIONAL REFERENCES

Chung EK: Artificial Cardiac Pacing: A Practical Approach. Second Edition. Baltimore, Williams & Wilkins Co., 1984

Donovan KD: Cardiac pacing in intensive care. Anaesth Intensive Care 1985; 13:41

Donovan KD, Lee KY: Indications for and complications of temporary transvenous cardiac pacing. Anaesth Intensive Care 1985; 13:63

Luceri RM, Myerburg RJ: Indications for and management of cardiac pacemakers. DM 1985; 31:1

PULSUS PARADOXUS

RATIONALE 31-e

Pulsus paradoxus is an exaggeration of the normal decrement in arterial pressure during inspiration. Although for this condition to be present the inspiratory decrement should be 10 mm Hg or greater. Healthy subjects have almost no respiratory excursion in arterial pressure and, therefore, any detectable variation in arterial pressure should be noted carefully. Arterial pressure is decreased when left ventricular filling is compromised in inspiration by (1) torsion of a tense pericardium during diaphragmatic descent, (2) retardation of forward blood flow in pulmonary veins with negative intrathoracic pressures, and (3) encroachment of the right ventricle on the left ventricle when inspiration enhances right heart filling within a restrictive pericardium. This nonparadoxical "paradox" is associated with pericardial tamponade or constriction, vena caval obstruction, and with severe cardiomyopathy. It is seen commonly in chronic obstructive lung disease, upper airway obstruction, pulmonary embolization, and acute bronchial asthma when the excursions of intrathoracic pressures with breathing are exaggerated. In asthma the magnitude of pulsus paradoxus correlates with the severity of airway obstruction and is a valuable vital sign. In pneumonia, pulsus paradoxus may be observed when labored breathing causes exaggerated excursions in intrathoracic pressure, but it is an uncommon finding. In hypovolemic hypotension pulsus paradoxus is common, is associated with low rather than high venous pressures, and is corrected by intravascular volume augmentation.

REFERENCES

Cohn JN, Pinkerson AL, Tristani FE: Mechanism of pulsus paradoxus in clinical shock. J Clin Invest 1967; 46:1744

Fowler NO: Cardiac Diagnosis and Treatment. Second Edition. Maryland, Harper and Row, 1976, pp 862-865

Hurst JW, Schlant RC: Examination of the arteries and their pulsations. In: The Heart. Fourth Edition. Hurst JW (Ed). New York, McGraw-Hill Book Company, 1978, pp 191-192

Spodick DH: Acute cardiac tamponade: Pathologic physiology, diagnosis and management. Prog Cardiovasc Dis 1967; 10:64

Stein L, Shubin H, Weil MH: Recognition and management of pericardial tamponade. In: Critical Care Medicine. Weil MH, Shubin H (Eds). Maryland, Harper and Row, 1976, pp 83-89

RATIONALE 32-a

Normally there is slight fluctuation in arterial pressure during inspiration and expiration. A fall in pressure during inspiration is exaggerated with forced respiratory effort, cardiac failure, and cardiac tamponade and is termed pulsus paradoxus.

The mechanisms explaining pulsus paradoxus involve (1) the drop in pleural pressure during inspiration, and (2) the increase in venous return relating to this change.

Left ventricular afterload is determined by peripheral resistance and the transmural pressure affecting the ventricle. Any drop in pleural pressure will proportionately increase left ventricular afterload. At the same time, the drop in pleural pressure promotes venous return which increases right ventricular preload and shifts the interventricular septum toward the left. This effect is more pronounced at higher baseline venous pressures. The overall effect, therefore, is a drop in left ventricular filling, an increase in left ventricular afterload and a decrease in pulse pressure.

REFERENCES

Buda AJ, Pinsky MR, Ingels NB, et al: Effect of intrathoracic pressure on left ventricular performance. N Engl J Med 1979; 301:453

McGregor M: Pulsus paradoxus. N Engl J Med 1979; 301:480

Shabetai R: Diseases of the pericardium. In: The Heart. Sixth Edition. Hurst JW (Ed). New York, McGraw-Hill Book Company, 1986, pp 1249-1275

SHOCK

RATIONALE 33-e

Cefotaxime sodium is a semisynthetic, broad-spectrum cephalosporin antibiotic. Penicillin allergic patients may develop clinical hypersensitivity reactions to cephalosporins with a frequency of 5%-10%. Anaphylaxis is a Type I hypersensitivity reaction (Gell-Coombs). IgE mediated mast cell degranulation with release of potent vasoactive mediators represents the underlying pathophysiology. Reactions to radiographic contrast media (anaphylactoid reactions) cause direct mast cell degranulation and are not IgE mediated. Epinephrine remains the mainstay of therapy in anaphylactic and anaphylactoid reactions. The dosage of epinephrine is 0.2 - 0.5 cc of a 1:1,000 solution given IM or 2 - 5 cc of a 1:10,000 solution given iv. The dose is repeated every 15-20 minutes as needed. Airway management and volume expansion are certainly appropriate. Corticosteroids are also used but have a delayed onset of action. Bronchodilators and antihistamines have also been used.

Pulmonary fat embolization is a relatively uncommon clinical disorder occurring in patients who have sustained extensive fracture trauma. Signs and symptoms of this disorder usually appear 12-72 hours following trauma. These include among others: a petechial rash, tachycardia, tachypnea, fever, fat globules in the retinal vessels, neutral fat in the urine, progressive arterial hypoxemia and a diffuse infiltrate seen on chest radiography.

REFERENCES

Austen KF: Systemic anaphylaxis in the human being. N Engl J Med 1974; 291:661

Lahiri B, ZuWallack R: The early diagnosis and treatment of fat embolism syndrome: A preliminary report. J Trauma 1977; 17:956

Levine BB: Antigenicity and cross-reactivity of penicillins and cephalosporins. J Infect Dis 1973; 128:364

Lockey RF, Bukanty SC: Allergic emergencies. Med Clin North Am 1974; 58:147

Roitt IM: Essential Immunology. Fourth Edition. Boston, Blackwell Scientific Publications, 1981

Slavin R: Hyperimmune states. In: Critical Care: State of the Art. Vol 1. Shoemaker WC, Thompson WL (Eds). Fullerton, CA, Society of Critical Care Medicine, 1980, pp I(J):1-21

Section 4

34. The diagnosis of dysbarism (decompression sickness) is made in a 30-year-old scuba diver. Which ONE of the following statements regarding this disorder is FALSE?

a. Symptoms usually appear within the first hour but may be delayed for up to 36 hours.
b. An immediate redive utilizing SCUBA equipment is as effective as chamber recompression therapy in the treatment of this disorder.
c. Nitrogen bubbles in the microvasculature may produce endothelial surface changes that initiate intravascular coagulation.
d. Because nitrogen is much more soluble in lipid than in water, its concentration tends to be greatest in lipid rich tissues such as the central nervous system.
e. Treatment is more likely to be effective the sooner that it commences after the onset of symptoms.

35. Which of the following may predispose an individual to heat stroke?

a. Advanced age
b. Diabetes mellitus
c. Diuretic use
d. Ethyl alcohol ingestion
e. All of the above

36. Which of the following statements about accidental exposure-induced hypothermia (core temperature less than 35°C) is TRUE?

a. Osborn ("J") waves are frequently seen on the electrocardiogram.
b. The profoundly hypothermic heart in ventricular fibrillation is relatively unresponsive to electrical countershock.
c. The hematocrit is generally elevated at temperatures less than 27°C.
d. Active external rewarming may cause paradoxical central cooling.
e. All of the above

37. All of the following are frequently seen in the hypothermic patient (core temperature of 27°C) EXCEPT:

a. EKG abnormalities including sinus bradycardia, T-wave inversions, J-waves, and atrial and ventricular tachydysrhythmias
b. Hyperglycemia
c. Decreased urine flow
d. Hemoconcentration

38. A 10 kg, two-year-old child is found lying face down in a backyard swimming pool. He is brought to the Emergency Room by the EMS and appears to be awake but lethargic with a somewhat dusky color. He is taken to the ICU for subsequent management. Which ONE of the following statements concerning near-drowning in children is CORRECT?

a. Prophylactic antibiotics significantly improve the chance of survival in near-drowning victims.
b. Hypothermia, hyperventilation and hypotension can all be used to improve the cerebral survival in near-drowning victims.
c. Early use of corticosteroids improves the chance of survival in this setting.
d. Any patient with near-drowning, including those who are awake and alert on initial evaluation, should be admitted to the hospital for observation.

ENVIRONMENTAL INJURY

ANSWERS

34-b 35-e 36-e 37-c 38-d

==

DYSBARISM

==

RATIONALE 34-b

Nitrogen is far more soluble in lipid than in water. Its concentration, therefore, tends to be highest in highly vascular lipid rich tissue such as the central nervous system, bone marrow, and various fat deposits. If a SCUBA diver ascends too rapidly from a dive, nitrogen bubbles may form in these tissues in the intra and extravascular space.

Symptoms usually appear rapidly but may be delayed as long as 36 hours. Musculoskeletal pain (bends) is common and is caused by nitrogen bubbles in the muscles, joints, periarticular tissues, and bones. Nitrogen emboli in the pulmonary microcirculation may cause cough, dyspnea, and chest pain (chokes). Severe vascular occlusion may cause a reduction in cardiac output and even circulatory shock.

CNS involvement may present as lethargy, mood changes, focal deficits, and seizures. Spinal cord involvement is common.

Nitrogen bubbles may produce microvascular endothelial changes and initiate disseminated intravascular coagulation.

The first line of treatment in decompression sickness is prompt hyperbaric chamber recompression. Treatment delayed as long as several days may, however, be beneficial. The futility of in-water recompression is well known. Steroids may be beneficial in selected patients with neurologic symptoms.

REFERENCES

Bryan-Brown CW: Gas transport and delivery. In: Critical Care: State of the Art. Vol 1. Shoemaker WC, Thompson WL (Eds). Fullerton, CA, Society of Critical Care Medicine, 1980, pp I(E):1-36

Kizer KW: Delayed treatment of dysbarism: A retrospective review of 50 cases. JAMA 1982; 247:2555

Kizer KW: Diving medicine. Emerg Med Clin North Am 1984; 2:513

Rubenstein E: Water-related accidents. Sci Am 1983; 8:1

Strauss RH: Diving Medicine. New York, Grune & Stratton Inc., 1976

HYPERTHERMIA

RATIONALE 35-e

Individuals with autonomic dysfunction have imparied mechanisms for heat dissipation. Diabetics and the aged are at particular risk. Dehydration of any etiology decreases the efficiency of cooling by evaporation. Diuretics, therefore, may predispose to heat stroke. Alcohol, likewise, may cause diuresis and increase metabolic heat production.

REFERENCES

Clowes GH Jr, O'Donnell TF Jr: Heat stroke. N Engl J Med 1974; 291:564

Exertional heat injury. Med Lett Drugs Ther 1985; 27:55

Geiss P, Marr JJ: Management of heat injury syndromes. In: Critical Care: State of the Art. Vol 3. Shoemaker WC, Thompson WL (Eds). Fullerton, CA, Society of Critical Care Medicine, 1982, pp III(K):1-24

Levine JA: Heat stroke in the aged. Am J Med 1969; 47:251

Olson KR, Benowitz NL: Environmental and drug-induced hyperthermia: Pathophysiology, recognition and management. Emerg Med Clin North Am 1984; 2:459

Tucker LE, Stanford J, Granes B, et al: Classical heatstroke: Clinical and laboratory assessment. South Med J 1985; 78:20

Wheeler M: Heat stroke in the elderly. Med Clin North Am 1976; 60:1289

HYPOTHERMIA

RATIONALE 36-e 37-c

Hypothermia, defined as a core temperature less than 35°C, may have a significant morbidity and mortality, especially if unrecognized. All body systems are affected. A variety of electrocardiographic changes have been described, including sinus bradycardia, interval prolongation, the pathognomic "J" (Osborn) wave as well as atrial and ventricular tachydysrhythmias. The profoundly hypothermic heart is relatively unresponsive to electrical countershock. Countershock in the presence of ventricular fibrillation is worthwhile, but if unsuccessful, cardiopulmonary resuscitation should be continued until the core temperature is raised. Renal tubular oxidative activity decreases with the low temperature causing a "cold diuresis" with reduced sodium and water resorption. At core temperatures less than 27°C, plasma loss and splenic contraction cause elevation of the hematocrit.

REFERENCES

Gunton RW, Scott JW, et al: Changes in cardiac rhythm and in the form of the electrocardiogram resulting from induced hypothermia in man. Am Heart J 1956; 52:419

Kanter GS: Hypothermic hemoconcentration. Am J Physiol 1968; 214:856

Mayer JH, Morris G, et al: Hypothermia: I. Effect on renal hemodynamics and on excretion of water and electrolytes in dog and man. Ann Surg 1957; 145:26

Reuler JB: Hypothermia: Pathophysiology, clinical settings and management. Ann Intern Med 1978; 89:519

Schwab RH, Lewis DW, et al: Electrocardiographic changes occurring in rapidly induced deep hypothermia. Am J Med Sci 1964; 248:290

Trevino A, Razi B, Beller BM: The characteristic electrocardiogram of accidental hypothermia. Arch Intern Med 1971; 127:470

EDITORIAL COMMENT

Warming techniques in the hypothermic patient are controversial. Both external and internal techniques have been advocated. External warming may cause peripheral vasodilation with shunting of cold blood to the core and subsequent paradoxical decrease in core temperature.

Internal warming techniques are clearly favored in severe hypothermia (30°C or less) and refractory life-threatening ventricular arrhythmias. This may be accomplished by one or several of the methods listed below:

- Heart-lung bypass
- Hemodialysis
- Peritoneal dialysis with warmed fluid
- Warmed iv fluid (approx. 45°C)
- Heated humidified oxygen (at or below 40°C)
- Gastric lavage
- Bladder lavage
- Open thoracotomy with warm saline lavage

The most effective warming technique is extracorporeal circulation (heart-lung bypass) which not only warms but also supports oxygenation and circulation in the arrested patient. If the expertise is available, this technique should be considered for severely hypothermic patients. A quick and efficient method of warming resuscitation solutions has been described utilizing a microwave oven.

ADDITIONAL REFERENCES

Bangs CC: Hypothermia and frostbite. Emerg Med Clin North Am 1984; 2:475

Best R, Syverud S, Nowak RM: Trauma and hypothermia. Am J Emerg Med 1985; 3:48

Ferguson J, Epstein F, van de Leuv J: Accidental hypothermia. Emerg Med Clin North Am 1983; 1:619

Leaman PL, Martyak GG: Microwave warming of resuscitation fluids. Ann Emerg Med 1985; 14:876

Sturm JT, Logan MA: Microwave aids in external rewarming of hypothermia patients (letter). Ann Emerg Med 1985; 14:277

Zell SC, Kurtz KJ: Severe exposure hypothermia: A resuscitation protocol. Ann Emerg Med 1985; 14:339

NEAR-DROWNING

RATIONALE 38-d

Drowning is a major cause of death and severe CNS injury in children and young adults. Any victim of near-drowning, which is any person who at least temporarily survives submersion suffocation, should be observed in a hospital for at least 24 hours, even if chest radiograph and neurologic exam are normal. Although there is some difference in pulmonary pathophysiology between fresh and salt water near-drowning, the major hallmark of both is severe hypoxemia. CNS injury can occur from hypoxemia-induced cerebral edema. Such maneuvers as hypothermia and hyperventilation may help decrease cerebral metabolism and swelling. However, the injured brain is much more sensitive to the damaging effects of hypotension, hypoglycemia and hypoxemia than is the normal brain.

Aspiration of water is usually not of such volume in near-drowning to cause major fluid shifts, but can produce pulmonary edema and resultant hypoxemia. Pulmonary aspiration of gastric contents and other substances such as soil, bacteria and organisms from the water may be a cause of major morbidity. Nevertheless, routine prophylactic treatment with antibiotics is not recommended until culture proven or obvious clinical infection is present. Corticosteroid use in this setting has not improved survival. Mechanical ventilation with positive end-expiratory pressure (PEEP) to distend and open collapsed alveoli continues to be a mainstay of pulmonary management.

REFERENCES

Conn AW, Montes GA, Barker GA, et al: Cerebral salvage in near drowning following neurological classification by triage. Can Anaesth Soc J 1980; 27:3

Modell JH: Biology of drowning. Annu Rev Med 1978; 29:1

Modell JH, Boysen PG: Respiratory crises. In: Critical Care: State of the Art. Vol 1. Shoemaker WC, Thompson WL (Eds). Fullerton, CA, Society of Critical Care Medicine, 1980, pp I(F):1-38

Modell JH, Graves SA, Kuck EJ: Near drowning: Correlation of level of consciousness and survival. Can Anaesth Soc J 1980; 27:3

Peterson B: Morbidity of near drowning. Pediatrics 1977; 59:364

Spyker DA: Submersion injury: Epidemiology, prevention, and management. Pediatr Clin North Am 1985; 32:113

Tabeling BB: Near drowning evaluation and management. Current Reviews in Clinical Anesthesia, Lesson 1, Vol 2, 1982

Section 5

39. A 40-year-old female with a history of insulin dependent diabetes mellitus is admitted to the ICU with right upper quadrant pain, nausea, and vomiting.

Temperature: 102.4°F, oral

Examination reveals right upper quadrant tenderness without rebound or guarding.

Laboratory:
Total bilirubin: 2.1
WBC: 13,500 - 75 segmented neutrophils, 20 lymphocytes, 5 bands

Which ONE of the items listed below is the best diagnostic test to evaluate this patient's right upper quadrant pain?

a. Oral cholecystogram
b. 2 hour urine amylase
c. Computed tomography (CT)
d. Tc-99m Disida hepatobiliary scintigram (Hida scan)
e. Intravenous cholangiogram

40. An acutely ill male patient was transferred to the ICU with heart failure, bronchospasm and melena. A nasogastric (NG) tube was inserted, an aspirate from which was hemoccult negative. The following therapy was instituted: furosemide, 40 mg intravenously; oxygen by nasal cannula at 2 liters/minute; enteral feeding by NG tube; and aerosolized beta agonists. A chest radiograph was obtained shortly after the patient arrived in the ICU (Fig. 3). Two hours later, the patient developed increasing shortness of breath and worsening hypoxemia.

Which ONE of the following is the MOST appropriate IMMEDIATE action?

a. Discontinue furosemide and give volume to increase preload.
b. Obtain ventilation/perfusion lung scintigraphy.
c. Increase intravenous furosemide dose to 80 mg.
d. Discontinue enteral feedings.
e. Discontinue the beta agonist aerosol therapy.

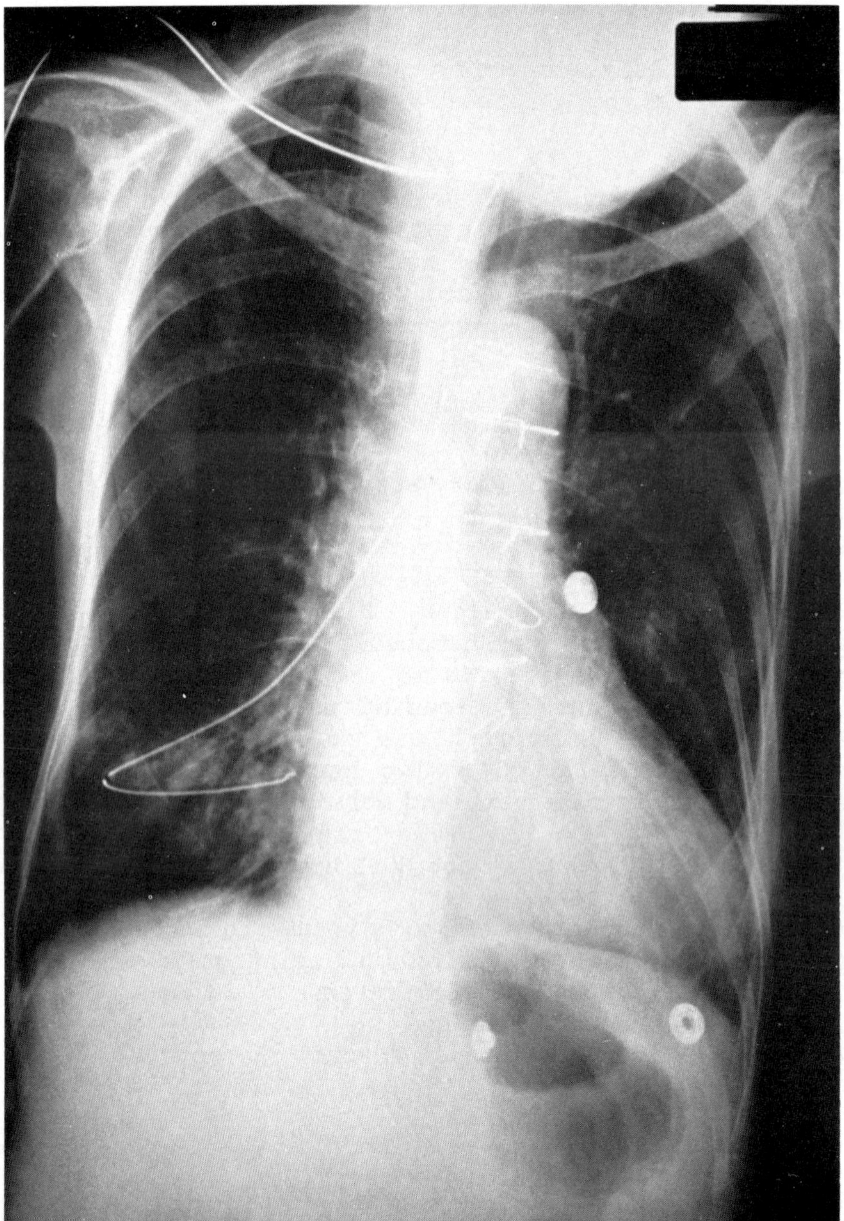

Figure 3

41. A patient with cirrhosis and esophageal varices developed an upper GI bleed. Vasopressin infusion was unsuccessful in controlling the bleeding. A Sengstaken-Blakemore (SB) tube was inserted and the gastric balloon (only) was inflated. Brisk bleeding continued. A chest radiograph following the SB tube insertion is shown in Figure 4.

Which ONE of the following options regarding management of this case is MOST correct?

a. Inflate the esophageal balloon.
b. Reposition the SB tube.
c. Reposition the left chest tube.
d. Obtain a left lateral decubitus chest radiograph.

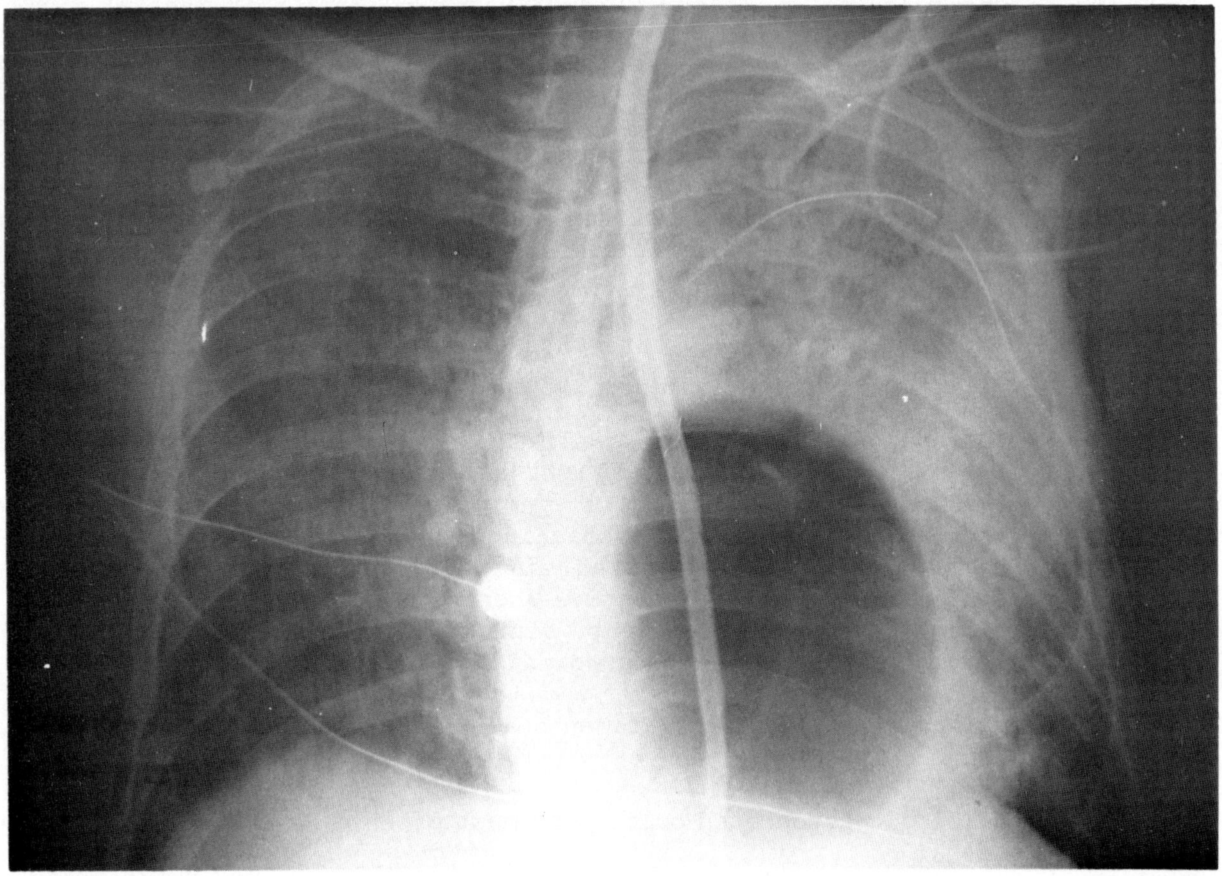

Figure 4

42. A 36-year-old man develops fever and abdominal tenderness. He has had regional enteritis for 5 years and has several fistulae between loops of bowel. You suspect he has peritonitis caused by anaerobic bacteria from his colon. Which ONE of the following antibiotics is LEAST likely to be effective?

a. Carbenicillin
b. Cefoxitin
c. Cephalothin
d. Chloramphenicol
e. Clindamycin

43. Which of the following statements regarding generalized bacterial peritonitis is/are CORRECT?

a. Generalized bacterial peritonitis resulting from a perforated duodenal ulcer has a better prognosis than bacterial peritonitis that develops following breakdown and leakage of a colonic anastomosis.
b. The classical physical signs of peritonitis are less reliable in postoperative patients.
c. Patients whose operative therapy is performed more than 24 hours after the onset of peritonitis have a higher mortality than those operated upon within the first 24 hours of symptoms.
d. Generalized bacterial peritonitis secondary to a perforated viscus is most often a polymicrobial infection.
e. All of the above

44. Which ONE of the following statements concerning radiological procedures for evaluation of a potential intra-abdominal abscess is FALSE?

a. Ultrasound is preferable to CT as the initial radiological procedure for left upper quadrant and right lower quadrant abscess detection.
b. Localized abdominal signs or symptoms make ultrasound or CT scan preferable to radionuclide scanning.
c. In the absence of localizing signs or symptoms, ultrasound and CT scan are usually more effective when guided by radionuclide scan.
d. In the postoperative patient, search for abscesses should be guided by knowledge of suspected surgical complications.

45. Which ONE of the following statements about antibiotic-associated colitis is TRUE?

a. Antibiotic-associated colitis is most often caused by Staphylococcus aureus.
b. Antibiotic-associated colitis is best diagnosed with stool cultures.
c. Common causative agents are ampicillin and clindamycin.
d. The treatment of choice is intravenous vancomycin.

ANSWERS

39-d 40-d 41-b 42-c 43-e 44-a 45-c

CHOLECYSTITIS

RATIONALE 39-d

The patient most likely has acute cholecystitis as the cause of her right upper quadrant pain, nausea, and vomiting. Hepatobiliary scintigraphy has proved to be of greatest value in the diagnosis of acute cholecystitis. If one were to pathologically examine the gallbladders from patients with acute cholecystitis, over 95 percent would have cystic duct obstruction. In this group of patients, radiopharmaceuticals secreted into the bile by the liver cannot enter the inflamed gallbladder. This fact provides the theoretical basis for employing Technetium-99m hepatobiliary agents to diagnose the disease. In several large series, accuracy has been greater than 95 percent. Additionally, this imaging modality is usually unaffected by modest levels of jaundice.

Computed tomography and ultrasonography may demonstrate the presence of gallstones, however, these imaging modalities are unable to consistently diagnose cystic duct obstruction. The use of an oral cholecystogram or intravenous cholangiogram is not justified in the acute setting. The symptom complex does not suggest acute pancreatitis.

REFERENCES

Freitas JE: Cholescintigraphy in acute and chronic cholecystitis. Semin Nucl Med 1982; 12:18

Weismann HS, Badia J, Sugarmen LA, et al: Spectrum of cholescintigraphic patterns in acute cholecystitis. Radiology 1981; 138:167

Weismann HS, Frank M, Rosenblatt R, et al: Cholescintigraphy, ultrasound, and computerized tomography in the evaluation of biliary tract disorders. Semin Nucl Med 1979; 9:22

ENTERAL TUBES

RATIONALE 40-d

The chest radiograph in Figure 3 demonstrates NG tube placement in the right mainstem bronchus. The patient's shortness of breath and hypoxemia were secondary to the intrabronchial infusion of the feeding solution. Discontinuation of the feeding and removal of the tube is the most appropriate initial therapy. Although insertion of a large-bore NG tube into the bronchial tree is unusual, it is certainly possible, particularly in debilitated patients. Elderly debilitated patients may have very little cough reflex upon stimulation of the upper tracheal bronchial tree. Bronchial placement is more likely with the smaller enteral feeding tubes. It is imperative that a radiograph be obtained to verify position of enteral feeding tubes prior to administration of solution. Careful review of the chest radiograph demonstrated in this patient should have prevented this complication.

REFERENCES

Culpepper JA, Veremakis C, Guntupalli KK, et al: Malpositioned nasogastric tube causing pneumothorax and bronchopleural fistula. Chest 1982; 81:389

Ratzlaff HC, Heaslip JE, Rothwell ES: Factors affecting nasogastric tube insertion. Crit Care Med 1984; 12:52

Sweatman AJ, Tomasello PA, Longhead MG, et al: Misplacement of nasogastric tubes and esophageal monitoring devices. Br J Anaesth 1978; 50:389

ESOPHAGEAL VARICES

RATIONALE 41-b

The chest radiograph in Figure 4 demonstrates a left hemithoracic location of the SB tube gastric balloon.

Treatment of bleeding esophageal varices with balloon tamponade may be effective but is associated with significant complications. Numerous cases of esophageal rupture following balloon tamponade have been reported. Intra-esophageal inflation of the gastric balloon is the most common cause of esophageal rupture in this setting. Excessive traction on the tube has also been associated with distal esophageal perforation.

Balloon esophageal perforation may be associated with abrupt cardiovascular collapse or may take a more subacute course. In the latter case, pleural effusions may develop and suggest the diagnosis.

Rapidly progressive hemodynamic compromise with balloon esophageal perforation may warrant urgent surgical exploration.

REFERENCES

Burcharth F, Malmstrom J: Experiences with the Linton-Nachlas and Sengstaken-Blakemore tubes for bleeding esophageal varices. Surg Gynecol Obstet 1976; 142:529

Conn HO, Simpson JA: Excessive mortality associated with balloon tamponade of bleeding varices. JAMA 1967; 202:587

Johansen TS, Baden H: Re-appraisal of Sengstaken-Blakemore balloon tamponade for bleeding esophageal varices: Results in 91 patients. Scand J Gastroenteral 1973; 8:181

Rubin SA, Winsett MA, Diner WC: Intrathoracic gastric balloon: Radiographic recognition of esophageal perforation. Gastrointest Radiol 1982; 7:311

PERITONITIS

RATIONALE 42-c

All of the antibiotics listed, except cephalothin, have satisfactory efficacy against anaerobic organisms. Carbenicillin has an anaerobic spectrum similar to a penicillin G except that it is usually effective against Bacteroides fragilis. In one study, involving 9 patients with intra-abdominal sepsis due to anaerobic flora, 8 isolates were susceptible to carbenicillin.

Cefoxitin is a second generation cephalosporin with a spectrum of activity that, unlike cephalothin, includes B. fragilis and most other anaerobes. It is bactericidal, and an acceptable alternative to chloramphenicol or clindamycin after bowel trauma or surgery.

Chloramphenicol is bacteriostatic, but has an outstanding spectrum for all anaerobes. Clindamycin is usually bactericidal, and has a broad anaerobic spectrum that includes B. fragilis. For this reason, it may be considered in preference to penicillin when this organism is suspected. For sepsis, including septic shock secondary to an intra-abdominal focus, the combination of clindamycin with an aminoglycoside, usually gentamicin, may be the chemotherapy of choice. The major drawback of clindamycin is development of pseudomembranous enterocolitis by some patients due to overgrowth of Clostridia.

REFERENCES

Fass RJ, Ruiz DE, Gardner WG, et al: Clindamycin and gentamicin for aerobic and anaerobic sepsis. Arch Intern Med 1977; 137:28

Kislak JW: The susceptibility of Bacteroides fragilis to 24 antibiotics. J Infect Dis 1972; 125:295

Meny R, Webb CD, Fiedelman W: Carbenicillin therapy of anaerobic infections. Curr Therapeut Res 1975; 17:478

Neu HC: The penicillins. I. Overview of microbiology. NY State J Med 1977; 77:768

Neu HC: The new beta-lactamase-stable cephalosporins. Ann Intern Med 1982; 97:408

Sutter VL, Finegold SM: Susceptibility of anaerobic bacteria to carbenicillin, cefoxitin, and related drugs. J Infect Dis 1975; 131:417

RATIONALE 43-e

Mortality from generalized bacterial peritonitis is extremely high in certain groups of patients. Peritonitis secondary to perforation of a duodenal ulcer or appendix may have a mortality of 10% while peritonitis secondary to breakdown and leakage of a colonic anastomosis has a mortality as high as 60% in some series.

Because of sedation, narcotic analgesia or incisional pain, the classical physical findings of generalized peritonitis may be obscured in the post-surgical patient and are less reliable than in the preoperative state.

The mortality rate in individuals who underwent delayed surgery (i.e., surgery performed more than 24 hours after the onset of symptoms) was threefold that of individuals who underwent early surgery in a series of 176 patients with generalized peritonitis published by Bohnen.

Peritonitis secondary to a perforated viscus is usually due to infection with mixed bowel flora including anaerobes. Broad-spectrum antibiotics are warranted in this setting.

REFERENCES

Bohnen J, Boulanger M, et al: Prognosis in generalized peritonitis. Arch Surg 1983; 118:285

Fry DE, Garrison RN: Determinants of death in patients with intraabdominal abscess. Surgery 1980; 88:517

Sabiston DC (Ed): Textbook of Surgery. Twelfth Edition. Philadelphia, WB Saunders Co., 1981

Stephen M, Loewenthal J: Generalized infective peritonitis. Surg Gynecol Obstet 1978; 147:231

RATIONALE 44-a

Occasionally, conventional radiographic studies provide objective evidence of intra-abdominal abscess by virtue of abnormal gas collections or mass displacement of bowel loops. More often, however, they are unrevealing. Even if conventional radiographic studies are suggestive, further anatomic detail is often required to select the optimal treatment. Ultrasonography and/or computed tomography are now utilized to provide confirmatory and complementory anatomic data. Radionuclide scanning plays a secondary role in most cases except in patients with persistent fever and absence of localizing signs. In such cases, a positive gallium scan may serve to focus subsequent examination techniques.

Certain guidelines should be followed. A search for an abscess should be guided by localizing signs, symptoms, laboratory data, and from consideration of the most likely site in a given area. When there are localized findings referable to the right upper quadrant or pelvis, ultrasonography is a reasonable choice, particularly in patients who are critically ill and difficult to move. Computed tomography, although technically more difficult in the critically ill, is complementary to ultrasound as it tends to provide valuable data in areas other than right upper quadrant and pelvis.

REFERENCES

Altemeier WA, Culbertson WR, Fullen WD, et al: Intraabdominal abscesses. Am J Surg 1973; 25:70

Ferrucci JT Jr, Vonsonnenberg E: Role of ultrasound and computed tomography in the diagnosis and treatment of intraabdominal abscess. In: Current Clinical Topics in Infectious Diseases. Remington JS, Swartz MN (Eds). New York, McGraw-Hill Book Company, 1982, pp 136-159

Knochel JQ, et al: Diagnosis of abdominal abscesses with computed tomography, ultrasound and in leukocyte scans. Radiology 1980; 137:425

Levitt RG, et al: Computed tomography and Ga citrate radionuclide imaging for evaluating suspected abdominal abscess. Am J Roentgenol 1979; 132:529

Nichols RL: Intraabdominal sepsis: Characterization and treatment. J Infect Dis 1977; 135:S54

PSEUDOMEMBRANOUS ENTEROCOLITIS

RATIONALE 45-c

Colitis is one of the more serious drug reactions associated with antimicrobial agents. There is a wide spectrum of disease. In mild cases, the mucosa may appear normal and the symptoms are minimal. In severe disease, the mucosa may be covered with pseudomembranes and the associated diarrhea is severe. Clostridium difficile is associated with 15%-20% of cases of simple diarrhea and 95% of cases of pseudomembranous colitis. Stool cultures for C. difficile are difficult to perform and are less specific than the toxin assay.

There are several approaches to therapy. One consists of treating the C. difficile directly with oral (not intravenous) vancomycin. The dosage is 100-125 mg four times daily. Relapse occurs in about 20% of the cases. The major disadvantage of vancomycin is its high cost ($125-$500 for a 10-day course). Metronidazole and bacitracin also appear to be effective in treatment of C. difficile colitis.

Cholestyramine, an ion exchange resin, binds the toxin and has been shown to improve symptoms. It has not, however, been shown to eliminate the toxin and therefore is not recommended as replacement therapy for antibiotics.

REFERENCES

Bartlett JG: Antibiotic-associated colitis. DM 1984; 30:1

Bartlett JG: Antimicrobial agents implicated in Clostridium difficile toxin associated diarrhea or colitis. Johns Hopkins Med J 1981; 149:6

Bartlett JG: New developments in infectious diseases for the critical care physicians. Crit Care Med 1983; 7:566

Bartlett JG, Tedesco FJ, Shull S, et al: Relapse following oral vancomycin therapy of antibiotic-associated pseudomembranous colitis. Gastroenterology 1979; 78:431

Chang TW, Lauerman M, Bartlett JG: Cytotoxicity assay in antibiotic-associated colitis. J Infect Dis 1979; 140:765

Cherry RD, Portnoy D, Jabbari M, et al: Metronidazole: An alternate therapy for antibiotic-associated colitis. Gastroenterology 1980; 78:431

Tedesco FJ, Napier J, Gamble H, et al: Therapy of antibiotic-associated pseudomembranous colitis. J Clin Gastroenterol 1979; 1:51

Trnka YM, Lamont JT: Clostridium difficile colitis. Adv Intern Med 1984; 29:85

Section 6

Questions 46-49: For each numbered statement, select the one lettered heading that is most closely associated with it. Each lettered heading may be selected once, more than once, or not at all.

a. Plasminogen
b. Antithrombin III
c. Platelets
d. Tissue thromboplastin
e. Fibrin monomer

46. Streptokinase activates ____________.

47. Bleeding following massive transfusion is most likely secondary to decreased ____________.

48. ____________ activates the extrinsic system.

49. The primary substrate for factor XIII is ____________.

50. You are treating a young man with multiple gunshot wounds. In the first hour of resuscitation you must give him 40 units of banked whole blood as rapidly as possible. Which ONE of the following complications of such massive transfusions is LEAST likely to be found at the end of the first hour of care?

a. Metabolic acidosis with increased unmeasured anions ("anion gap")
b. Metabolic alkalosis due to sodium citrate metabolism
c. Coagulation abnormalities
d. Hyperkalemia
e. Increased affinity of hemoglobin for oxygen

51. Transfusion reactions:

a. Are likely to first become manifest about one to two hours after the initiation of transfusion if due to an ABO incompatibility
b. Are sometimes heralded by the appearance of DIC, particularly in the surgical patient
c. Are usually due to an error in cross-matching minor determinants
d. Are less likely to be fatal if of the septic rather than hemolytic variety

52. Which ONE of the following items is MOST likely to cause a bleeding diathesis following massive blood transfusion (greater than 20 units of packed red blood cells)?

a. A decrease in serum calcium concentration
b. Disseminated intravascular coagulation
c. Hypofibrinogenemia
d. Dilutional thrombocytopenia
e. Fibrinolysis

53. Many abnormalities may develop in banked blood. In the previously healthy trauma victim, which ONE of the abnormalities listed below is MOST important in the production of immediate problems during rapid, massive transfusion.

a. Acidosis
b. Hypothermia
c. Hyperkalemia
d. Hypocalcemia
e. Citrate intoxication

HEMATOLOGIC

ANSWERS

46-a 47-c 48-d 49-e 50-b 51-b 52-d 53-b

COAGULATION

RATIONALE 46-a 47-c 48-d 49-e

A detailed discussion of the coagulation scheme is beyond the scope of this program. An excellent review of bleeding and clotting disorders by Dr. George Rodman can be found in Volume 1, Critical Care: State of the Art, 1980. Other general references are cited below.

Normally the tendency for clot formation is balanced by the tendency for clot dissolution. Removal of blood clots is the primary function of the fibrinolytic system. Streptokinase and urokinase stimulate the formation of plasmin from plasminogen. Plasmin acts on fibrin and fibrinogen yielding "fibrin split products" and subsequent clot lysis.

Massive transfusion of banked blood may result in deficiencies in platelets and Factors V and VIII. The majority of patients who manifest uncontrolled bleeding following massive blood transfusion are controlled with platelet transfusion.

Factor VII in the presence of tissue thromboplastin and calcium activates the extrinsic coagulation system.

Thrombin acts on fibrinogen to form fibrin monomer. In the presence of fibrin stabilizing factor (Factor XIII) fibrin monomer polymerizes to form tough stable fibrin strands.

REFERENCES

Bowie EI, Sharp AA (Eds): Hemostasis and Thrombosis. London, Butterworths, 1985

Collins JA: Problems associated with massive transfusion of stored blood. Surgery 1974; 75:274

Ellison N: Diagnosis and management of bleeding disorders. Anesthesiology 1977; 47:171

Nemerson Y: Diagnosis of hemorrhagic disorders. Med Clin North Am 1973; 57:531

Rice CL, Moss GS: Blood and blood substitutes: Current practice. Adv Surg 1979; 13:93

Rodman GH: Bleeding and clotting disorders. In: Critical Care: State of the Art. Vol 1. Shoemaker WC, Thompson WL (Eds). Fullerton, CA, Society of Critical Care Medicine, 1980, pp I(G):1-35

TRANSFUSIONS

RATIONALE 50-b

Metabolic alkalosis does not occur in the first hours after massive transfusions. These patients are hypovolemic and have a metabolic acidosis that may be worsened by transfusion of old stored blood containing acidotic plasma and anticoagulants. Banked blood is deficient in clotting factors, and massive transfusions often aggravate coagulopathies by dilution of existing procoagulants. Coagulopathies are, of course, seen in patients receiving massive transfusions. Hyperkalemia is an uncommon complication of massive transfusion, but may occur because stored whole blood and packed cells contain larger than normal amounts of potassium in plasma--up to 15 mEq/L of stored blood. Hypokalemia is a more frequent late complication as potassium depleted older transfused cells take up potassium from the recipient. Banked blood develops an increased affinity for oxygen primarily because the 2,3-DPG levels are decreased, and this increases the affinity of hemoglobin for oxygen.

Massive transfusions can result in a significant number of problems, either volume related or rate and volume related, as completely reviewed by Collins in 1974. Because critical care providers often deal with patients requiring large quantities of blood replacement, an understanding of these problems, real or suspected, is important.

Disease can be transmitted by transfusion and always poses a problem. Adequate donor selection minimizes this occurrence. Mismatch can be a major problem and the risk for major mismatch increases as more units are demanded. Obviously, one cannot check for all minor factors and, thus, immunization of the recipient can occur.

Metabolic derangements and associated abnormalities are far more common events with less mortality risk. When blood with high oxygen affinity is mixed with normal blood, the resulting effective affinity is intermediate. The exact cardiovascular effects of this are ill-defined. It is apparent, however, that a greater cardiac output is required to supply the same quantity of oxygen when affinity increases. Critically ill hypovolemic patients are acidotic because of poor perfusion. When the vascular space is filled and all the "leaks" closed, this metabolic acidosis is corrected readily by normal homeostatic mechanisms. One should be careful in correcting the acute acidosis of massive transfusion by rapid systemic alkalinization because this may further increase the oxyhemoglobin affinity and lead later to severe metabolic alkalosis.

Massive infusion of cold bank blood can cause systemic hypothermia--this may be mildly protective by decreasing oxygen demand but also increases oxygen affinity. As the patient warms, it is necessary to fill the vascular space as the vasoconstriction of hypothermia abates.

Microembolization may be a problem with massive transfusions. The use of blood filters is debatable. While they may prevent microembolization, they also slow infusion rates, may become occluded after four to five units of blood, and may actually begin to shed larger particles.

New additives and red cell preservatives may have a toxicity of their own; inosine and adenine are vasodilators. In sufficient quantities, they may increase the intravascular space.

REFERENCES

Benson RE, Isbister IP: Massive blood transfusion. Anaesth Crit Care 1980; 8:152

Bowen J, Fleming WH: Increased oxyhemoglobin affinity after transfusion of stored blood: Evidence for circulatory compensation. Ann Surg 1974; 180:760

Collins JA: Problems associated with the massive transfusion of stored blood. Surgery 1977; 75:274

Lim R Jr, Olcott C 4th, Robinson AJ, et al: Platelet response and coagulation changes following massive blood replacement. J Trauma 1973; 13:577

Lovric VA: Alterations in blood components during storage and their clinical significance. Anaesth Intensive Care 1984; 12:246

Miller RD: Complications of massive blood transfusions. Anesthesiology 1973; 39:82

Schweizer O, Howland WS: Potassium levels, acid-base balance and massive blood resplacement. Anesthesiology 1962; 23:735

Sugerman HJ, Davidson DT, Vibul S, et al: The basis of defective oxygen delivery from stored blood. Surg Gynecol Obstet 1970; 131:733

Wilson RF, Mammen E, Walt AJ: Eight years of experience with massive blood transfusions. J Trauma 1971; 11:275

RATIONALE 51-b

Transfusion reactions in the postsurgical patient are becoming less frequent with improved blood banking and stricter indications for use. The reaction caused by contaminated blood, a septic transfusion, has the highest mortality of all transfusion reactions. The hemolytic transfusion reaction is usually a result of ABO incompatibility and has a mortality of about 10%. Intraoperatively, the only sign of its occurrence may be generalized oozing as a result of DIC. The onset of a hemolytic transfusion reaction is usually rapid, occurring with the first 50 cc's of transfusion in most cases. The most common cause of mismatched transfusion is a bookkeeping error and not faulty laboratory technique.

REFERENCES

Collins JA: Use of blood and blood components. In: Manual of Surgical Intensive Care. Philadelphia, WB Saunders Co., 1977, pp 132-135

Mollison PL: Blood transfusion. In: Clinical Medicine. Sixth Edition. Philadelphia, JB Lippincott Co., 1979

Rodman GH: Bleeding and clotting disorders. In: Critical Care: State of the Art. Vol 1. Shoemaker WC, Thompson WL (Eds). Fullerton, CA, Society of Critical Care Medicine, 1980, pp I(G):1-35

RATIONALE 52-d

A bleeding diathesis is frequently observed in patients receiving multiple transfusions of stored blood. A wide range of coagulation defects has been implicated. Although a decrease in serum calcium may occur with massive transfusion, it is usually associated with myocardial depression and not coagulation defects. Disseminated intravascular coagulation is not likely to result from uncomplicated transfusions but may occur with ABO incompatibility.

Dilution of intrinsic clotting factors and platelets is the usual etiology of coagulation defects developing from massive blood transfusion. The latter is of primary concern if a clinical coagulopathy develops. Dilutional thrombocytopenia occurs following the short term administration of greater than 10 units of bank blood. In this instance, a minimum of 6 to 10 units of platelets should be given for each 20 units of blood. Clinically significant fibrinolysis or hypofibrinogenemia is uncommon with transfusion of compatible blood.

REFERENCES

Advanced Trauma Life Support Manual. Amer Coll Surg Committee on Trauma, 1981, p 169

Hewson JR, Neame PB, Kumar N, et al: Coagulopathy related to dilution and hypotension during massive transfusion. Crit Care Med 1985; 13:387

Miller RD, Robbins, TO, Tong MJ, et al: Coagulation defects associated with massive blood transfusions. Ann Surg 1973; 174:794

Rodman GH: Bleeding and clotting disorders. In: Textbook of Critical Care. Shoemaker WC, Thompson WL, Holbrook PR (Eds). Philadelphia, WB Saunders Co., 1984, pp 730-732

RATIONALE 53-b

Blood is usually stored in an acid-citrate-dextrose (ACD) solution. It is cold, has an acid pH, and may contain 10-15 mEq/L of potassium. Practically all of the ionized calcium is bound by the large amount of citrate. The most important problem for a previously healthy patient undergoing rapid, massive transfusion is hypothermia. Cold blood, if pumped rapidly into the central circulation, may produce ventricular fibrillation. Thus, the blood should be warmed in a warming oven or passed through a warming coil. The low pH and increased potassium rarely cause problems. The large amount of citrate is also well tolerated, except in those patients with severe liver disease.

Evidence indicates that symptomatic hypocalcemia may develop in patients given ACD blood at rapid rates (> 100 cc/min or 1 unit of blood every 5 minutes). Hypocalcemia may be prevented by the simultaneous intravenous administration of calcium chloride. Two cc of a 10% solution is given for each 500 ml of blood transfused, not to exceed 2 grams. In the majority of cases, blood is not given at these rates and, therefore, supplemental calcium is not indicated.

REFERENCES

Advanced Trauma Life Support Manual. Amer Coll of Surg Comm on Trauma, 1981, pp 169-1970

Cooper N, Brazier JR, Hohenisott C, et al: Myocardial depression following citrated blood transfusion. Arch Surg 1973; 107:756

Walker CW: Blood donors, blood and transfusion. Manual of Pre- and Post-operative Care. Second Edition. Amer Coll of Surg, Committee on Pre- and Postoperative Care. Philadelphia, WB Saunders Co., 1971, pp 139-156

Section 7

54. The LEAST correct statement about thrombi caused by radial arterial cannulae is:

a. May result in skin slough over the cannulation site
b. Increase in frequency with long duration of cannulation
c. Are asymptomatic in most patients if ulnar artery blood flow is adequate
d. Are formed as often with 20 gauge as with 18 gauge catheters
e. May embolize to the cerebral circulation with rapid injection of 5 ml of flush solution

55. Which ONE of the following statements is TRUE regarding complications related to arterial cannulation?

a. Complications are less frequent when the radial artery is used.
b. Complications are more frequent with percutaneous insertion rather than with insertion by cutdown under direct visualization.
c. Complications are as frequent with 18 gauge as with 20 gauge catheters.
d. Complications may involve retrograde flow with cerebral embolism.

56. Which ONE of the following is FALSE regarding arterial monitoring of infants and children in the intensive care setting?

a. Significant morbidity from arterial lines in children can come from embolization proximal to the cannulation site.
b. Retrograde flow into the central circulation from radial-arterial line flushing is dependent upon the volume of flush used with respect to the patient's height.
c. Upon removal of radial-arterial lines in children, there is a high (70%) incidence of temporary arterial obstruction.
d. In children under 5 years of age, 2 cc of flush in the radial artery line can be used safely without fear of the flush producing retrograde flow into the central circulation.

57. The Fick Principle relates:

a. Right atrial pressure to pulmonary wedge pressure
b. Arterial oxygen tension to hemoglobin saturation
c. Cardiac output and oxygen consumption to arteriovenous oxygen contents
d. Myocardial diastolic fiber length to stroke work
e. Colloidal osmotic pressure and hydrostatic pressure to fluid transudation

58. In measurement of blood flow by thermodilution, which of the following errors will cause a falsely low reading of blood flow:

a. A leak at the syringe-catheter junction permitting some of the injected solution to spill on the bed
b. Allowing the syringe of indicator solution to warm in the hand prior to injection
c. Injecting chilled indicator solution through a long "extension" tubing rather than directly into the correct lumen
d. All of the above
e. None of the above

59. Which ONE of the following equations is INCORRECTLY stated?

a. Fick Equation:

$$\dot{V}O_2 = \frac{\dot{Q}_T}{CaO_2 - C\bar{v}O_2}$$

b. Henderson-Hasselbalch Equation:

$$pH = pKa + \log \frac{[HCO_3^-]}{[H_2CO_2]}$$

c. Intrapulmonary Shunt Fraction:

$$\frac{\dot{Q}_S}{\dot{Q}_T} = \frac{Cc'O_2 - CaO_2}{Cc'O_2 - C\bar{v}O_2}$$

where $Cc'O_2$ equals the oxygen content of end capillary blood.

d. Physiologic Dead Space to Tidal Volume Ratio:

$$\frac{V_D}{V_T} = \frac{PaCO_2 - P_ECO_2}{PaCO_2},$$

where P_ECO_2 equals the partial pressure of expired CO_2.

Questions 60-62 refer to the following patient: During a right subclavian catheterization attempt, a 35-year-old female patient became tachypneic, tachycardiac, hypotensive and hemiplegic. Auscultation of the chest revealed breath sounds to be present and symmetrical in all areas. Heart sounds were obscured by a "crunching" murmur that had not previously been present.

60. Which ONE of the following represents the MOST appropriate initial maneuver?

    a. Immediate pericardiocentesis
    b. Left lateral decubitus and Trendelenburg positioning
    c. Surgical exploration of the right subclavian artery
    d. Immediate systemic heparinization
    e. Chest radiography

61. Which ONE of the following is LEAST likely to result?

    a. Hypotension
    b. Elevation in central venous pressure
    c. Hemiparesis
    d. Hemoptysis

62. Which of the following statements regarding this condition is/are TRUE?

    a. Obstruction to blood flow occurs at the pulmonary outflow tract.
    b. Right to left intracardiac shunting may occur.
    c. Serious cardiac dysrhythmias are likely.
    d. Myocardial ischemia is common.
    e. All of the above

Questions 63-64 refer to the following patient: A pulmonary artery catheter has recently been placed by a right subclavian approach in an ICU patient. A short while later, the patient develops sudden new onset of large amounts of frank hemoptysis.

63. What event has MOST likely occurred?

    a. Embolus from the pulmonary artery catheter tip
    b. Rupture of the pulmonary artery
    c. Puncture of the trachea with the introducer needle at the time of insertion of the guide wire
    d. Sudden incease in filling pressure secondary to volume infusion

64. Which ONE of the following is MOST likely to predispose the above patient to this condition?

    a. Ruptured balloon
    b. Improper flushing technique
    c. Distal positioning of the pulmonary artery catheter
    d. Aortic stenosis

Questions 65-66 refer to the following patient: A 44-year-old female with hypoxemia and suspected cardiac failure had a pulmonary artery catheter inserted. The following morning (12 hours after catheter insertion) a portable AP chest radiograph was obtained and is shown in Figure 5).

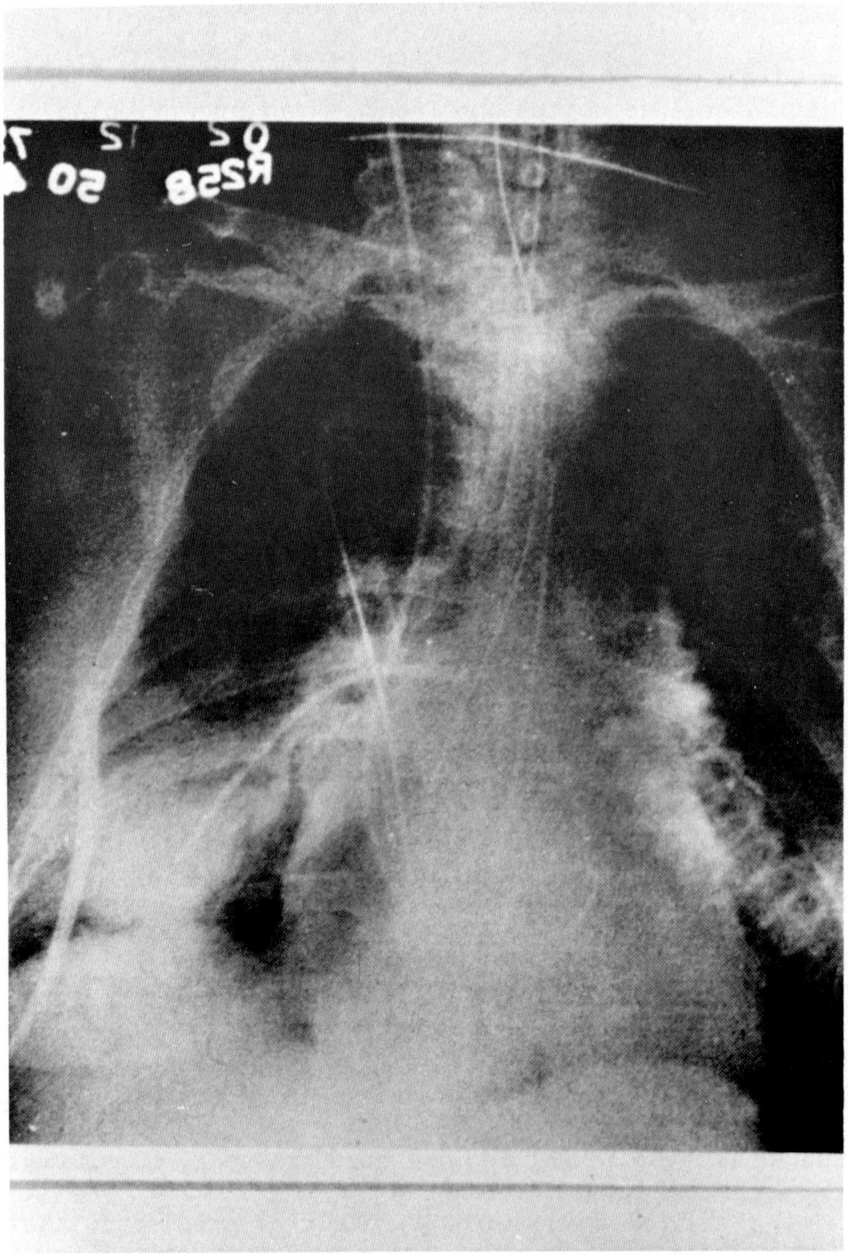

Figure 5

65. Which ONE of the following tracings was MOST likely obtained through the distal port of the pulmonary artery catheter at the time of the chest radiograph?

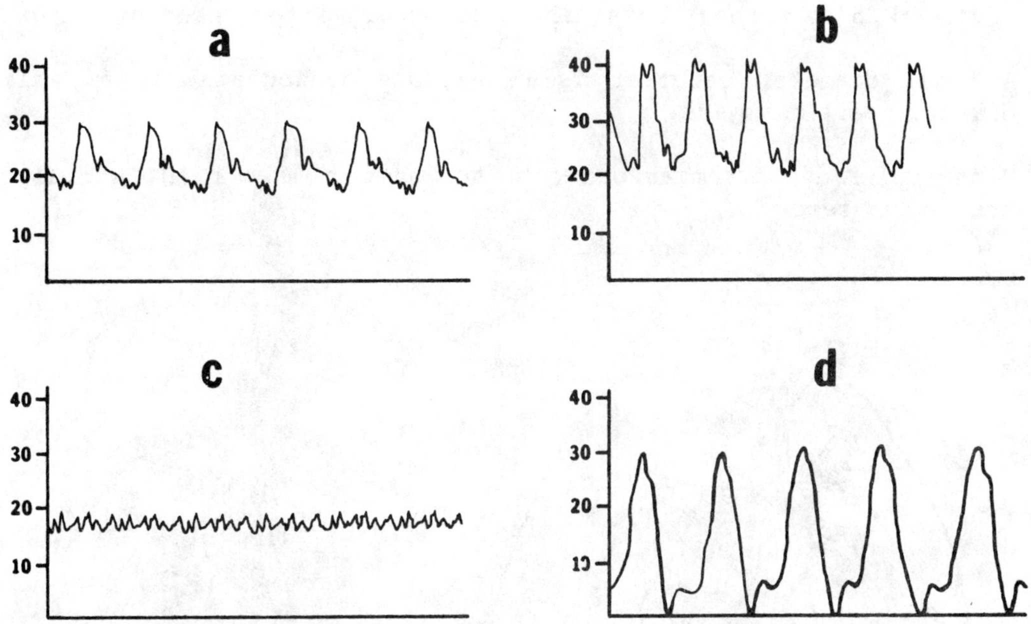

66. Which ONE of the following is the MOST likely etiology of the abnormal radiographic finding in the right lower lung field of Figure 5?

a. Lung abscess
b. Pulmonary infarction
c. Bacterial pneumonia
d. Small cell carcinoma of the lung
e. Viral pneumonia

67. Which ONE of the following statements regarding flow-directed pulmonary artery catheters is INCORRECT?

a. Catheter knotting is more likely to occur with larger rather than small diameter catheters.
b. Noninfectious thrombotic lesions of the right atrial endocardium, tricuspid valve, chordae tendinae and pulmonic valve may occur during catheterization.
c. The incidence of pulmonary artery rupture during catheterization is less than 1%.
d. The incidence of the right bundle branch block during catheterization is higher in patients with pre-existing left bundle branch block than in patients without this condition.
e. Right-sided infective endocarditis may occur as a consequence of flow-directed pulmonary artery catheterization.

tions 68-71: Match each of the following situations with the MOST appropriate diagram (a-d). Each of the diagrams must be used once and only once.

68. Eight hours have passed since an uneventful catheter insertion.

69. After a right ventricular pressure tracing is obtained, the catheter is advanced 25 cm without obtaining a pulmonary artery pressure tracing.

70. A small diameter catheter is repeatedly manipulated in a patient with dilated heart chambers.

71. Ventricular dysrhythmias occur at the same time a right atrial pressure tracing is recorded.

a

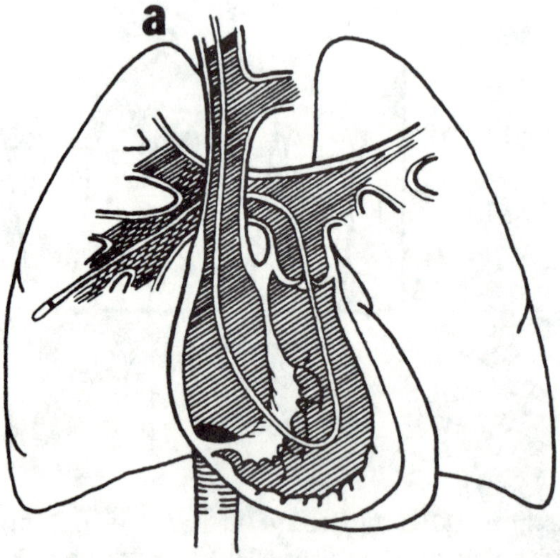

b

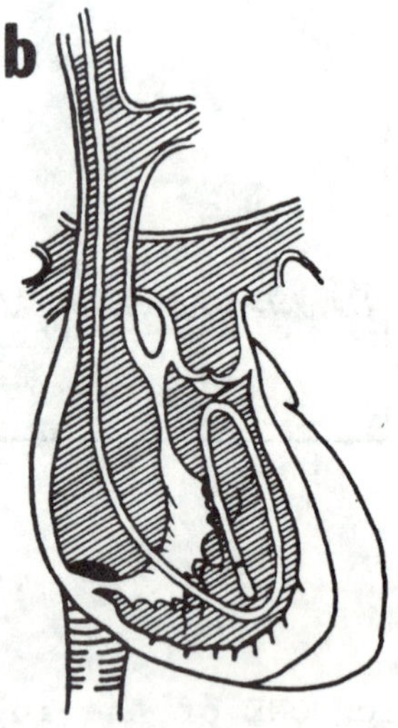

c

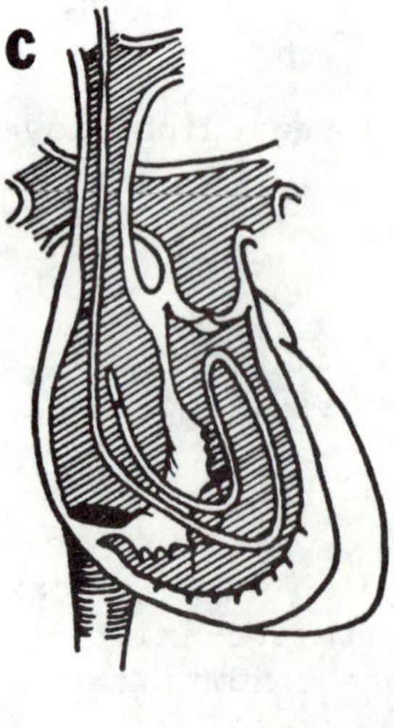

d

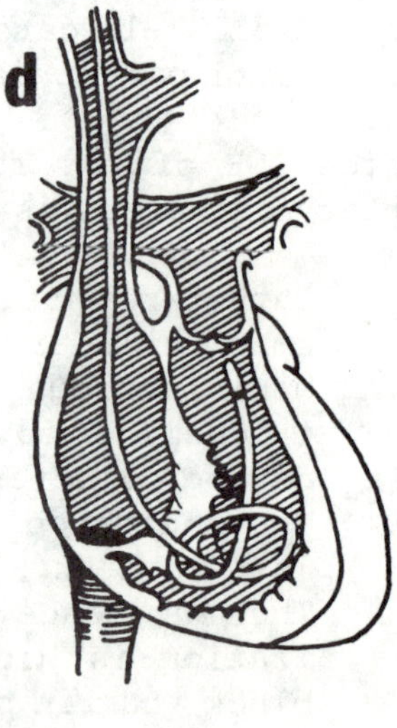

Questions 72-75: Match the following hemodynamic profiles (a-d) with the appropriate condition below. The profiles may be used once, more than once, or not at all.

a.	HR - 120	PAOP - 6 mm Hg	lactic acid - 3 mMol/L
	BP - 85/60 mm Hg	C.I. - 1.8 $L/min \bullet m^2$	
	$\overline{RA}$ - 2 mm Hg	$P\bar{v}O_2$ - 25 mm Hg	
	PA - 20/10 mm Hg	SVRI - 3,200 $dyne \bullet sec/cm^5$	
b.	HR - 110	PAOP - 8 mm Hg	lactic acid - 4 mMol/L
	BP - 85/60 mm Hg	C.I. - 1.8 $L/min \bullet m^2$	
	$\overline{RA}$ - 8 mm Hg	$P\bar{v}O_2$ - 25 mm Hg	
	PA - 20/9 mm Hg	SVRI - 2,900 $dyne \bullet sec/cm^5 \bullet m^2$	
c.	HR - 110	PAOP - 8 mm Hg	lactic acid - 3 mMol/L
	BP - 85/60 mm Hg	C.I. - 4.4 $L/min \bullet m^2$	
	$\overline{RA}$ - 8 mm Hg	$P\bar{v}O_2$ - 35 mm Hg	
	PA - 20/9 mm Hg	SVRI - 1,200 $dyne \bullet sec/cm^5 \bullet m^2$	
d.	HR - 110	PAOP - 8 mm Hg	lactic acid - 6 mMol/L
	BP - 100/60 mm Hg	C.I. - 3.0 $L/min \bullet m^2$	
	$\overline{RA}$ - 8 mm Hg	$P\bar{v}O_2$ - 40 mm Hg	
	PA - 20/9 mm Hg	SVRI - 1,800 $dyne \bullet sec/cm^5$	

72. Splanchnic ischemia

73. Malignant pericardial effusion

74. Barbiturate overdose

75. Fractured pelvis

76. You are presented a patient with the following hemodynamic profile:

PAOP - 10 mm Hg; $\overline{RA}$ - 8 mm Hg; C.O. - 8.4 L/min

SVR - 800 $dyne \bullet sec/cm^5$; $P\bar{v}O_2$ - 43 mm Hg

The differential diagnosis given these parameters includes:

a. A patient with early septic shock
b. A patient receiving chronic hemodialysis
c. A patient with 7 gm/dl of hemoglobin
d. A patient with liver disease
e. All of the above

77. Which ONE factor LEAST influences dissociation of oxygen from hemoglobin?

a. Temperature
b. Intraerythrocytic pH
c. Intraerythrocytic potassium concentration
d. Intraerythrocytic ATP concentration
e. Intraerythrocytic 2,3-DPG concentration

78. A decreased P_{50} is seen with:

a. Chronic sideropenic anemia
b. Cyanotic congenital heart disease
c. Hypophosphatemia
d. None of the above
e. All of the above

79. Normal hemoglobin in healthy patients is 50% and 75% saturated with oxygen at tensions of:

a. 10 and 28 mm Hg
b. 10 and 40 mm Hg
c. 27 and 40 mm Hg
d. 27 and 70 mm Hg
e. 40 and 70 mm Hg

80. Which ONE of these statements is LEAST correct concerning the numerical values of partial pressure (PO_2) in mm Hg and hemoglobin saturation with oxygen (SO_2) in percent?

a. In venous blood PO_2 is greater than SO_2.
b. Acidosis causes a decrease in SO_2 at constant PO_2.
c. Hypothermia increases SO_2 at constant PO_2.
d. Methemoglobin decreases SO_2 at constant PO_2.
e. Carbon monoxide exposure decreases SO_2 at constant PO_2.

81. Which ONE of the following shifts the oxyhemoglobin dissociation curve to the left?

a. Acidosis
b. Increased carbon dioxide tension
c. Increased 2,3-diphosphoglycerate
d. Decreased body temperature

82. You are treating a 40-year-old patient with multiple injuries after a motorcycle accident. His lungs become congested, he has increased hypoxemia, and you decide to perform endotracheal intubation and start controlled volume-cycled ventilation with 5 cm H_2O of positive end-expiratory pressure. You observe this treatment to decrease oxygen transport.

Which ONE of the following factors is MOST likely to have caused this decreased oxygen transport?

a. Decreased arterial PO_2
b. Decreased hemoglobin content
c. Increased oxygen consumption
d. Decreased ventricular filling
e. Increased venoarterial admixture

83. You are treating a patient with severe respiratory distress. Oxygen delivery to tissues is LEAST reduced if which ONE of the following physiological variables is reduced to half of its current value?

a. Hemoglobin of 15 g/dl
b. Stroke volume of 60 ml
c. Oxygen saturation of 97%
d. Heart rate of 140
e. Arterial oxygen tension of 200 mm Hg

84. Which ONE of the following changes is LEAST likely to INCREASE myocardial oxygen consumption?

a. Increased contractility
b. Increased heart rate
c. Increased aortic systolic pressure
d. Increased ventricular volume
e. Decreased arterial oxygen tension

85. Which ONE of the following statements concerning evaluation of mixed venous blood samples is TRUE?

a. Available data suggest there is a critical $P\bar{v}O_2$ (34 mm Hg) below which anaerobic metabolism occurs resulting in hyperlactatemia.
b. $P\bar{v}O_2$ is a better indicator of tissue oxygenation than is cardiac output.
c. The $P\bar{v}O_2$ in a patient with cirrhosis is usually decreased.
d. An increase in $P\bar{v}O_2$ reflects a decrease in overall reserve O_2 transport.

86. From the following set of data: Hemoglobin 10 gm/dl, PaO_2 60 mm Hg, $P\bar{v}O_2$ 35 mm Hg, and cardiac output 4.0 L/min, oxygen delivery is improved greatest by which of the following variable changes (assuming other variables remain constant)? Assume a normal oxyhemoglobin disassociation curve.

a. Increase in PaO_2 to 90 mm Hg
b. Increase in cardiac output to 5.5 L/min
c. Increase in hemoglobin to 14 gm/dl
d. Increase in $P\bar{v}O_2$ to 40 mm Hg

Questions 87-90: Use the information shown below to answer the questions. This data was simultaneously collected on a 65-year-old female in the Intensive Care Unit.

Height	62 inches
Weight	156 pounds
Body Surface Area	1.72 $meters^2$
Temperature	37.5°C
Heart Rate	114 beats/minute
Mean Arterial Pressure (MAP)	60 mm Hg
Systolic Pulmonary Artery Pressure	40 mm Hg
Diastolic Pulmonary Artery Pressure	20 mm Hg
Pulmonary Artery Occlusive Pressure	18 mm Hg
Central Venous Pressure (CVP)	10 mm Hg
Cardiac Output (Thermodilution)	4.0 liters/minute
Hemoglobin	10.0 grams %
FIO_2	0.8
PEEP	0
pH (arterial)	7.39
$PaCO_2$	40 mm Hg
PaO_2	70 mm Hg
Arterial Hb Saturation	95%
$P\bar{v}O_2$ (mixed venous O_2)	28 mm Hg
Mixed Venous Hb Saturation	75%

(Assume 1.34 ml of O_2 per gram Hb at 100% sat.)

87. Which ONE of the following answers is closest to the correct cardiac index ($L/min \cdot m^2$)?

    a. 1.8
    b. 2.3
    c. 2.8
    d. 3.4
    e. 6.8

88. Which ONE of the following answers is closest to the correct systemic vascular resistance ($dyne \cdot sec/cm^5$)?

    a. 530
    b. 998
    c. 1522
    d. 1919
    e. 2241

89. Which ONE of the following answers is closest to the correct arterial oxygen content (ml O_2 per 100 ml blood)?

    a. 5.1
    b. 8.3
    c. 10.1
    d. 12.9
    e. 16.8

90. Which ONE of the following answers is closest to the correct oxygen transport value (ml O_2/min)?

a. 134
b. 241
c. 338
d. 450
e. 518

91. Which ONE of the following sets of hemodynamic variables is sufficient to permit construction of a ventricular function curve (Frank-Starling relationship)?

a. Central venous pressure, pulmonary artery occlusive pressure, and heart rate
b. Stroke index, heart rate, and mean arterial pressure
c. Stroke index, pulmonary artery occlusive pressure, and mean arterial pressure
d. Stroke work, heart rate, and cardiac output
e. Mean arterial pressure, heart rate, and central venous pressure

92. Which ONE of the following disorders is MOST likely to increase central venous pressure and simultaneously DECREASE pulmonary artery occlusive (wedge) pressure?

a. Left ventricular myocardial infarction
b. Excessive infusion of intravenous fluids
c. Rupture of a mitral valve papillary muscle
d. Acute pulmonary embolization
e. Acute dissecting aneurysm with aortic regurgitation

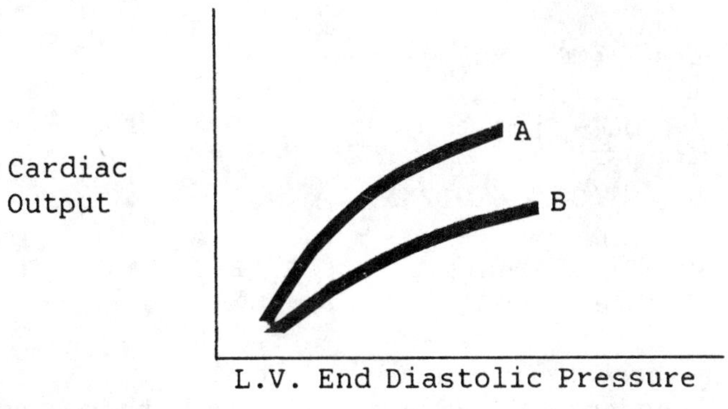

93. A cardiac function curve is shown above. A shift from Curve A to Curve B may reflect a change in:

a. Left ventricular afterload
b. Heart rate
c. Left ventricular compliance
d. Left ventricular contractility
e. All of the above

94. Myocardial compliance is usually INCREASED by which ONE of the following?

a. Digitalis
b. Dobutamine
c. Nitroglycerin
d. Right ventricular dilation and overload

95. A 55-year-old woman with hypertensive cardiovascular disease develops chest pain. Subsequently, EKG changes suspicious for an infero-lateral myocardial infarction are seen and creatine kinase isoenzymes show a trend consistent with a moderate amount of myocardial necrosis. Shortly after admission to the Coronary Care Unit, a pulmonary arterial catheter is inserted.

Which ONE of the following statements is TRUE?

a. The best pulmonary artery occlusive pressure (PAOP) for this patient is 15-20 mm Hg.
b. Clinical assessment of hemodynamic status with stethoscope and chest radiograph allows estimation of "wedge" pressure and cardiac index accurately enough to place the patient in the proper Forrester classification less than 20% of the time.
c. Clinical assessment of hemodynamic status with stethoscope and chest radiograph allows estimation of "wedge" pressure and cardiac index accurately enough to place the patient in the proper Forrester classification approximately 40% of the time.
d. Left ventricular end-diastolic volume can be calculated using radionuclide angiography to determine the left ventricular ejection fraction and thermodilution determination of stroke volume.

96. The relationship between pulmonary vascular resistance (Rpv) in dyne•sec/cm^5, cardiac output (CO) in liters/minute, pulmonary artery mean pressure ($P\overline{pa}$) in mm Hg and pulmonary (capillary) wedge pressure ($P\overline{pc}$) in mm Hg is best expressed as:

a. $Rpv = (P\overline{pa} - P\overline{pc}) / (CO \times 80)$
b. $Rpv = 80 \times (P\overline{pa} - P\overline{pc}) \times CO$
c. $Rpv = 80 \times CO / (P\overline{pa} - P\overline{pc})$
d. $Rpv = CO / (P\overline{pa} - P\overline{pc})$
e. $Rpv = (P\overline{pa} - P\overline{pc}) / (CO \times 0.0125)$

97. Which of the following statements is/are TRUE? A rise in the pulmonary artery occlusive pressure (PAOP):

a. May reflect an increase in venous return
b. May occur secondary to changes in intrathoracic pressure and accompany a drop in venous return
c. May result from readings measured at different phases of the respiratory cycle
d. May reflect no change in the "true" (transmural) filling pressure of the heart
e. All of the above

Questions 98-101: Match the following pulmonary artery catheter problems with the most likely etiology (a-d). Use each answer (a-d) only once.

a. Air in system
b. Catheter tip totally occluded by vessel wall or balloon
c. Balloon ruptured
d. Distal migration of catheter

98. No longer able to obtain wedge tracing with injection of air into the balloon and no resistance to injection

99. Low straight line on oscilloscope

100. Volume of air to inflate balloon is less than previously required

101. Significant decrease in systolic pressure reading and minimal change in diastolic pressure reading compared to previous measurement at same site (damping)

102. Which ONE of the following factors predisposes to a West Zone 1 or 2 pulmonary artery catheter tip placement (as opposed to a Zone 3)?

a. More dependent catheter position by cross table lateral chest radiograph
b. Decreased mean airway pressure
c. Hypovolemia
d. Left subclavian introducer placement

Questions 103-107: Shown below (A-D) are diagrams of 4 pressure transducers with attached stopcocks and tubing. Match the following statements with the MOST appropriate diagram. Each diagram may be used once, more than once, or not at all.

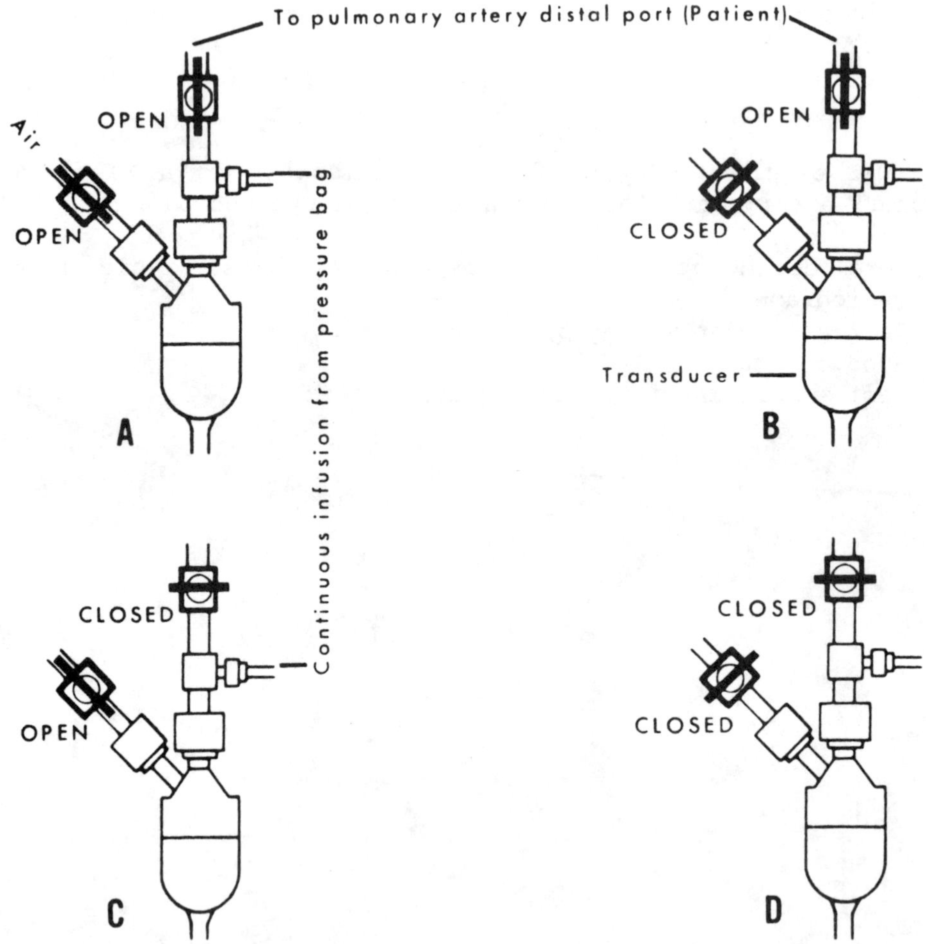

B 103. A pulmonary artery pressure tracing is displayed.

C 104. Allows mechanical zeroing

A 105. Allows blood to enter the transducer dome

D 106. A pressure equivalent to that of the high pressure infusion bag is displayed.

B 107. Allows a pulmonary artery occlusion pressure to be displayed following balloon inflation

108. In order to calculate the actual amount of venoarterial admixture (pulmonary shunt), blood sample must be obtained from which ONE of the following sets of sites:

a. Antecubital vein and central aorta
b. Antecubital vein and pulmonary artery
c. Antecubital vein, central aorta, and radial artery
d. Pulmonary artery, central aorta, and radial artery
e. Pulmonary and radial arteries

109. A 32-year-old female undergoing chemotherapy treatment for acute myelogenous leukemia develops fever, acute respiratory distress and is noted to have diffuse infiltrates on her chest radiograph. Her urine output has markedly decreased and there has recently been a question of myocardial dysfunction. Her respiratory rate is 42 and arterial blood gases while breathing 60% oxygen are PO_2 40 mm Hg, PCO_2 24 mm Hg, and pH 7.54. Her platelet count is 20,000. The decision to intubate her trachea and to insert a pulmonary artery catheter has been made. Of the choices given below, which is the MOST appropriate?

a. Nasotracheal intubation and internal jugular vein catheter placement
b. Nasotracheal intubation and antecubital vein catheter placement by cutdown
c. Orotracheal intubation and subclavian vein catheter placement
d. Orotracheal intubation and antecubital vein catheter placement by cutdown
e. Nasotracheal intubation and femoral vein catheter placement

ANSWERS

54-d	55-d	56-d	57-c	58-e	59-a	60-b	61-d
62-e	63-b	64-c	65-c	66-b	67-a	68-a	69-b
70-d	71-c	72-d	73-b	74-a	75-a	76-e	77-c
78-c	79-c	80-a	81-d	82-d	83-e	84-e	85-b
86-c	87-b	88-b	89-d	90-e	91-c	92-d	93-e
94-c	95-d	96-e	97-e	98-c	99-b	100-d	101-a
102-c	103-b	104-c	105-a	106-d	107-b	108-e	109-d

ARTERIAL CATHETERS

RATIONALE 54-d

Skin over the radial artery is supplied with blood only from the radial artery, with little ulnar anastomotic flow. Pathological examination of such skin after radial arterial catheterization may reveal mild ischemia of epidermis and dermis, but overt necrosis is uncommon. Thrombi in the radial artery are not symptomatic if ulnar arterial blood flow is adequate. If possible, ulnar flow should be evaluated before radial arterial catheterization by elevating the arm, occluding both radial and ulnar arteries, and observing the fingers for flushing as the ulnar arterial occlusion is released. Flushing of radial arterial catheters with as little as 3 ml of saline can cause cerebral embolization. Such syringe flushing should be avoided. Continuous flow of flush solution at slow rates (3 ml/hour) will maintain patency with only occasional controlled rapid flushing of fluid passed through a millipore filter to eliminate bubbles and other emboli. The frequency of thrombotic occlusion of the radial artery is related to both catheter size and duration of catheterization. The frequency increases greatly after 20-40 hours of catheterization with 18 gauge catheters and after 72 hours of catheterization with 20 gauge catheters.

REFERENCES

Bedford RF: Long-term radial artery cannulation: Effects on subsequent vessel function. Crit Care Med 1978; 6:64

Lowenstein E, Little JW III, Lo HH: Prevention of cerebral embolization from flushing radial-artery cannulas. N Engl J Med 1971; 285:1414

Wyatt R, Glaves I, Cooper DJ: Proximal skin necrosis after radial-artery cannulation. Lancet 1974; 1:1135

RATIONALE 55-d

Major complications related to arterial cannulation include thrombosis, embolism, hemorrhage and infection. No studies have ever proven the superiority of one site over another. The frequency of arterial thrombosis increases as the diameter of the catheter increases. In radial artery studies comparing 18 gauge catheters with 20 gauge catheters, a marked increase in thrombosis was seen with the large catheters. Other studies have shown that retrograde flow causing cerebral embolization may occur when flushing radial arterial monitoring systems. Infection is always a risk with indwelling arterial or venous catheters. Insertion by surgical cutdown increases the risk of infection ninefold over percutaneously placed catheters.

REFERENCES

Adler DC, Bryan-Brown CW: Use of axillary artery for intravascular monitoring. Crit Care Med 1973; 1:148

Band J, Maki D: Infections caused by arterial catheters used for hemodynamic monitoring. Am J Med 1979; 67:735

Bedford R: Radial artery cannulation with 18 and 20 gauge catheters. Anesthesiology 1977; 47:37

DeAngelis J: Axillary arterial monitoring. Crit Care Med 1976; 4:205

Gardner R, et al: Percutaneous indwelling radial artery catheters for monitoring cardiovascular function. N Engl J Med 1974; 290:1227

RATIONALE 56-d

Extensive monitoring of patients in the intensive care setting is commonplace in today's clinical practice. EKG with a rate meter, temperature (core or peripheral) and urine output compromise the major noninvasive monitors. However, there is no substitute for an observant, well-trained nurse or physician at the bedside.

Invasive monitoring may be accomplished by insertion of central venous, pulmonary artery and arterial catheters. Not only can pressure readings be of significant value, but blood samples to determine mixed venous oxygen tension and content and arterial samples to determine arterial blood gas values can be extremely valuable. However, the use of these catheters is associated with a small but significant patient risk. The critical care practitioner should be cognizant of the possible complications prior to catheter insertion and/or manipulation. The common and sometimes too lightly taken arterial line is associated with a high (71%) incidence of obstruction of the radial artery upon removal. However, recannulization usually occurs within 14 days. When the arterial line is flushed with excessive volume, there is significant risk of retrograde flow of the flush to the central circulation with possible embolization of air bubbles and/or clots. The volume of flush causing retrograde flow seems to correlate most closely with the patient's height.

REFERENCES

Edmonds JF, Barker GA, Conn AW: Current concepts in cardiovascular monitoring in children. Crit Care Med 1980; 8:548

Lowenstein E, Little JW, Lo HH: Prevention of cerebral embolization from flushing radial-artery cannulas. N Engl J Med 1971; 285:1414

Miyasaka K, Edmonds JF, Conn AW: Complications of radial artery lines in the pediatric patient. Can Anaesth Soc J 1976; 23:9

EDITORIAL COMMENT

Complications associated with arterial catheters are legion. Common problems include bleeding, arterial obstruction and infection. If the catheters are properly inserted and maintained, the morbidity associated with their use is acceptable.

Cooper and Hopkins recently reported an interesting technique designed to aid in rapid diagnosis of catheter-associated infection. They found that Gram stain of the catheter tip was 100% sensitive and 97% specific for the detection of catheter tip colonization if greater than one organism was seen per high power field. In the septic patient this simple and inexpensive test may help direct antibiotic therapy many hours before semi-quantitative culture results are known.

ADDITIONAL REFERENCE

Cooper GL, Hopkins CC: Rapid diagnosis of intravascular catheter-associated infection by direct Gram staining of catheter segments. N Engl J Med 1985; 312:1142

CARDIAC OUTPUT

RATIONALE 57-c

The Fick Principle relates the loss (or gain) of an indicator from blood and the consumption (or production) of indicator within a vascular network to the volume flow of blood in that network. When applied to the whole subject, with oxygen as the indicator, the loss of indicator (oxygen) from arteries to veins and the total oxygen consumption rate can be related to the total blood flow (cardiac output):

$$\text{Cardiac Output} = \frac{\text{Oxygen Consumption}}{\text{Arteriovenous Oxygen Content Difference}}$$

REFERENCES

Franch RH: Cardiac catheterizations. In: The Heart. Fourth Edition. Hurst JW (Ed). New York, McGraw-Hill Book Company, 1978, pp 491-493

Levine HJ: Clinical cardiac physiology. In: Clinical Cardiovascular Physiology. Levine HJ (Ed). New York, Grune & Stratton, 1976, p 646

Neville WE: Care of the Surgical Cardiopulmonary Patient. Chicago, Year Book Medical Publishers Inc., 1971, pp 42-44

RATIONALE 58-e

To measure the plasma volume, a known amount of labeled albumin is injected; after mixing has occurred, the concentration of the indicator is measured. The dilution of the indicator is inversely proportional to the distribution volume of indicator:

$$\text{Volume} = \frac{\text{Amount of Indicator Injected}}{\text{Concentration of Indicator}}$$

The same principle is applied for indicator dilution measurement of solvent flow. The amount of indicator must be known, it must mix adequately in the solvent, and the detector must measure over time the concentration of indicator. If there is a large flow, the concentration-time curve (i.e., area under the curve) will be small.

$$\text{Flow} = \frac{\text{Amount of Indicator Injected}}{\text{Concentration of Indicator}}$$

If by accident the amount of indicator injected is less than planned, then the indicator concentration will be falsely low and the volume (or blood flow) calculated on assuming the full amount of indicator will be falsely large. If some of the solution is not injected, if the solution is not adequately chilled, or if the cold solution is warmed by injection through long tubing or held in the hand, then the amount of indicator is falsely low and the apparent volume (or flow) will be falsely high.

Moral: Indicator dilution techniques require precise quantitation of both amount of indicator injected and the indicator concentration. Using fixed volumes of iv solutions equilibrated at 0°C is a convenient technique, but it requires careful attention to the volume of injectate, the equilibrium temperature of solution, and the method of injection.

REFERENCE

Franch RH: Cardiac catheterizations. In: The Heart. Fourth Edition. Hurst JW (Ed). New York, McGraw-Hill Book Company, 1978, pp 493-495

RATIONALE 59-a

The FICK EQUATION states that oxygen consumption per unit time ($\dot{V}O_2$) is equal to the oxygen extracted from the blood per unit time. Correctly stated:

$$\dot{V}O_2 = \dot{Q}_T\,(CaO_2 - C\bar{v}O_2) \text{ or } \dot{Q}_T = \frac{\dot{V}O_2}{CaO_2 - C\bar{v}O_2}$$

The other equations are correct.

REFERENCES

Berk JL, Sampliner JE (Eds): Handbook of Critical Care. Second Edition. Boston, Little, Brown and Co., 1982

West JB: Respiratory Physiology: The Essentials. Second Edition. Baltimore, Williams & Wilkins Co, 1979

COMPLICATIONS

RATIONALE 60-b 61-d

Air embolization occurring with central venous catheterization is a well described phenomenon. Of all the complications associated with central venous catheterization, air embolism is one of the most dangerous, yet it is also one of the most preventable. It may occur during the insertion of the catheter, during a catheter disconnect, secondary to cracks in the catheter hub or secondary to an improperly functioning infusion pump. Proper catheter insertion technique, patient positioning, the use of a Luer-lock connection between catheter and tubing and careful catheter care may help prevent this complication.

Almost all patients with significant air embolism demonstrate sudden respiratory difficulty. Many experience severe cardiovascular compromise. Obstruction by air of the right ventricular outflow tract and the pulmonary vasculature accounts for most of the cardiopulmonary dysfunction. A wide variety of neurologic symptoms may occur which include seizures, hemiplegia and coma. Cerebral air embolism through a patent foramen ovale was reported by Ponsky and Paries. There are also reported cases of cerebral air embolism in patients with no demonstrable cardiac defects. It is postulated that air traverses from vein to artery through intrapulmonary arteriovenous anastomoses.

The volume of air necessary to cause significant problems in man is not known. Ordway suggested that the injection of 20 ml/sec of air is associated with symptoms and 75 ml/sec with death in most patients.

Treatment of this condition requries prompt recognition. Positioning the patient in the left lateral decubitus position in steep Trendelenberg causes the pulmonary outflow tract to assume an inferior position with respect to the body of the right ventricle. Air may subsequently be displaced to the more superior position and the obstruction to blood flow decreased. Aspiration of air may be attempted but because of variability in catheter tip position this procedure is often unsuccessful.

REFERENCES

Baskin SE, Woznials RF: Air embolism occurring during hemodialysis. N Engl J Med 1975; 293:184

Lambert MJ: Air embolism in central venous catheterization: Diagnosis, treatment and prevention. South Med J 1982; 75:1189

Menkin M, Schwartzman RJ: Cerebral air embolism: Report of five cases and review of the literature. Arch Neurol 1977; 34:168

Ordway CB: Air embolus via CVP catheter without positive pressure. Ann Surg 1974; 179:479

Peters JL, Armstrong R: Air embolism occurring as a complication of central venous catheterization. Ann Surg 1978; 197:375

Ponsky JL, Paries WJ: Paradoxical cerebral air embolism. N Engl J Med 1971; 284:985

Sink JD, Comer PB, James PM, et al: Evaluation of catheter placement in the treatment of venous air embolism. Ann Surg 1976; 1983:58

RATIONALE 62-e

Venous air embolism may obstruct blood flow from the right to the left side of the heart. This obstruction occurs primarily at the pulmonary artery outflow tract of the right ventricle. Air bubbles may also occlude the pulmonary microvasculature. Pulmonary vasoconstriction and the mechanical obstruction mentioned above cause an acute increase in pulmonary artery and right-sided heart pressures. Severe hypoxemia may result from ventilation-perfusion mismatching and intrapulmonary shunting. Large air emboli may result in cardiac dysrhythmias, myocardial ischemia, systemic hypotension, and death. Cerebral air embolism may occur by right-to-left intracardiac shunting of air through a patent foramen ovale or by passage of air through intrapulmonary AV shunts.

Hyperventilation, hypovolemia, and obstructive lung disease may be associated with large intrapleural pressure changes. The markedly negative intrapleural pressure that occurs during inspiration in this group of patients places them at greater risk for air embolism during central venous cannulation and various surgical procedures.

Specific treatment of air embolism consists of placing the patient on the left side in a head down position. Aspiration of air from the right ventricle is occasionally effective. Air emboli are composed of 80% nitrogen. The air may diffuse down a concentration gradient from the pulmonary capillary into the alveolus. This diffusion is facilitated by the administration of 100% oxygen.

REFERENCES

Berglund E, Josephson S, Ovenfors CO: Pulmonary air embolism: Physiological aspects. Progr Respir Res 1970; 5:259

Flanagan J, Gradishar I, Gross R, et al: Air embolism: A lethal complication of subclavian venipuncture. N Engl J Med 1969; 281:488

Gottlib J, Ericsson J, Sweet R: Venous air embolism: A review. Anesth Analg 1965; 44:773

Hybels C: Venous air embolism in head and neck surgery. Laryngoscope 1980; 90:946

Lambery MI: Air embolism in central venous catheterization: Diagnosis, treatment and prevention. South Med J 1982; 75:1189

Munson E: Effect of nitrous oxide on the pulmonary circulation during venous air embolism. Anesth Analg 1971; 50:785

O'Quin RJ, Lakshminarayan S: Venous air embolism. Arch Intern Med 1982; 142:2173

RATIONALE 63-b 64-c

Rupture of the pulmonary artery as a complication of catheter placement may be due to vessel puncture by the catheter tip or more likely due to overinflation of the balloon relative the the diameter of the pulmonary artery. It is an uncommon but disastrous occurrence. Predisposing factors include:

a. placement of the catheter far distal into small diameter branches of the pulmonary artery,
b. pulmonary artery hypertension (decreased diameter of vessel), and
c. overinflation of the balloon (usually against resistance).

Prompt hemoptysis usually results. The most immediate concern is airway control, and intubation may be necessary. If the catheter is found to be far distal on the chest radiograph, it should be pulled back. A fan-shaped infiltrate representing bleeding into lung parenchyma may be seen on the chest film. The need to withdraw the catheter entirely is debatable, as the addition of this complication to the patient's pre-existing illness may make hemodynamic data even more necessary. Some advocate pulling the catheter back to the proximal pulmonary artery and partially inflating the balloon to decrease blood flow to the rupture site. The patient should be placed with the bleeding side down. Additional measures such as isolation of the bleeding lung segment utilizing a Fogarty catheter or emergent surgery may be necessary, depending upon the amount and duration of hemorrhage.

A thromboembolus from the catheter tip is unlikely to occur immediately after insertion. Puncture of the trachea with the needle at the time of insertion is very unlikely with proper subclavian technique. It is more likely to occur with internal jugular approaches. Hemoptysis in this setting is usually immediate.

Although mitral stenosis has been reported to cause frank hemoptysis, it would not be expected to occur in a patient with aortic stenosis. A ruptured balloon is usually associated with an inability to wedge the catheter or withdraw air, and it is occasionally associated with air embolism. Hemoptysis has been reported with flushing of the catheter in the wedged position. This condition, however, is usually associated with small amounts of hemoptysis only.

REFERENCES

Krantz EM, Viljoen JF: Hemoptysis following insertion of a Swan Ganz catheter. Br J Anaesth 1979; 51:457

Ohn KC, Cottsell JE, Turndorf H: Hemoptysis from a pulmonary artery catheter. Anesthesiology 1979; 51:485

Rosenbaum L, Rosenbaum SH, Askanazi J, Hyman AI: Small amounts of hemoptysis as an early sign of pulmonary artery rupture by a pulmonary arterial catheter. Crit Care Med 1981; 9:319

Wolfe JD, Simmons DH: Hemoptysis: Diagnosis and management. West J Med 1977; 127:383

EDITORIAL COMMENT

Introduction of air into the venous or arterial circulation can cause cerebral air embolization which is associated with a variety of neurological deficits. Murphy et al. recently reported successful treatment with hyperbaric oxygen of 16 patients with cerebral air embolism. Eight of the patients had complete resolution of neurologic symptoms, five had partial relief and three had no benefit.

ADDITIONAL REFERENCES

Gronert GA, Messick JM, Cucchiara RF, et al: Paradoxical air embolism from a patent foramen ovale. Anesthesiology 1979; 50:548

Michel L, Poskanzer DC, McKusick KA, et al: Fatal paradoxical air embolism to the brain: Complication of central venous catheterization. J Parent Enter Nutr 1982; 6:68

Murphy BP, Harford FJ, Cramer FS: Cerebral air embolism resulting from invasive medical procedures: Treatment with hyperbaric oxygen. Ann Surg 1985; 201:242

RATIONALE 65-c 66-b

Figure 5 demonstrates a wedge-shaped infiltrate located at the tip of the pulmonary artery catheter. This finding is associated with a pulmonary infarction and can be seen with far distal catheter placement, overzealous flushing, and/or with failure to deflate the catheter balloon after occlusion pressure measurement. The catheter position in this patient is extremely distal. Of the options shown, a wedged tracing is most likely. This patient is also at risk for pulmonary artery rupture.

REFERENCES

Boyd KD, Thomas SL, Gold I, et al: A prospective study of complications of pulmonary artery catheterization in 500 consecutive patients. Chest 1983; 84:245

Elliott C, Zimmerman GA, Clemmer TP: Complications of pulmonary artery catheterization in the care of critically ill patients: A prospective study. Chest 1979; 76:647

Grose R, Strain J, Cohen MV: Pulmonary arterial V waves in mitral regurgitation clinical and experimental observations. Circulation 1984; 69:214

Hannah AT, Brown M, Bigman O: Pulmonary artery catheter induced hemorrhage. Chest 1984; 85:129

Slung HB, Scher KS: Complications of the Swan-Ganz catheter. World J Surg 1984; 8:76

Widemann HP, Matthay MA, Matthay RA: Cardiovascular-pulmonary monitoring in the intensive care unit (Part 1). Chest 1984; 85:537

RATIONALE 67-a

Catheter knotting occurs more frequently with small diameter catheters, particularly when an excessive length of catheter is inserted. This may result in catheter coiling and subsequent knotting in the right ventricle. After entering the right ventricle, pulmonary artery (PA) pressures are usually obtained following insertion of no more than 15 cm of catheter. If a PA pressure tracing is not obtained, the balloon should be deflated, the catheter withdrawn and the attempt repeated.

Infective endocarditis, aseptic thrombotic endocarditis, valvular damage and chordae rupture have all been reported with PA catheter use.

The incidence of pulmonary artery rupture is less than 1%. Cough, hemoptysis, dyspnea or shock may warn of this complication. It has been associated with excessive lengths of catheter insertion, distal migration of the catheter and with prolonged balloon inflation. Patients with pulmonary artery hypertension and those receiving anticoagulants appear to be at increased risk for this complication.

The incidence of catheter induced temporary right bundle branch block has been variably reported from less than 0.1% to 6% and is related to direct trauma of the HIS bundle. The incidence of this complication has been reported in up to 23% of patients with pre-existing left bundle branch block. Temporary transvenous ventricular pacing has been advocated by some prior to catheter insertion in patients with left bundle branch block.

REFERENCES

Daily EK, Schoeder JS: Techniques in Bedside Hemodynamic Monitoring. Third Edition. St. Louis, CV Mosby Co., 1985

Elliott CG, Zimmerman GA, Clemmer TP: Complications of pulmonary artery catheterization in the care of critically ill patients. Chest 1979; 76:647

Greene JF, Cummings KC: Aseptic thrombotic endocardial vegetations: A complication of indwelling pulmonary artery catheters. JAMA 1973; 225:1525

Lipp H, O'Donoghue K, Resenkov L: Intracardiac knotting of a flow-directed balloon catheter. N Engl J Med 1971; 284:220

Pace NL, Horton W: Indwelling pulmonary artery catheters: Their relationship to aseptic thrombotic endocardial vegetations. JAMA 1975; 233:893

Rowley KM, Clubb KS, Smith GJW, et al: Right-sided infective endocarditis as a consequence of flow-directed pulmonary-artery catheterization: A clinicopathological study of 55 autopsied patients. N Engl J Med 1984; 311:1152

Sprung CL (Ed): The Pulmonary Artery Catheter: Methodology and Clinical Applications. Baltimore, University Park Press, 1983

RATIONALE 68-a 69-b 70-d 71-c

Catheter knotting (Diagram d) occurs most often with small diameter catheters. Repeated manipulations or catheter advancement without balloon inflation predisposes to this condition. Knot formation may be suggested radiographically or if resistance is encountered during catheter withdrawal.

Kinking and looping (Diagrams b and c) are caused by insertion of excessive catheter length. If after a right ventricular pressure tracing is obtained, the catheter is advanced greater than 15 cm without demonstrating a pulmonary artery pressure tracing, looping in the right ventricle should be suspected. Advancing the catheter further may cause the tip to re-enter the right atrium.

As the catheter warms and softens, it may migrate to a more distal location in the pulmonary artery (Diagram a). A wedged tracing is likely to be displayed in this setting. Radiographic confirmation of catheter position is recommended immediately following catheter insertion and may also be advisable 4-8 hours later.

REFERENCES

Fibuch EE, Tuohy GF: Intracardiac knotting of a flow-directed balloon tipped catheter. Anaesth Analg 1980; 59:217

Schwartz KV, Garcia EG: Entanglement of Swan-Ganz catheter around an intracardiac structure. JAMA 1977; 237:1198

Sprung CL (Ed): Complications of pulmonary artery catheterization. In: The Pulmonary Artery Catheter. Baltimore, University Park Press, 1983, pp 87-89

EDITORIAL COMMENT

Use of flow-directed pulmonary artery catheters is commonplace in most ICUs. Few topics in medicine, unfortunately, have demanded more printers ink than the never-ending list of complications associated with pulmonary artery catheterization.

Most would agree that our ability to clinically assess accurately hemodynamic status in the critically ill is poor. What remains to be proven, however, is that this fact makes any difference. We have yet to adequately study which groups of critically ill patients demonstrate improved survival because of pulmonary artery catheter use.

ADDITIONAL REFERENCES

Connors AF, McCaffree DR, Gray BA: Evaluation of right heart catheterization in the critically ill patient without myocardial infarction. N Engl J Med 1983; 308:263

Robin ED: The cult of the Swan-Ganz catheter: Overuse and abuse of pulmonary flow catheters. Ann Intern Med 1985; 103:445

HEMODYNAMIC PROFILE

RATIONALE 72-d 73-b 74-a 75-a

The shock syndromes have been classified by Drs. Schubin and Weil into four basic categories: (1) oligemic or hypovolemic shock, (2) cardiogenic shock, (3) obstructive shock, and (4) distributive shock. Hypoperfusion, generalized or regional, is characteristic of all shock states. Elevated lactic acid levels reflect the increase in anaerobic metabolism and/or the decrease in lactate metabolism by the liver and kidney. The partial pressure of oxygen in mixed venous blood is indicative of oxygen utilization and debt. Levels below 28 mm Hg are associated with elevated lactic acid levels.

Profile A is a patient with low ventricular filling pressures, low cardiac index, low $P\bar{v}O_2$, and elevated vascular resistance. This is typical of oligemic shock. A fractured pelvis results in significant hemorrhage into the surrounding tissues and retroperitoneal space.

Profile A is also the hemodynamic profile found in patients with barbiturate overdose, an example of distributive shock. Barbiturates cause venodilatation, relative hypovolemia, decreased venous return and a low cardiac output. Vascular resistance is normal or high.

Profile B is a patient with low filling pressures, low cardiac index, low $P\bar{v}O_2$, and elevated vascular resistance. In addition, there is equalization of RA, PA diastolic and PAOP pressures. This is characteristic of pericardial tamponade, an obstructive form of shock.

Profile C reveals a patient with low to normal filling pressures, high cardiac output, low $P\bar{V}O_2$ and low vascular resistance. This is characteristic of early or warm septic shock, which is another form of distributive shock. With sepsis, the distributive defect involves both the venous (venodilatation with pooling) system and the arterial (regional hypoperfusion/hyperperfusion, AV shunts) system. Since the amount of arteriovenous shunting is variable, mixed venous oxygen saturations may be high, normal or low.

Profile D is a patient with normal filling pressures, normal blood pressure, normal cardiac index and normal mixed venous oxygen. However, the patient has a high lactic acid level. Lactic acidosis in the absence of obvious circulatory failure may be caused by hypoxemia, grand mal seizures, chronic ethanol abuse, hypoglycemia, leukemia, phenformin and salicylate intoxication. Although a biochemical explanation can be offered in most cases, there remains a group of patients with lactic acidosis and no obvious etiology. Such patients have been said to have "spontaneous" or "idiopathic" lactic acidosis, an almost uniformly fatal disorder. Huckabee, in 1963, first described this entity and postulated that the acidosis might be due to tissue hypoxia secondary to clinically inapparent regional hypoperfusion. Numerous authors refer to the metabolic/lactic acidosis associated with regional obstruction to blood flow, but offer little documentation. Isolated reports describe lactic acidosis and normal cardiac function in patients who subsequently respond to efforts raising or redistributing blood flow. Indeed, the category "distributive shock" implies the co-existence of normally and abnormally perfused vascular beds in the presence of normal to high cardiac outputs. Patient D has "idiopathic" lactic acidosis secondary to regional hypoperfusion and tissue hypoxia. Since the mixed venous oxygen tension is the average of the venous blood from all capillary beds, limited areas of hypoperfusion would have little impact on the final value.

REFERENCES

Bergan J, Yao J: Visceral ischemic syndromes. In: Textbook of Surgery. Sabiston D (Ed). Philadelphia, WB Saunders Co., 1981, pp 1995-2000

Fulop M, Hoberman H: Is lactic acidosis "spontaneous"? NY State J Med 1977; 77:24

Gaspar M: Mesenteric arterial disease. In: Peripheral Arterial Disease. Gaspar M, Barker W (Eds). Philadelphia, WB Saunders Co., 1981

Kaswitz P, et al: Mixed venous oxygen tension and hyperlactatemia. JAMA 1976; 236:570

Kreisberg RA: Lactate homeostasis and lactic acidosis (Part I). Ann Intern Med 1980; 92:227

Sobel B: Cardiac and noncardiac forms of acute cardiovascular collapse. In: Heart Disease. Braunwald E (Ed). Philadelphia, WB Saunders Co., 1980, pp 590-629

Taradash M, Jacobson L: Vasodilator therapy of idiopathic lactic acidosis. N Engl J Med 1975; 293:468

Weil M, Schubin H: Shock associated with barbiturate intoxication. JAMA 1971; 215:263

RATIONALE 76-e

The hemodynamic profile shown is that of a hyperdynamic state with adequate tissue oxygenation and without cardiac decompensation. A reduced afterload is the primary mechanism by which the normal heart increases cardiac output. Heart rate also increases in hyperdynamic states but is usually less than 110. Thyrotoxicosis, beriberi, anemia, systemic arteriovenous fistulas, liver disease, Paget's disease, carcinoid syndrome and pregnancy are all consistent with the hemodynamic parameters listed. Septic shock with or without segmental hypoperfusion may also present early with high cardiac output and low vascular resistance.

REFERENCE

Fowler N: High cardiac output states (hyperkinetic or hyperdynamic states). In: The Heart. Hurst JW (Ed). New York, McGraw-Hill Book Company, 1982

OXYGEN TRANSPORT

RATIONALE 77-c

The affinity of hemoglobin for oxygen is increased at low temperatures, alkaline pH, and when intraerythrocytic ATP and 2,3-DPG concentrations are reduced. Intraerythrocytic potassium concentrations have a minimal effect, although potassium depletion may be associated with metabolic alkalosis. When hemoglobin affinity for oxygen is increased, the delivery of the required volume of oxygen to tissues is accomplished only at lower tissue oxygen tensions, and this may diminish diffusion of oxygen. This effect may be especially important in severe hypothermia and in patients with extreme hypophosphatemia (e.g., ethanol abusers) during treatment of diabetic ketoacidosis, and in patients with inappropriate parenteral feeding.

REFERENCES

Harkness DR: The regulation of hemoglobin oxygenation. Adv Intern Med 1971; 17:189

Kilmartin JV: Molecular mechanism of the Bohr effect. In: Oxygen Affinity of Hemoglobin and Red Cell Acid Base Status. Fourth Edition. Rorth M, Astrup P (Eds). New York, Academic Press, 1972, pp 93-100

Lenfant C, Bellingham AJ, Detter JC: Physiological factors influencing the hemoglobin affinity for oxygen. In: Oxygen Affinity of Hemoglobin and Red Cell Acid Base Status. Fourth Edition. Rorth M, Astrup P (Eds). New York, Academic Press, 1972, pp 736-747

RATIONALE 78-c

If the affinity of hemoglobin for oxygen is increased, more oxygen is associated with hemoglobin at any oxygen tension. Normally hemoglobin is half-saturated with oxygen (0.67 ml/gm) at PO_2 = 27 mm Hg. The oxygen tension at half-saturation of hemoglobin with oxygen is termed "P_{50}." A decreased P_{50} is associated with INCREASED affinity of hemoglobin for oxygen, as at lower oxygen tension MORE oxygen is associated with hemoglobin. Such increased oxygen affinity (decreased P_{50}) is seen in hypophosphatemia in association with decreased concentrations of 2,3-DPG in the erythrocyte. In chronic iron-deficient anemia and cyanotic heart disease the opposite effect is observed; oxygen affinity is decreased, P_{50} is increased, and tissues are delivered the requisite volumes of oxygen at higher tissue oxygen tensions.

Tissue oxygenation is dependent upon delivery of adequate volumes of oxygen at adequate tensions. Increased hemoglobin affinity for oxygen may compromise tissue oxygenation even though the product of blood flow and arterial oxygen content is unchanged. Many blood gas laboratories do not measure directly hemoglobin saturation with oxygen, but calculate it from equations representing normal hemoglobins at standard conditions. Such "derived parameters" may be misleading, especially if the patient has an abnormal hemoglobin, severe acidosis or alkalosis, hypophosphatemia, chronic anemia or cyanosis.

REFERENCES

Fitzgerald F: Clinical hypophosphatemia. Annu Rev Med 1978; 29:177

Licthman MA, Miller DR, Cohen J, et al: Reduced red cell glycolysis, 2,3-diphosphoglycerate and adenosine triphosphate concentration, and increased hemoglobin-oxygen affinity caused by hypophosphatemia. Ann Intern Med 1971; 74:562

Metcalfe J, Dhindsa DS: The physiological effects of displacements of the oxygen dissociation curve. In: Oxygen Affinity of Hemoglobin and Red Cell Acid Base Status. Fourth Edition. Rorth M, Astrup P (Eds). New York, Academic Press, 1972, pp 613-628

Sheldon GF: Hyperphosphatemia, hypophosphatemia, and the oxyhemoglobin dissociation curve. J Surg Res 1973; 14:367

Travis SF, Sugerman HJ, Ruberg RL, et al: Alterations of red-cell glycolytic intermediates and oxygen transport as a consequence of hypophoshatemia in patients receiving intravenous hyperalimentation. N Engl J Med 1971; 285:763

RATIONALE 79-c

The shape of the curve relating the volume of oxygen bound to hemoglobin to oxygen tension has been defined repeatedly. Saturation of 25%, 50% and 75% occurs at oxygen tensions of about 10, 28 and 40 mm Hg.

REFERENCE

Roughton FJW, Deland EC, Kemohan JC, et al: Some recent studies of the oxyhaemoglobin dissociation curve of human blood under physiological conditions and the fitting of the Adair equation to the standard curve. In: Oxygen Affinity of Hemoglobin and Red Cell Acid Base Status. Fourth Edition. Rorth M, Astrup P (Eds). New York, Academic Press, 1972, pp 73-81

RATIONALE 80-a

Oxygen tension in normal mixed venous blood is about 40 mm Hg with an oxygen saturation of 75%. As additional oxygen is extracted from capillary blood in response to tissue needs, oxygen tension and saturation decline further. At an oxygen saturation of 50%, oxygen tension is about 27 mm Hg and this value of oxygen tension is termed the P_{50} value. Acidosis results in a shift of the normal oxyhemoglobin dissociation curve to the right (Bohr effect) that causes a decrease in oxygen saturation at a constant oxygen tension. A similar change is caused by an increase in temperature. Hypothermia causes a shift of the oxyhemoglobin dissociation curve to the left, reflected in an increase in oxygen saturation at a constant oxygen tension.

Methemoglobin and carboxyhemoglobin affect the oxyhemoglobin dissociation curve. In addition to binding hemoglobin and making it unavailable for oxygen transport, thus reducing total oxygen saturation, the remaining available hemoglobin is altered in its oxygen binding function and resulting in a shift of the oxyhemoglobin dissociation curve to the left, reducing oxygen delivery to the tissues. Another way of expressing this function is that the P_{50} value of hemoglobin available for oxygen transport is reduced in blood containing methemoglobin and carboxyhemoglobin.

The oxygen tension at which normal hemoglobin, hemoglobin A1, is half-saturated under normal conditions (pH 7.40, temperature 37°C, base excess 0), in the presence of normal values for intracellular components, is referred to as standard P_{50}. The standard P_{50} in healthy subjects is about 27 mm Hg. A decreased oxygen affinity (high PO_2) of hemoglobin facilitates oxygen unloading from hemoglobin at tissue sites. Similarly, a decreased standard P_{50} implies an increased oxygen affinity of hemoglobin. The presence of carboxyhemoglobin, methemoglobin, or sulfhemoglobin in association with red cells containing hemoglobin A1 results in a decrease in the amount of hemoglobin available for oxygen transport. These abnormal hemoglobin species are stable compounds and cannot be converted to hemoglobin A1 except by therapeutic interventions or natural clearance mechanisms. Because of the decrement in available hemoglobin, the presence of the stable abnormal hemoglobin species directly affects the calculations of arteriovenous oxygen difference, oxygen consumption and pulmonary venous admixture. Based upon the work of Roughton and Darling, expressions may be derived for defining the effect of carboxyhemoglobin and methemoglobin on the oxyhemoglobin dissociation curve, and these effects may be quantitated for calculation of oxygen transport functions. Knowledge of these values is particularly useful and important in the presence of toxic ingestions, smoke inhalation, drug therapy, and methylene chloride exposure where elevations in carboxyhemoglobin and methemoglobin may be significant.

REFERENCES

Bodansky O: Methemoglobinemia and methemoglobin-producing compounds. Pharmacol Rev 1951; 3:144

Cohn JD, Engler PE: Effects of carboxyhemoglobin, methemoglobin and sulfhemoglobin on oxyhemoglobin dissociation and heme-heme interaction. Clin Res 1977; 25:415A

Cohn JD, Engler PE: Shunt effect of carboxyhemoglobin. Crit Care Med 1979; 7:54

Collier CR: Oxygen affinity of human blood in presence of carbon monoxide. J Appl Physiol 1976; 40:487

Finch CA, Lenfant C: Oxygen transport in man. N Engl J Med 1972; 286:407

Roughton FJW, Darling RC: The effect of carbon monoxide on the oxyhemoglobin dissociation curve. Am J Physiol 1974; 141:17

Severinghaus JW: Blood gas calculator. J Appl Physiol 1966; 21:1108

Valeri CR: Oxygen transport function of preserved cells. Clin Haematol 1974; 3:649

RATIONALE 81-d

The oxyhemoglobin dissociation curve displays the variation in degree of oxygen saturation of hemoglobin at different partial pressures of oxygen. The ability of the hemoglobin molecule to bind oxygen and later release it to the tissues is determined by the oxidation state of the heme iron, the presence of defects in the hemoglobin molecule and by numerous other physiologic factors.

The partial pressure of oxygen at which hemoglobin is 50% saturated (P_{50}) is 27 mm Hg for normal hemoglobin at a pH of 7.4. An oxyhemoglobin dissociation curve that is shifted to the right (increased P_{50}) results in decreased "onloading" of oxygen onto the hemoglobin molecule (at a given PO_2) in the pulmonary capillaries but increased "offloading" of oxygen to the tissues. A "right shifted" curve occurs with a decrease in pH, an increase in pCO_2 and an increase in body temperature. Changes in these physiologic variables in the opposite direction shift the curve to the left.

The binding of 2,3-diphosphoglycerate to the beta chain of the hemoglobin molecule confers stability of the deoxygenated molecule. Increased binding of 2,3-diphosphoglycerate to hemoglobin therefore shifts the oxyhemoglobin dissociation curve to the right.

In the setting of cardiopulmonary insufficiency the clinical significance of altered affinity of hemoglobin for oxygen is controversial. One might postulate, however, that an increased affinity of hemoglobin for oxygen (left shifted curve) may be detrimental to efficient tissue oxygenation.

REFERENCE

Bryan-Brown CW: Oxygen transport and the oxyhemoglobin dissociation curve. In: Handbook of Critical Care. Berk JL, Sampliner JE (Eds). Boston, Little, Brown and Co., 1982, pp 557-578

RATIONALE 82-d

Controlled ventilation with positive end-expiratory pressure increases intrathoracic pressure. In a patient with multiple injuries, associate hypovolemia is likely, so that a reduction in venous return to the heart is probable, and cardiac output is reduced as the relative filling pressure of the heart is reduced. Another mechanism that may cause a reduction of left ventricular fillings is the increased pulmonary vascular resistance that is exaggerated in hypovolemic states with an increase in intra-alveolar pressure. The condition is correctable by volume loading of the circulation to restore the central blood volume, monitoring pulmonary arterial pressures and mixed venous blood gases.

The PaO_2 is likely to be increased. If hemoglobin is reduced, there will be a reduction of the oxygen carrying capacity of the blood. This can result in lowering of mixed venous oxygen saturation. Pulmonary arterial PO_2 will be lowered to a greater extent by pulmonary arteriovenous admixture.

The usual compensation for a low hemoglobin content is an increased cardiac output. Increased oxygen consumption does occur in the recovery phase from trauma, but this does not reduce oxygen transport. Oxygen transport requires cardiac output, hemoglobin and oxygenation of blood in the lungs. The treatment is to support this triad, and each component should be monitored.

REFERENCES

Barcroft J: On anoxaemia. Lancet 1920; 2:485

Downs JB, Douglas ME, Sanfelippo PM, et al: Ventilatory pattern, intrapleural pressure and cardiac output. Anesth Analg (Cleve) 1977; 56:88

Gallagher TJ, Civetta JM, Kirby RR: Terminology update: Optimal PEEP. Crit Care Med 1978; 6:323

Guyton AC, Jones CE, Coleman TG: Circulatory Physiology: Cardiac Output and its Regulation. Second Edition. Philadelphia, WB Saunders Co., 1973, pp 406-407

Powers SR Jr, Mannal R, Neclerio M, et al: Physiologic consequences of positive end-expiratory pressure (PEEP) ventilation. Ann Surg 1973; 178:265

Shoemaker WC, Montgomery ES, Kaplan E, et al: Physiologic patterns in surviving and nonsurviving patients: Use of sequential cardiorespiratory variables in defining criteria for therapeutic goals and early warning of death. Arch Surg 1973; 106:630

Suter PM, Fairley HB, Isenberg MD: Optimum end-expiratory airway pressure in patients with acute pulmonary failure. N Engl J Med 1975; 292:284

RATIONALE 83-e

Oxygen delivery to the tissues is defined as the product of arterial oxygen content (ml/dl) and cardiac output (L/min) multiplied by a factor, 10, that converts the units to ml/min. This value, oxygen delivery, is expressed under standard conditions of temperature and pressure (760 mm Hg, 0°C, dry). Cardiac output is defined as the product of stroke volume and pulse rate, so halving either of these two variables would result in a reduction of oxygen delivery by exactly 50%.

Arterial oxygen content is the sum of the oxygen bound to hemoglobin and the oxygen dissolved in whole blood. Oxygen bound to hemoglobin is the product of hemoglobin concentration (g/dl), saturation, and the factor 1.39 ml O_2/g Hb. This represents the volume of oxygen at standard conditions that combines with each gram of normal hemoglobin. Thus, halving hemoglobin concentration or oxygen saturation results in a reduction in oxygen delivery of about 50%.

Dissolved oxygen is expressed as the product of oxygen tension and the oxygen solubility for blood divided by the factor 7.60 which converts the volume of oxygen to ml/dl, at standard conditions. Substituting the appropriate constant, the value for the oxygen solubility coefficient may be calculated to be 0.0031 ml/dl•torr. Hence, reduction in arterial oxygen tension from 200-100 torr results in a reduction in dissolved oxygen from 0.62 - 0.31 ml/dl. The corresponding change in saturation reflected by the decrease in arterial oxygen tension is from 99.5% to 98% as shown by Severinghaus. Thus, there is a reduction in total arterial oxygen content from 21.38 to 20.76 ml/dl due to the reduction in arterial oxygen tension from 200-100 torr.

Assessment of oxygen delivery may be particularly important in patients receiving positive-pressure ventilation. Under these circumstances, cardiac output is often reduced by the effect of positive pressure breathing and positive end-expiratory pressure. Whereas beneficial effects may be noted in arterial oxygen tension and venoarterial admixture, the decrement in cardiac output may exceed the benefits of the rise in arterial oxygen tension resulting in yet further deterioration in oxygen delivery. Often times, a more optimum value for oxygen delivery may be achieved by manipulating end-expiratory pressure, volume replacement and cardiotonic agents. Use of cardiac output measurements and arterial blood gas analyses provide a rapid means to define optimum oxygen delivery and facilitate ventilator management.

REFERENCES

Cohn JD, Engler PE: Molecular weight and oxygen binding capacity of human hemoglobin variants. Clin Res 1977; 25:662A

Kirby RR, Downs JB, Civetta JM, et al: High level positive end-expiratory pressure (PEEP) in acute respiratory insufficiency. Chest 1975; 67:156

Kumar A, Falke KJ, Geffin B, et al: Continuous positive-pressure ventilation in acute respiratory failure: Effects on hemodynamics and lung function. N Engl J Med 1970; 283:1430

Lozman J, Powers SR Jr, Older T, et al: Correlation of pulmonary wedge and left atrial pressures: A study in the patient receiving positive end expiratory pressure ventilation. Arch Surg 1974; 109:270

Lutch JS, Murray JF: Continuous positive-pressure ventilation: Effects on systemic oxygen transport and tissue oxygenation. Ann Intern Med 1972; 76:193

Severinghaus JW: Blood gas calculator. J Appl Physiol 1966; 21:1108

Suter PM, Fairley HB, Isenberg MD: Optimum end-expiratory airway pressure in patients with acute pulmonary failure. N Engl J Med 1975; 292:284

Thomas LJ Jr: Algorithms for selected blood acid-base and blood gas calculations. J Appl Physiol 1972; 33:154

RATIONALE 84-e

In 1907, Barcroft and Dixon related the oxygen consumption of the heart to external work, the product of aortic pressure and flow. Heart rate was added to this equation in 1912 and, by 1915, contractility was added as the fourth component. Evans and Matsuoka reported that volume work was less demanding of oxygen consumption than pressure work, and they noted that the tension in the wall of the heart increased exponentially with increments in ventricular volume. The indices of myocardial oxygen consumption often are described as products of ventricular or aortic pressure and heart rate ("tension-time index").

Arterial oxygen tension does not directly regulate myocardial oxygen consumption, though it limits it. The heart extracts a large fraction of oxygen from the coronary circulation. Coronary sinus oxygen tension is often 20 mm Hg with only 30% saturation of hemoglobin with oxygen. This maintains a myoglobin oxygen saturation of about 85% because of the hyperbolic relation of myoglobin oxygen content to tension. Were arterial oxygen tensions, or coronary flow, to diminish, myocardial oxygen requirements might not be met and myocardial oxygen consumption may then decline, not increase.

REFERENCES

Barcroft J, Dixon WE: The gaseous metabolism of the mammalian heart: Part I. J Physiol (Lond) 1907; 35:182

Evans CL, Matsuoka Y: The effect of various mechanical conditions on the gaseous metabolism and efficiency of the conditions on the gaseous metabolism and efficiency of the mammalian heart. J Physiol (Lond) 1915; 49:378

Forster RE: Oxygenation of the muscle cell. Circ Res 1967; 20(Suppl 1):115

Sarnoff SJ, Braunwald E, Welch GH Jr, et al: Hemodynamic determinants of oxygen consumption of the heart with special reference to the tension-time index. Am J Physiol 1958; 192:148

Schlant RC: Metabolism of the heart. In: The Heart. Fourth Edition. Hurst WC, Logue RB, Schlant RC, et al (Eds). New York, McGraw-Hill Book Company, 1978, pp 107-118

RATIONALE 85-b

The single most reliable physiologic parameter for monitoring the overall balance between O_2 supply and demand is the mixed venous oxygen tension ($P\bar{v}O_2$). Studies have indicated that other measurements including cardiac output and $C(a-v)O_2$ are not as valid an indicator of the adequacy of tissue oxygenation as is the $P\bar{v}O_2$. Available data indicates that anaerobic metabolism and hyperlactatemia occur at a $P\bar{v}O_2$ less than 28 mm Hg. Sustained levels below this point are associated with a very high mortality. Disease states with an altered regional perfusion make analysis of $P\bar{v}O_2$ difficult. Because of the "shunting phenomena" seen in sepsis and cirrhosis, the $P\bar{v}O_2$ is frequently elevated. Without exception, however, a drop in $P\bar{v}O_2$ reflects a decrease in oxygen transport reserve.

REFERENCES

Kasnitz P, Druger GI, Yorra F, et al: Mixed venous oxygen tension and hyperlactatemia. JAMA 1976; 236:570

Krauss XH, Verdouw PD, Hugenholt PG, et al: On monitoring of mixed venous oxygen saturation after cardiothoracic surgery. Thorax 1975; 30:636

Martini GA, Baltzer G, Arndt H: Some aspects of circulatory disturbances in cirrhosis of the liver. In: Progress in Liver Diseases. New York, Grune & Stratton, 1972, p 231

Simmons DH, Alpas AP, Tashkin ET, et al: Hyperlactatemia due to arterial hypoxemia or reduced cardiac output or both. J Appl Physiol 1978; 45:195

Snyder JV, Carroll GC: Tissue oxygenation: A physiologic approach to a clinical problem. Curr Probl Surg 1982; IX:11

Stanley TH, Isern-Amaral J: Periodic analysis of mixed venous oxygen tension to monitor the adequacy of perfusion during and after cardiopulmonary bypass. Can Anaesth Soc J 1974; 21:454

RATIONALE 86-c

Using the formula O_2 content/dl = 1.36 x Hgb x Hgb O_2 saturation + .0031 x PaO_2, baseline O_2 content above = 12.4 ml O_2/dl. Multiplying then x 40 (CO x 10) = total O_2 delivery of 497 ml/min. Increasing the PaO_2 to 90 increases the saturation from .90 to .95 and therefore increases the O_2 content to 13 ml O_2/dl and the O_2 delivery to 524 ml/min. Increasing the CO to 5.5 L/min increases the O_2 delivery to 683 ml/min without changing the O_2 content. Increasing the Hgb to 14.0 increases the O_2 content to 19 ml/dl and the O_2 delivery to 769 ml/min.

$P\bar{v}O_2$ has no direct effect on O_2 content or delivery except as it may effect PaO_2 via saturation of shunted blood. In some situations, however, it may reflect adequacy of O_2 delivery (decreasing with decreased oxygen delivery), assuming that oxygen consumption remains constant.

This problem is an excellent example of the minor contribution of PaO_2 to O_2 delivery as the PaO_2 increases above 60 mm Hg and the significant benefit of raising Hgb and increasing CO where there is leadway to do so. In those patients with low Hgb and decreased CO, gains in this area may be most beneficial to the patient.

REFERENCES

Clemmer TP: Oxygen transport. Present Concepts 1974; 7:1

Finch CA, LenFant C: Oxygen transport in man. N Engl J Med 1972; 286:407

Kandel GK, Aberman A: Mixed venous oxygen saturation. Arch Intern Med 1983; 143:1400

Miller MJ: Tissue oxygenation in clinical medicine: An historical overview. Anesth Analg 1982; 61:527

RATIONALE 87-b 88-b 89-d 90-e

A systematic evaluation of hemodynamic, respiratory and oxygen transport variables may aid in evaluation and therapy of critically ill patients. Hand-held calculators and microcomputers now make calculation and storage of this information very easy. Appropriate evaluation of these calculated parameters, however, demands a thorough understanding of their derivation.

Cardiac Index = Cardiac Output/Body Surface Area

Systemic Vascular Resistance = (MAP - CVP) 79.9/Cardiac Output

Arterial Oxygen Content = (Hb x 1.34) Arterial Hemoglobin Saturation + (PaO_2 x 0.003)

Oxygen Transport = Cardiac Output x Arterial Oxygen Content x 10

REFERENCES

Berk JL, Sampliner JE (Eds): Handbook of Critical Care. Second Edition. Boston, Little, Brown and Co., 1982

Snyder JV, Carroll GC: Tissue oxygenation: A physiologic approach to a clinical problem. Curr Probl Surg 1982; XIX:11

PRELOAD

RATIONALE 91-c

Starling's law of the heart states that the volume of blood returned to the heart (preload) is a main determinant of the volume pumped by the heart. Therefore, as the volume of blood returned to the heart increases, the volume of blood pumped by the heart also increases up to a limit. The Frank-Starling phenomenon is a direct result of the biochemical and ultrastructural design of the myocardium.

To construct a ventricular function curve, one plots some measure of cardiac pumping action (cardiac output, stroke volume, stroke index, or stroke work) against a simultaneous measure of the volume returned to the heart such as pulmonary artery occlusion pressure (PAOP) or left ventricular end-diastolic pressure (LVEDP). CVP can be used to measure right ventricular preload and PAOP is an approximation of left ventricular preload. PAOP may not correlate with LVEDP in patients with high levels of positive end-expiratory pressure, mitral stenosis, or very severe left ventricular dysfunction. It is important to realize that the right and left ventricle have quite different function curves, and substantial errors can be made if measures of right ventricular end-diastolic pressure are used to estimate left ventricular function.

A change in preload causes a ventricle to move upward or downward along a given ventricular function curve. Changes in the other two main determinants of cardiac function, contractility and afterload, cause the ventricle to operate on a different ventricular function curve. For example, if the patient is given a drug that increases cardiac contractility, there will be a greater stroke index at the same preload.

Ventricular function curves can be used as a means of assessing ventricular performance and the effect of pathological processes on ventricular performance. They are also useful means of directing and evaluating therapeutic interventions in the critically ill patient. This can be done in two ways - the preload may be altered by volume infusion or diuresis to move to a different point on a ventricular function curve, or the ventricle may be shifted to a new ventricular function curve by altering contractility and/or afterload.

REFERENCES

Crexells C, Chatterjee K, Forrester JS, et al: Optimal level of filling pressure in the left side of the heart acute myocardial infarction. N Engl J Med 1973; 289:1263

Guyton AC: Circulatory Physiology: Cardiac Output and its Regulation. Philadelphia, WB Saunders Co., 1963, pp 140-160

Pace NL: A critique of flow directed pulmonary arterial catheterization. Anesthesiology 1977; 47:455

Sonnenblick EH: Myocardial ultrastructure in the normal and failing heart. In: The Myocardium: Failure and Infarction. Braunwald E (Ed). New York, HP Publishing Co., 1974, pp 1-13

Vinocur B, Sampliner JE, Artz JS: Hemodynamic monitoring. In: Handbook of Critical Care. Berk JL, Sampliner JE, Artz JS, et al (Eds). Boston, Little, Brown and Co., 1976, pp 127-129

RATIONALE 92-d

Central venous pressure (CVP) is a measure of the preload of the right ventricle and a reflection of the functional state of the right side of the heart. The pulmonary artery occlusion pressure (PAOP) estimates the left atrial pressure and left ventricular end-diastolic pressure in many clinical settings and, thus, serves as a measure of left ventricular preload and the functional state of the left ventricle. There is poor correlation between the CVP and PAOP in seriously ill patients because right and left ventricular function may differ, especially in patients with cardiopulmonary disease. In these patients, not only the absolute CVP but even changes in the CVP often are unreliable and misleading estimates of left heart filling. In acute pulmonary embolization, there may be disparate ventricular function. The obstruction of the pulmonary vascular bed by an embolus increases right ventricular afterload. In response to this increased demand, the right heart fails or moves upward on its ventricular function curve; either of these actions increases CVP. The decrement in right ventricular output that follows a major pulmonary embolus decreases volume return to the left ventricle causing a fall in left ventricular preload that may be reflected by a decrease in PAOP.

Left ventricular myocardial infarction, excessive infusions of intravenous fluids, rupture of a mitral valve papillary muscle, and acute aortic regurgitation are all situations that increase PAOP. Left ventricular myocardial infarction causes a decrease in left ventricular contractility and an increase in left ventricular end-diastolic pressure. Excessive infusions of intravenous fluids, rupture of the mitral valve, or acute aortic regurgitation all result in an increased left ventricular end-diastolic volume. Because the pressure developed in the left ventricle during diastole is exponentially related to its volume, an increased left ventricular end-diastolic pressure and, thus an increase in the PAOP. Rupture of a mitral valve papillary muscle can be diagnosed by the characteristic giant V waves seen in the pulmonary artery tracing.

REFERENCES

Buchbinder N, Ganz W: Hemodynamic monitoring: Invasive techniques. Anesthesiology 1976; 45:146

Forrester JS, Diamond G, McHugh TH, et al: Filling pressures in the right and left sides of the heart in acute myocardial infarction: A re-appraisal of central-venous-pressure monitoring. N Engl J Med 1977; 285:190

Moser KM: Pulmonary embolism-state-of-the-art. Am Rev Respir Dis 1977; 115:829

Pace NL: A critique of flow directed pulmonary arterial catheterization. Anesthesiology 1977; 47:455

RATIONALE 93-e

The cardiac function curve is a limited clinical tool. A shift from Curve A to Curve B may be caused by any or all of the mentioned alternatives. If the y axis represents stroke volume, then changes in heart rate have no effect. If the y axis represents left ventricular stroke work, then afterload does not influence the curve. Because some index of function is plotted against filling pressure rather than end-diastolic volume, acute changes in ventricular compliance shift the curve. When afterload, compliance, and heart rate are constant, only then does a shift in the cardiac function curve reflect a change in contractility.

REFERENCES

Ayres SM: Ventricular function. In: Critical Care: State of the Art. Vol 1. Shoemaker WC, Thompson WL (Eds). Fullerton, CA, Society of Critical Care Medicine, 1980, pp I(C):1-42

Braunwald E, Sonnenblick EH, Ross J: Contraction of the normal heart. In: Heart Disease. Second Edition. Braunwald E (Ed). Philadelphia, WB Saunders Co., 1984, pp 409-446

Goldberg HS, Rabson J: Control of cardiac output by systemic vessels. Am J Cardiol 1981; 47:696

RATIONALE 94-c

Inotropic agents such as dobutamine or digitalis improve the contractile state of the myocardium therefore making the ventricular muscle stiffer. Increased compliance occurs when ventricular muscle is poorly contractile as in congestive cardiomyopathy. The simple relief of ischemia by nitroglycerin can increase compliance; and even if there is no myocardial ischemia, nitroglycerin causes reduction in ventricular wall tension as it decreases preload.

REFERENCES

Armstrong PW, Walker DC, et al: Vasodilator therapy in acute myocardial infarction: A comparison of sodium nitroprusside and nitroglycerin. Circulation 1975; 52:1118

Brodie BR, Grossman W, et al: Effects of sodium nitroprusside on left ventricular diastolic pressure-volume relations. J Clin Invest 1977; 59:59

Franciosa JA, Guiha NH, Limas CJ, et al: Improved left ventricular function during nitroprusside infusion in acute myocardial infarction. Lancet 1972; 1:650

Myers ML, Finley R, et al: The influence of the right on the left ventricle in human adult respiratory distress syndrome. Annals of the Royal College of Physicians and Surgeons of Canada 1981; 14:174

Sibbald WJ, et al: Right and left ventricular preload and diastolic ventricular compliance: Implications for therapy in critically ill patients. In: Critical Care: State of the Art. Vol 3. Shoemaker WC, Thompson WL (Eds). Fullerton, CA, Society of Critical Care Medicine, 1982, pp III(F):1-33

RATIONALE 95-d

The optimal pulmonary artery occlusion pressure (PAOP) for a patient is found in the vicinity of the shoulder of the left ventricular function curve (Frank-Starling relationship). This point differs from patient to patient and from day to day in an individual patient. Increasing PAOP beyond this point results in little improvement of cardiac output and increased risk of pulmonary edema. The pulmonary artery occlusion pressure does not predict with accuracy left ventricular preload in critically ill patients with cardiac disease. However, 80%-85% of patients presenting with myocardial infarction may be placed in the appropriate Forrester classification using a clinical assessment of hemodynamic status. Clinical hemodynamic status accurately predicts PAOP in patients without myocardial infarction only 42% of the time and the cardiac index only 44% of the time. Left ventricular end-diastolic volume (LVEDV) can be calculated in milliliters per meter^2 by the following formula:

$$\text{LVEDV} = \frac{\text{stroke volume index}}{\text{left ventricular ejection fraction}}$$

REFERENCES

Calvin JE, Driedger AA: Does the pulmonary capillary wedge pressure predict left ventricular preload in critically ill patients? Crit Care Med 1981; 9:437

Conners AF, McCaffree DR, Gray BA: Evaluation of right-heart catheterization in the critically ill patient without acute myocardial infarction. N Engl J Med 1983; 308:263

Forrester JS, Diamond GA, Swan HJC: Correlative classification of clinical and hemodynamic function after acute myocardial infarction. Am J Cardiol 1977; 39:137

PULMONARY VASCULAR RESISTANCE

RATIONALE 96-e

Vascular resistance is the ratio of pressure difference to fluid flow. Ohm's law is written: $R = P/F$. Thus the numerator must be the difference between pressures on the inflow and outflow sides of the vascular network or, in this case, the pulmonary artery pressure minus the pulmonary artery occlusive pressure. The denominator must be the blood flow or, in this case, the cardiac output. To convert from the usual units of pressure (mm Hg) and the usual units of blood flow (liters/minute) to the cgs units yielding dyne•sec/cm^5 one must multiply the pressures by 1333 and multiply the cardiac output by 1000/60 (to convert to ml/sec). Thus 1333/(1000/60) = 80. One "resistance unit," the ratio of pressure (mm Hg) to flow (L/min), is 80 dyne•sec/cm^5. In the examples given, only answers "a" and "e" have the proper ratio of pressure to flow, but answer "a" gives resistances 6400 times too small.

REFERENCES

Franch RH: Cardiac catheterizations. In: The Heart. Fourth Edition. Hurst JW (Ed). New York, McGraw-Hill Book Company, 1978, pp 498-499

Guyton AC: Textbook of Medical Physiology. Fifth Edition. Philadelphia, WB Saunders Co., 1976, pp 229-232

PULMONARY ARTERY CATHETER

RATIONALE 97-e

The pulmonary artery occlusive pressure (PAOP) is the best clinically available estimate of left ventricular filling pressure. However, its interpretation is not simple. Generally, a rise in PAOP reflects a rise in venous return and/or an increase in left ventricular pressure and volume. Changes in intrathoracic pressure alter the meaning of a given PAOP. When intrathoracic pressure rises the transmural filling pressure may stay the same or decrease in spite of a rise in the PAOP. These considerations must be taken into account in a patient who is dyspneic, tachypneic, or on positive pressure ventilation and PEEP.

REFERENCES

Buda A, et al: Effect of intrathoracic pressure on left ventricular performance. N Engl J Med 1979; 301:453

Jardin F, Farcott JC, et al: Influence of PEEP on left ventricular performance. N Engl J Med 1981; 304:421

Pick RA, Handler JB: The cardiovascular effects of positive end-expiratory pressure. Chest 1982; 82:345

Robotham J: Cardiovascular disturbances in chronic respiratory failure. Am J Cardiol 1981; 47:941

Snyder JV, Carroll GC: Tissue oxygenation: A physiologic approach to a clinical problem. Curr Probl Surg 1982; XIX:11

RATIONALE 98-c 99-b 100-d 101-a

If the oscilloscope does not show a pulmonary artery occlusion pressure tracing when air is injected into the balloon, possible causes include (1) an incorrect amount of air in the balloon, (2) the balloon may be ruptured (no resistance is met), or (3) the catheter is no longer in pulmonary artery. A low straight line on the oscilloscope implies that the transducer is not securely attached to the catheter or, more commonly, that catheter tip is totally occluded by clot, wall of vessel, or by overinflation of the balloon itself. If the volume of air required to inflate the balloon is less than was initially needed at the time of flotation, the most likely reason is distal migration of the catheter. A significant decrease in systolic reading and minimal change in diastolic pressure reading when compared to previous measurements at the same site is called damping and may be due to partial occlusion of the distal port. This may be secondary to a clot in the system, kinking of the catheter lumen or abutting of the catheter tip against the vessel wall. However, the most common etiology of damping is air in the system.

REFERENCES

Civetta JM: Pulmonary catheter insertion. In: The Pulmonary Artery Catheter: Methodology and Clinical Applications. Sprung CL (Ed). Baltimore, University Park Press, 1983, pp 27-29

Wiedemann HP, Matthay MA, Matthay RA: Cardiovascular pulmonary monitoring in intensive care unit (Part I). Chest 1984; 85:537

Woods SL: Monitoring pulmonary artery pressures. Am J Nurs 1976; 76:1765

RATIONALE 102-c

The pulmonary artery occlusion pressure approximates the pulmonary venous pressure only if the catheter tip is in a West Zone 3 position in the lung. Only in this position is pulmonary venous pressure greater than airway pressure. In Zones 1 and 2, as described by West, mean airway pressure is greater than pulmonary venous pressure and there no longer exists an uninterrupted column of blood between the catheter and the pulmonary veins. In these situations, the catheter reflects airway pressure more than pulmonary venous pressure. Airway pressure tends to be higher than vascular pressure in the uppermost lung areas. It follows, therefore, that more dependent catheter positions are more likely to be in West Zone 3 areas. Decreases in mean airway pressure also increase the West Zone 3 area of the choices listed. Only hypovolemia, which decreases vascular pressure, decreases Zone 3. Left subclavian introducer placement has no effect on zone placement of the PA catheter tip.

REFERENCES

Moser KM, Spragg RG: Use of the balloon-tipped pulmonary artery catheter in pulmonary disease. Ann Intern Med 1983; 98:53

O'Quin R, Marini JJ: Pulmonary artery occlusion pressure: Clinical physiology, measurement, and interpretation. Am Rev Respir Dis 1983; 128:319

Wiedemann HP, Matthay MA, Matthay RA: Cardiovascular pulmonary monitoring in intensive care unit (Part I). Chest 1984; 85:537

RATIONALE 103-b 104-c 105-a 106-d 107-b

When the transducer is being used to measure pulmonary artery pressure or the pulmonary artery occlusion pressure through the distal port, the catheter port is opened to the transducer dome and the atmospheric port is closed (B). The pressure bag allows a slow continuous infusion through the line to ensure patency. When mechanical zeroing is accomplished, the catheter port is closed and the atmospheric port is open (C). If both ports of the transducer dome are closed at the same time, the pressure in the transducer dome increases until it reaches the infusion bag pressure (D). This will likely damage the diaphragm of the transducer. Opening both the pulmonary artery catheter port to the transducer dome and the transducer dome to air allows blood to enter the transducer dome.

REFERENCES

Civetta JM: Pulmonary artery catheter insertion. In: The Pulmonary Artery Catheter. Sprung CL (Ed). Baltimore, University Park Press, 1983, pp 21-32

Morris AH, Chapman RH, Gardner RM: Frequency of technical problems encountered in the measurement of pulmonary artery wedge pressure. Crit Care Med 1984; 12:164

Morton BC: Basic equipment requirements for hemodynamic monitoring. CMA J 1979; 121:879

SHUNT

RATIONALE 108-e

In order to calculate the pulmonary shunt, blood must be obtained from the pulmonary artery and a systemic artery. The shunt is the fraction of cardiac output that is not oxygenated at the alveolar-capillary membrane. It is determined by examining the oxygen contents of alveolar capillary (CAO_2) mixed venous ($C\bar{v}O_2$) and systemic arterial blood (CaO_2). The relationship is given by the formula:

$$\text{shunt fraction} = (CAO_2 - CaO_2)/CAO_2 - C\bar{v}O_2).$$

The oxygen content of blood is the sum of the dissolved oxygen and the oxygen combined with hemoglobin. The dissolved oxygen is proportional to PO_2 and is usually a relatively small amount. The amount of oxygen dissolved in blood at 37°C is about 0.003 ml/100 ml blood per mm Hg. The amount of oxygen combined with hemoglobin is determined by multiplying the amount of oxygen carried by hemoglobin at complete saturation by the fractional saturation. Each gram of hemoglobin has the capacity to carry about 1.34 ml of oxygen. The oxygen content of alveolar capillary blood is taken as the content at alveolar PO_2. If the shunt is to be measured at an FIO_2 of 1.0, the alveolar PO_2 equals approximately the barometric pressure minus 47 torr (the vapor pressure at H_2O at 37°C), minus the $PaCO_2$. In order to measure the shunt with an FIO_2 of less than 1.0, a more complex equation for determining the PaO_2 must be used.

It is not necessary to obtain blood from the central aorta as radial arterial blood has the same oxygen content. Blood from the antecubital vein may have a different oxygen content than mixed venous blood and should not be used in the shunt calculation. The oxygen content of mixed venous blood, withdrawn from the pulmonary artery, represents the true oxygen content of blood entering the alveolar capillary system.

REFERENCES

Bushnell LS: Acute respiratory failure in the surgical patient: Physiology and management. In: Intensive Care. Skillman JJ (Ed). Boston, Little, Brown and Co., 1975, p 204

Vinocur B, Artz JS, Sampliner JE: Monitoring of respiratory status. In: Handbook of Critical Care. Berk JL, Sampliner JE, Artz JS, et al (Eds). Boston, Little, Brown and Co., 1976, p 72

RATIONALE 109-d

This patient has marked intrapulmonary shunting and ventilation/perfusion abnormalities. The respiratory rate of 42 indicates decreased lung compliance and an increased work of breathing. Based on these parameters, she is clearly a candidate for intubation and mechanical ventilation.

Although hemodynamic monitoring is indicated in this setting, the patient is at risk for a bleeding complication because of a low platelet count. This also makes the risk of nasopharyngeal hemorrhage significant with nasotracheal intubation. Although infusion of platelets followed by insertion of a pulmonary artery catheter at a central puncture site might seem appropriate, the safest method of catheter insertion is a cutdown where hemostasis can be directly and visually maintained.

Orotracheal intubation, although associated with decreased patient comfort and less secure stabilization, is less likely to cause hemorrhage and is the method of choice in this case. Although femoral vein catheterization is an alternative, realizing the possibility of inadvertent femoral arterial puncture, its pairing with nasotracheal intubation makes it an incorrect choice. One must realize that, although a cutdown for line placement decreases the chance of severe hemorrhage, it also increases the chance of infection. Another alternative for line placement in this patient would be the external jugular vein, utilizing the Seldinger technique.

REFERENCES

Civetta JM: Pulmonary artery catheter insertion. In: The Pulmonary Artery Catheter. Sprung CL (Ed). Baltimore, University Park Press, 1983, pp 21-32

Liebson PR: Postoperative hemodynamic monitoring. In: Intensive Care of the Surgical Patient. Goldin MD (Ed). Chicago, Year Book Medical Publishers, 1981, p 10

Section 8

110. A 26-year-old male is admitted to your intensive care unit. He admits to intravenous drug abuse and a five-month history of depression, weight-loss, and anorexia. A chest radiograph shows bilateral infiltrates. The patient is febrile, hypoxemic, and appears toxic. Pneumocystis carinii pneumonia is suspected. The patient is started on trimethoprim-sulfamethoxazole (TMP-SMX), tobramycin, and piperacillin. After three days of therapy, the patient begins to feel better. Five days after initiation of therapy, the patient develops a maculopapular rash, an elevated serum creatinine, and leukopenia.

Which ONE of the following agents is MOST likely to be the cause of this patient's adverse reaction?

a. Tobramycin
b. An illicit drug surreptitiously injected intravenously by the patient's twice-daily visitor
c. Piperacillin
d. Trimethoprim-sulfamethoxazole
e. None of the above

111. Which of the following groups is/are at greater risk than the general population for the development of the acquired immune deficiency syndrome (AIDS)?

a. Hemophiliacs
b. Intravenous drug abusers
c. Homosexual males
d. Haitian nationals
e. All of the above

112. The drug LEAST likely to impair ventilation in myasthenia gravis or botulism is:

a. Procainamide
b. Gentamicin
c. D-tubocurarine
d. Guanidine
e. Succinylcholine

113. Which ONE of the following findings is MOST helpful in distinguishing botulism from Guillain-Barre' syndrome?

a. Blood cultures are sterile.
b. Cerebrospinal fluid is normal at onset of symptoms.
c. Swallowing and breathing are affected early.
d. Two other family members have similar illness.
e. No response to edrophonium (Tensilon)

114. A 44-year-old patient treated for Hodgkins disease is receiving parenteral hyperalimentation. The morning of admission to the ICU, the patient becomes confused, tachypneic, and febrile. Examination reveals macronodular lesions over the trunk and lower extremities. Ophthalmoscopic exam reveals an endophthalmitis with cottonball-like lesions.

Which ONE of the following statements concerning this condition is TRUE?

a. Intravenous trimethoprim/sulfamethoxazole have proven efficacious.
b. Proper therapy may cause hypokalemia.
c. A lung biopsy provides the best means of diagnosis.
d. Venous blood cultures provide a higher yield than arterial blood cultures.

115. The diagnosis of Candida sepsis is BEST made by which ONE of the following?

a. Awaiting blood culture results
b. Observing Candida mycelial forms in the urine
c. Awaiting serum precipitin or agglutinin titers
d. Finding white, raised retinal lesions on fundoscopic exam
e. Culturing Candida albicans from the nasopharynx of the patient

116. You are treating a child brought to the hospital by anxious parents because of difficulty breathing. It appears likely that the child has either croup (viral laryngotracheobronchitis) or acute epiglottitis.

Which ONE of the following findings MOST likely indicates that the problem is croup?

a. The child is 8 years old.
b. The rectal temperature is 40.5°C.
c. The child is anxious and appears "toxic."
d. The child is sitting up and drooling.
e. The child has had symptoms of upper respiratory infection with noisy breathing for 3 days.

117. Which of the following statements regarding acute epiglottitis in children is TRUE?

a. Nasotracheal intubation is contraindicated.
b. The most common etiologic organism is influenza A.
c. Children with acute epiglottitis may be safely managed without an artificial airway if closely observed.
d. Direct pharyngoscopy is contraindicated.
e. None of the above

118. A 25 kg, 5-year-old girl awakens her parents at 11:30 p.m. with crying, a sore throat, high fever and inspiratory stridor. By the time she arrives at the Emergency Room, she appears toxic with a pulse of 140, shallow respirations at 40/minute and a rectal temperature of 104°F. She is sitting at the side of the bed with her mouth open and tongue protruding. She is unable to swallow her saliva which drools down her chin.

Appropriate initial management of this patient includes:

a. Starting antibiotics, intravenous fluids and steroids, and sending the patient to the ICU to be placed in a humidified oxygen hood for observation
b. Immediate transfer of the patient to the operating room, induction of the patient with halothane in the sitting position followed by endotracheal intubation
c. Immediate examination of the airway with a tongue blade in the Emergency Room to look for an enlarged epiglottis
d. Sending the patient to the Radiology department with a technician for lateral neck films and a chest radiograph

119. A 2-year-old male presents with a 3-day history of coryza with the onset of stridor over the last 24 hours. The child is restless. His rectal temperature is 101°. His respiratory rate is 50/minute and he has severe intercostal, subcostal, and supraclavicular retractions. His voice is hoarse.

Which ONE of the following statements is TRUE?

a. The slow onset of symptoms and hoarseness point to subglottitis (croup) rather than epiglottitis.
b. Antiobiotics are indicated.
c. If respiratory failure ensues and the child is intubated, the tube can probably be removed within 12 hours.
d. Nebulized racemic epinephrine is not indicated.
e. Iv steroid therapy is of definitive proven value.

120. Which ONE of the following statements regarding epiglottitis in children is FALSE?

a. A physician skilled in airway management should attend the child at all times.
b. Racemic epinephrine mist should be used.
c. Elective intubation is best performed in the operating room with tracheostomy standby capability.
d. Antibiotics are indicated.

121. Which ONE of the following statements concerning infectious endocarditis is TRUE?

a. A murmur of aortic stenosis is characteristic.
b. Four blood cultures will identify the causative organism less than 50% of the time.
c. Gram negative organisms are the most likely etiologic agent.
d. A positive rheumatoid factor is common.

122. The antibiotic LEAST appropriate to use intravenously in management of enterococcal endocarditis is:

a. Sodium penicillin G
b. Vancomycin
c. Cephalothin
d. Gentamicin
e. Ampicillin

123. You are managing an 80-year-old man who has developed fever and Roth spots 1 week after prostatectomy. His urine contains Enterococci (Streptococcus faecalis) but antibiotic sensitivities are not yet available. He has received no antibiotics. You suspect endocarditis.

Which ONE of these antibiotics is MOST appropriate to include?

a. Cephalothin
b. Chloramphenicol
c. Clindamycin
d. Rifampin
e. Tobramycin

124. A 54-year-old man has a Hickman catheter for cancer chemotherapy which includes cis-platinum. He is admitted for a two-day history of chills and fever to 103°F and promptly defervesces after receiving antibiotics. His WBC is 11,000 with a left shift. Blood cultures subsequently grow Klebsiella pneumoniae. Last year, he developed a rash on the third day of a course of ampicillin for a urinary tract infection.

Which ONE of the following statements is TRUE?

a. The catheter must be discontinued.
b. Antibiotic therapy alone may be sufficient in the treatment of this disorder.
c. Aminoglycosides are contraindicated.
d. Cephalosporins are contraindicated.

125. Which ONE of the following statements concerning nosocomial infection in hospitalized patients is TRUE?

a. The most frequent significant site of nosocomial infection is the lung.
b. Gram-negative sepsis from the urinary tract is the nosocomial infection most frequently associated with death.
c. Handwashing is considered the single most important procedure in preventing nosocomial infection.
d. Antibiotic therapy for patients whose respiratory tract is colonized with gram-negative organisms decreases mortality from nosocomial infection.

Questions 126-130: Match the numbered organism (126-130) with the condition (a-e) it is most likely to be associated. The conditions (a-e) may be used once, more than once, or not at all.

a. Sickle-cell anemia
b. Toxic epidermal necrolysis
c. Reye syndrome
d. Epiglottitis
e. Croup

126. Influenza B

127. Streptococcus pneumoniae

128. Staphylococcus aureus

129. Hemophilus influenzae

130. Salmonella

131. Which ONE of the following statements about Rocky Mountain Spotted Fever is CORRECT?

a. The rash characteristically begins as an erythematous vesicular lesion of the chest and back.
b. Noncardiogenic pulmonary edema is usually responsible for the impaired gas exchange that often occurs in this disorder.
c. The rickettsia Coxiella burnetii is the causative organism.
d. The antibiotic of choice is cefoxitin.

132. In children, sepsis and death from Streptococcus pneumoniae occurs MOST commonly in association with:

a. Diabetes mellitus (juvenile onset)
b. Cystic fibrosis
c. Rheumatic mitral stenosis
d. Splenectomy
e. Juvenile rheumatoid arthritis

133. A 32-year-old male patient in the ICU has trismus with progression to generalized reflex spasms. He is having frequent ventricular dysrhythmias. Clostridium tetani is grown from a small wound on his foot.

Which ONE of the items listed below is NOT indicated in the management of this patient?

a. Tetanus immune globulin - 5000 units IM
b. Thiacetazone
c. D-tubocurarine as necessary
d. Morphine to control sympathetic overactivity
e. Wound debridement

134. A 28-year-old menstruating female presents to the hospital with vomiting, diarrhea, and fever. On examination she has a diffuse macular rash and conjunctival and pharyngeal erythema.

Vital signs include:

Temperature - 39°C (102.2°F)	Pulse - 95
Respiratory Rate - 20	BP - 90/60
Hct - 37	WBC - 11,000
Na^+ - 137 mEq/L	Cl^- - 98 mEq/L
HCO_3^- - 24 mEq/L	BUN - 40 mg/dl
K^+ - 3.8 mEq/L	

Which ONE of the following statements concerning the disease process is TRUE?

a. The disease causes renal and hepatic dysfunction.
b. Nafcillin 1 gm Q 4 hours reverses the acute disease process.
c. Alterations of consciousness are rare.
d. Blood cultures will probably be positive for Staphylococcus aureus.

INFECTIOUS DISEASE/IMMUNOLOGIC

ANSWERS

110-d	111-e	112-d	113-d	114-b	115-d	116-e	117-e
118-b	119-a	120-b	121-d	122-c	123-e	124-b	125-c
126-c	127-a	128-b	129-d	130-a	131-b	132-d	133-b
134-a							

ACQUIRED IMMUNODEFICIENCY

RATIONALE 110-d

This patient's disease process is compatible with the acquired immune deficiency syndrome (AIDS) and Pneumocystis carinii pneumonia (PCP). Major diagnostic clues are the weight loss and anorexia. This so-called "wasting syndrome" may precede the clinical presentation of AIDS by several months.

Another major clue is the patient's history of intravenous drug abuse. Seventeen percent of AIDS victims are intravenous drug abusers, making this the second most common risk factor after homo- or bisexuality.

The cause of the rash, elevated creatinine and leukopenia is TMP-SMX. This is seen in as many as 30% of patients with AIDS, compared with an incidence of 5% in patients without the syndrome. The drug reaction is seen as frequently with therapeutic as well as prophylactic doses. Although the aminoglycosides occasionally (5%) cause transient skin rashes and may certainly result in nephrotoxicity (2%-10%), the chance of this patient's abnormalities being due to tobramycin is much less than that resulting from the use of TMP-SMX. Piperacillin, a penicillin, could also cause these ontoward effects via a hypersensitivity reaction. The reported incidence of such reactions is 0.7% to 10% in different studies.

The surreptitious injection of an illicit drug is always a possibility in a drug abuser. The likelihood of this causing the above described problem, however, is low.

REFERENCES

Fauci AS: Acquired immune deficiency syndrome: Epidemiologic, clinical, immunologic, and therapeutic considerations. Ann Intern Med 1984; 100:92

Mandell GL, Sande MA: Penicillin and cephalosporins. In: The Pharmacologic Basis of Therapeutics. Goodman LS, Gilman AG (Eds). New York, Macmillan Publishing Co. Inc., 1980, pp 1126

Mildvan D: Acquired immune deficiency syndrome or an opportunistic infection. In: The Acquired Immune Deficiency Syndrome and Infections of Homosexual Men. Ma P, Armstrong D (Eds). New York, Yorke Medical Books, 1984, pp 240-252

Sande MA, Mandell GL: The Aminoglycosides. Sixth Edition. New York, Macmillan Publishing Co. Inc., 1980, pp 1162-1180

RATIONALE 111-e

Four groups of individuals are at increased risk for the development of AIDS. Of these, homosexual or bisexual males constitute the largest group, accounting for 71% of all reported cases in the United States. AIDS has also been noted in Haitians residing in the United States, who otherwise have no other known risk factors. Intravenous drug abusers comprise 17% of the total affected patient population. Hemophiliacs constitute the final group.

REFERENCES

Amman AJ, et al: Acquired immunodeficiency in an infant: Possible transmission by means of blood products. Lancet 1983; 1:767

Davis KC, et al: Acquired immunodeficiency syndrome in a patient with hemophilia. Ann Intern Med 1983; 3:284

Fauci, AS, et al: Acquired immunodeficiency syndrome: Epidemiologic, clinical, immunologic, and therapeutic considerations. Ann Intern Med 1984; 100:92

Fauci AS: The acquired immunodeficiency syndrome: The ever broadening clinical spectrum. JAMA 1983; 249:2375

EDITORIAL COMMENT

The acquired immunodeficiency syndrome (AIDS) has reached epidemic proportions. From June 1981 to February 1986, over 17,000 cases were reported in the United States and almost half of these patients have died. Diagnosed cases are projected to double over the next 12 months.

The acquired immunodeficiency syndrome is caused by the human T-cell lymphotrophic virus-III (HTLV-III). It has been isolated in blood, semen, saliva, tears, and other body fluids. A medical worker in England was infected with HTLV-III as a result of a needlestick, and two cases of probable exposure of health care workers by infected blood have recently been reported in the United States.

The risk to the critical care team seems small, however, all health care workers are encouraged to exercise extreme caution when coming into contact with the body fluids of patients with AIDS. The specific recommendations of the Centers for Disease Control and the U.S. Public Health Service should be carefully followed.

Difficult moral, ethical, and economic issues are raised in this cost-conscious time when allocation of expensive ICU resources to these patients is considered.

ADDITIONAL REFERENCES

Acquired immune deficiency syndrome (AIDS): Precautions for clinical and laboratory staffs. MMWR 1982; 31:577

Banks RA, Lindley KL, Pozniak AL: AIDS: A problem for intensive care. Intensive Care Med 1985; 11:169

Brandt EN: Implications of the acquired immunodeficiency syndrome for health policy. Ann Intern Med 1985; 103:771

Curran JW: The epidemiology and prevention of the acquired immuno-deficiency syndrome. Ann Intern Med 1985; 103:657

International Conference on Acquired Immunodeficiency Syndrome. Ann Intern Med 1985; 103:653

Needlestick transmission of HTLV-III from a patient infected in Africa (editorial). Lancet 1984; 2:1376

Prevention of acquired immune deficiency syndrome (AIDS): Report of inter-agency recommendations. MMWR 1983; 32:101

Update: Evaluation of human T-lymphotropic virus type III/lymphadenopathy-associated virus infection in health care personnel. United States MMWR 1985; 34:575

BOTULISM

RATIONALE 112-d

Myasthenia gravis is caused by circulating antibodies to acetylcholine receptors on the motor end plate and botulism is caused by decreased release of acetylcholine from the motor nerve endings. Patients with either illness are especially susceptible to other factors that compromise neuromuscular transmission. D-tubocurarine, procainamide, and gentamicin (and other aminoglycoside antibiotics such as streptomycin, neomycin, tobramycin, amikacin, etc.) inhibit acetylcholine effects at the motor end plate receptors. Succinylcholine mimics acetylcholine and depolarizes these receptors, making them unresponsive to the natural agonist. Guanidine, however, increases acetylcholine release and may be beneficial in the Eaton-Lambert syndrome, in which acetylcholine release is impaired, and in some patients with myasthenia gravis or botulism.

Many critically-ill patients have ventilatory insufficiency and administration of certain drugs may further compromise breathing and lead to crises. Thus, when ordering antidysrhythmic drugs (quinidine, procainamide, lidocaine), antibiotics (aminoglycosides, polymyxin B, colistin), quinine, etc., consider their effects on neuromuscular transmission.

REFERENCES

Cherington M, Ryan DW: Treatment of botulism with guanidine: Early neuro-physiologic studies. N Engl J Med 1970; 282:195

Long SS, Gajewski JL, Brown LW, et al: Clinical, laboratory and environmental features of infantile botulism in Southeastern Pennsylvania. Pediatrics 1985; 75:935

Merikangas JR, Johns RJ: The effect of guanidine on the muscle action potential. Johns Hopkins Med J 1968; 122:37

Schmidt JL, Vick NA, Sadove MS: The effect of quinidine on the action of muscle relaxants. JAMA 1963; 183:669

Seybold ME: Myasthenia gravis: A clinical and basic science review. JAMA 1983; 250:2516

Wright EA, McQuillen MP: Antibiotic-induced neuromuscular blockade. Ann NY Acad Sci 1971; 183:358

RATIONALE 113-d

The symptoms of botulism usually occur within 12-36 hours of ingestion of the toxin. Early symptoms include primarily bulbar dysfunction (blurred vision, diplopia, dizziness, dysarthria, and dysphagia), followed by descending paralysis, dyspnea, and respiratory paralysis. Botulism toxin interferes with acetylcholine release at nerve terminals, and rarely mild cases have been noted to have muscular fatigue-ability which was improved with edrophonium injection; however, this has no value as a diagnostic test. This illness usually occurs in epidemic fashion when several members of a party or a family ingest contaminated food.

In contrast, Guillain-Barre' syndrome (GBS) is a sporadically occurring illness after an infection or traumatic event, with gradual progressive deterioration in neurologic function. Most patients achieve maximum neurological deficit within 3 weeks of the onset of symptoms, rather than within 8-24 as observed with botulism. The initial symptoms in GBS are primarily paresthesias or motor weakness, with subsequent progressive ascending motor deficit. A descending pattern is not unusual, and cases involving initially primarily bulbar function have been reported. This illness is a result of segmental demyelination of the spinal nerve roots and proximal nerve segments, and the administration of edrophonium produces no improvement in the syndrome.

In both illnesses, blood cultures are sterile. In GBS, spinal fluid may be normal at the onset of symptoms, but demonstrates eventual elevation of protein to as high as 1300 mg/dl with minimal lymphocytic pleocytosis. The CSF is normal in botulism. Therefore, the history of two other members of a family affected by a similar illness would be the most valuable element in the history towards making a diagnosis of botulism.

REFERENCES

Cherington M: Botulism: Ten-year experience. Arch Neurol 1974; 30:432

Donadio JA, Gangarosa EJ, Faich GA: Diagnosis and treatment of botulism. J Infect Dis 1971; 124:108

Eisen A, Humphreys P: The Guillain-Barre' syndrome: A clinical and electro-diagnostic study of 25 cases. Arch Neurol 1974; 30:438

McFarland HR, Heller GL: Guillain-Barre' disease complex: A statement of diagnostic criteria and analysis of 100 cases. Arch Neurol 1966; 14:196

Merson MH, Hughes JM, Dowell VR, et al: Current trends in botulism in the United States. JAMA 1974; 229:1305

EDITORIAL COMMENT

Botulism has been reported in chronic iv and intranasal drug abusers. Skin lesions or the paranasal sinuses may harbor Clostridium botulinum, allowing for production and release of toxin.

ADDITIONAL REFERENCES

MacDonald KL, Rutherford GW, Friedman SM, et al: Botulism and botulism-like illness in chronic drug abusers. Ann Intern Med 1985; 102:616

Wound botulism associated with parenteral cocaine abuse. New York City MMWR 1982; 31:87

CANDIDIASIS

RATIONALE 114-b

An immunosuppressed patient receiving parenteral alimentation is at high risk to develop catheter induced sepsis. Bacterial and fungal sepsis is common. Authorities recommend daily ophthalmoscopic examinations on patients receiving hyperalimentation looking for the classic endophthalmitis of Candida sepsis. These retinal findings may be the only clue to a definitive diagnosis pending culture results. The patient in this question also has macronodular skin lesions consistent with disseminated Candidiasis. Arterial blood cultures provide a somewhat higher yield than venous blood cultures. The treatment of choice is intravenous amphotericin B. This potent polyene may cause nausea, vomiting, fever, chills, and bone marrow suppression. It also invariably causes some renal insufficiency, an incomplete distal renal tubular acidosis, and hypokalemia.

REFERENCES

Edwards JE: Candida endophthalmitis. In: Current Clinical Topics in Infectious Diseases. Remington JS, Schwartz MN (Eds). New York, McGraw-Hill Book Company, 1982, pp 381-397

Edwards JE (moderator): Severe candida infections. Ann Intern Med 1978; 89:91

Sen P, Louria D: Fungal infections in the compromised host. DM 1981; 27:1

RATIONALE 115-d

The only pathognomonic physical sign of systemic Candida infection is endophthalmitis. This is evidenced by multiple round, raised, white, cotton-like lesions on the chorioretina. These lesions are the result of hematogenous spread, and are frequently found if looked for diligently.

Blood cultures are a notoriously poor method of determining Candida sepsis. They not only take a great deal of time, but more importantly, autopsy data has shown that blood cultures were positive in only about one-half of the patients later found to have deep fungal infections. Moreover, if therapy is instituted after blood cultures become positive, the chance for recovery becomes less likely.

Serum precipitin and agglutinin tests for Candida are fraught with many false positives and false negatives and, therefore, are neither specific nor sensitive for the diagnosis of invasive Candidiasis.

Finding the BUDDING yeast form in the urine is supportive evidence, as it has been shown that nearly all patients with Candida septicemia will have Candiduria, but the reverse is not true.

Candida is opportunistic, and as such will colonize the upper respiratory and gastrointestinal tracts of the immunocompromised patient. This does not necessarily connote invasive Candidiasis. Positive cultures from three different sites are, however, in the opinion of many experts, an indication for parenteral therapy.

Perhaps the best answer, not listed, is a high index of suspicion in a patient at high risk for systemic Candidiasis.

Turner et al, have recently reviewed the consequences of candidemia for pediatric patients.

REFERENCES

Edwards JE, et al: Severe Candida infections: Clinical perspective, immune defense mechanisms, and current concepts of therapy. Ann Intern Med 1978 89:91

Edwards JE, Foos RY, Mongomerie JZ, et al: Ocular manifestations of Candida septicemia: Review of seventy-six cases of hematogenous Candida endophthalmitis. Medicine 1974; 53:47

Holder IA, Kozinn PJ, Law EJ: Evaluation of Candida precipitin and agglutinin tests for the diagnosis of systemic Candidiasis in burn patients. J Clin Microbiol 1977; 6:219

Solomkin JS, Flohr AB, Quie PG, et al: The role of Candida in intraperitoneal infections. Surgery 1980; 33:524

Solomkin JS, Simmons RL: Candida infection in surgical patients. World J Surg 1980; 4:381

Turner RB, Donowitz LG, Hendley O: Consequences of candidemia for pediatric patients. Am J Dis Child 1985; 139:178

Williams RJ, Chandler JG, Orloff MJ: Candida septicemia. Arch Surg 1971; 103:8

EDITORIAL COMMENT

Candida albicans is the most common pathogen associated with systemic candidiasis although other species do occasionally cause infection. Dick and associates recently reported a fatal case of candida sepsis in an immune compromised patient. The organism isolated was Candida guilliermondii which, interestingly, seems to be the least pathogenic in animal studies. This organism became resistant to amphotericin B during the course of therapy.

Practitioners should be aware that species other than C. albicans can cause serious systemic disease especially in the immune compromised host. Susceptibility testing should probably be performed on isolates recovered from immune compromised patients receiving polyene antibiotics.

ADDITIONAL REFERENCE

Dick JD, Rosengard BR, Merz WG, et al: Fatal disseminated candidiasis due to amphotericin-B resistant Candida guilliermondii. Ann Intern Med 1985; 102:67

CROUP/EPIGLOTTITIS

RATIONALE 116-e

Airway resistance increases inversely to the fourth power of the radius of the airway (Poiseuille's Law). The small pediatric airway is particularly susceptible to the effects of swelling via increased airway resistance, increased turbulence in the gas flow and decreased air movement. As the child exerts more effort to breathe in, he or she creates greater negative pressure in the chest which tends to collapse the extrathoracic airway further. The result is the inspiratory crowing and stridor characteristic of croup. As obstruction worsens, expiratory noise may occur as well.

Viral laryngotracheobronchitis (croup) is caused by a large number of viruses. Thus, croup symptomatology is a nonspecific response to swelling in the narrowest portion of the airway at the cricoid ring. Croup may be thought of as "common cold of the susceptible airway." It is more common in young children, less than 3 years of age, and is not usually characterized by high fever. The associated respiratory distress is not usually severe and the children do not usually appear toxic.

Epiglottitis is an acute inflammation of the supraglottic structures usually caused by Hemophilus influenzae. It is a malignant disease which may kill the patient quickly. It is found in patients of all ages. Cases in 2-month-old and 72-year-old patients have been reported, but the predominant age range is 3-8 years. Patients frequently have an accompanying bacteremia/sepsis and are usually toxic appearing.

Sitting and drooling may be found in either croup or epiglottitis. The difference is that the child with epiglottitis is doing so to protect his airway and will resist being put in the supine position, while the child with croup may be sitting up and playing.

Because viral laryngotracheobronchitis accompanies or is a part of the common cold, symptoms of URI usually precede the onset of croup symptomatology. Acute epiglottitis, on the other hand, progresses rapidly and prompts a visit to physician almost invariably within 24 hours.

REFERENCES

Baines DB, Wark H, Overton JH: Acute epiglottitis in children. Anaesth Intensive Care 1984; 13:25

Bass JW, Steele RW, Wiehe RA: Acute epiglottitis: A surgical emergency. JAMA 1974; 229:671

Davison FW: Acute laryngeal obstruction in children. JAMA 1959; 171:1301

Hannallah R, Rosales JK: Acute epiglottitis: Current management and review. Can Anaesth Soc J 1978; 25:84

Hawking DB, Miller AH, Sachs GB, et al: Acute epiglottitis in adults. Laryngoscope 1973; 83:1211

RATIONALE 117-e

The method of airway management in children with acute epiglottitis is highly controversial. Battaglia, Lockhart, and Diaz have reported high success rates with direct pharyngoscopy and nasotracheal intubation. Immediate tracheostomy has been advocated by Margolis while elective tracheostomy following initial tracheal intubation has been suggested by Fearon and Cinnamond. Raplain reported a retrospective analysis of children with epiglottitis. Twenty patients in this study were closely observed without an artificial airway. Four of these patients died and another nearly died during an emergency tracheostomy. Most authorities agree that some type of artificial airway is needed in this disorder.

The most common etiologic organism is Hemophilus influenzae - Type B.

REFERENCES

Battaglia JD, Lockhart CH: Management of acute epiglottitis by nasotracheal intubation. Am J Dis Child 1975; 120:334

Diaz JH, Lockhart CH: Early diagnosis and airway management of acute epiglottitis in children. South Med J 1982; 75:399

Fearon B, Cinnamond M: Tracheotomy in acute supraglottitis (epiglottitis): The treatment of choice. Laryngoscope 1977; 87:879

Margolis CZ, Ingram DC, Meyer JH: Routine tracheotomy in Hemophilus influenzae - Type B epiglottitis. J Pediatr 1972; 81:1150

Raplain RH: Tracheostomy in epiglottitis. Pediatrics 1973; 52:426

RATIONALE 118-b

Acute epiglottitis is a true medical emergency. The diagnosis can usually be made by the presenting history and clinical appearance, which include a previously well child who awakens in the middle of the night with a high fever, severe sore throat, difficulty swallowing, and toxic appearance. However, this disease is not limited to children and has been frequently described in adults. The infecting agent is usually Hemophilus influenzae, although other pathogens have been implicated. Further workup beyond the presenting history and physical appearance is often not needed until the airway is secured. However, should radiographs be needed, the child should always be accompanied by a clinician highly skilled in intubation, since the airway may obstruct at any time.

Many experts suggest that the patient be taken immediately to the operating room where a surgeon ready to do an emergency tracheostomy should be present. Gentle mask induction with oxygen and halothane is then accomplished with the patient in the sitting position. Only when the patient is deeply anesthetized should he or she be placed in a supine position. An endotracheal tube should be placed under direct visualization which will not only aid in securing the airway, but will also confirm the diagnosis. The size of the endotracheal tube is usually 1-2 sizes smaller than anticipated for a given child. The nasotracheal route is often more secure and better tolerated than oral intubation. The exact method of securing the airway remains controversial and there are some who advocate tracheostomy to secure the airway. In any case, the most important aspect is to SECURE the airway. The patient can then be transferred to the ICU where antibiotics and parenteral fluids can be given. Proper restraint of the child in the ICU to prevent accidental extubation cannot be overemphasized. The patient is usually able to be extubated within 48-72 hours and discharged from the hospital within 5-7 days of admission.

REFERENCES

Baines DB, Wark H, Overton JH: Acute epiglottitis in children. Anaesth Intensive Care 1984; 13:25

Selbst SM: Epiglottitis. Am J Emerg Med 1983; 3:342

RATIONALE 119-a

The preceding coryza, the onset of symptoms over 12 hours, the relatively low rectal temperature and hoarseness indicate a diagnosis of croup rather than epiglottitis. A lateral neck radiograph would show no epiglottic enlargement. As croup is a viral-induced process, antibiotics are of no value unless a site of bacterial infection is found. The patient with croup may require intubation and prolonged mechanical ventilation. Patients with epiglottitis, however, can frequently be extubated after 12-24 hours of antibiotic theraphy. Racemic epinephrine has been shown to be of value in croup. Although croup literally means noisy breathing, it is generally used to refer to the subglottic laryngitides which are viral-induced, as opposed to epiglottitis or supraglottitis caused by Hemophilus influenzae. There is no conclusive data to support using steroids in this situation.

REFERENCES

Adair JC, Ring WH: Management of epiglottitis in children. Anesth Analg 1975; 54:622

Bottenfield GW, Arcinue EL, Sarnaik A, et al: Diagnosis and management of acute epiglottitis - Report of 90 consecutive cases. Laryngoscope 1980; 90:822

Hannallah R, Rosales JK: Acute epiglottitis: Current management and review. Can Anaesth Soc J 1978; 25:84

RATIONALE 120-b

Epiglottitis is a fulminant disease often resulting in death within hours. If a child is strongly suspected of having epiglottitis, time should not be spent obtaining a lateral neck radiograph. A clinician capable of emergency airway management should be in attendance at all times. Racemic epinephrine has no therapeutic value, may irritate the airways, and is therefore contraindicated. Elective intubation is best performed in the operating room. Mask induction using halothane should be performed with the patient in a sitting position to optimize airway patency. Supine positioning may cause the epiglottis to move posteriorly and obstruct the airway. A physician skilled in the performance of tracheostomy should be present in the operating room in case intubation fails and tracheostomy is necessary. Hemophilus influenzae is the usual causative organism. Ampicillin and chloramphenicol are the antibiotics of choice pending cultures and sensitivities.

REFERENCES

Davis H: Acute upper airway obstruction: Croup and epiglottitis. Pediatr Clin North Am 1981; 28:859

Holbrook PE: Care of the critically ill child. In: Critical Care: State of the Art. Vol 1. Shoemaker WC, Thompson WL (Eds). Fullerton, CA, Society of Critical Care Medicine, 1980, pp I(R):26-27

Weibley RE, Holbrook PE: Proximal airway failure in children. In: Textbook of Critical Care. Shoemaker WC, Thompson WL, Holbrook PR (Eds). Philadelphia, WB Saunders Co., 1984, pp 245-246

EDITORIAL COMMENT

Epiglottitis is not only a disease of children, but occurs in adults as well. As previously mentioned, the infecting organism in children is usually H. influenza - Type B. Many organisms have been implicated in adults including H. parainfluenza, Streptococcus pneumoniae, Staphylococcus aureus, and beta hemolytic streptococcus. The disease presents as a fulminating illness in adults with acute onset, rapidly progressive course, and high mortality.

ADDITIONAL REFERENCES

Garfinkel HJ, Brown R, Kabins SA: Acute infectious epiglottitis in adults. Ann Intern Med 1969; 70:289

Kander PL, Richards SH: Acute epiglottitis in adults. J Laryngol Otal 1977; 91:295

Warner JA, Finlay WEI: Fulminating epiglottitis in adults. Anaesthesia 1985; 40:348

ENDOCARDITIS

RATIONALE 121-d

Careful auscultation for a new regurgitant murmur is important. Laboratory abnormalities are nonspecific and include mild anemia (usually normochromic and normocytic), a mildly elevated white blood cell count and microscopic hematuria. A positive rheumatoid factor in high titer is common. Blood cultures provide crucial laboratory information. A 90% accuracy is achieved after four blood cultures, and rarely are more than six required to obtain a positive culture. About 10%-20% of patients will have negative blood cultures. Most of these patients have received prior antibiotic therapy. Gram-negative organisms are unusual causes of infectious endocarditis and when present are usually in patients with prosthetic valves or in intravenous drug abusers.

REFERENCES

Csete ME: Infective endocarditis. In: Manual of Intensive Care Medicine. Rippe JM, Csete ME (Eds). Boston, Little, Brown and Co., 1983, pp 258-259

Pelletier LL, Petersdorf RG: Infective endocarditis: A review of 125 cases from the University of Washington Hospitals, 1963-1972. Medicine 1977; 56:287

Weinstein L: Infective endocarditis. In: Heart Disease: A Textbook of Cardiovascular Medicine. Braunwald E (Ed). Philadelphia, WB Saunders Co., 1980

RATIONALE 122-c

Enterococcal infections respond most frequently to a combination of a penicillin with an aminoglycoside antibiotic (streptomycin, gentamicin, tobramycin, amikacin, etc.), but some enterococci are sensitive to penicillin, ampicillin, or gentamicin alone. Vancomycin is a potent bactericidal antibiotic that is a second choice for treating enterococcal infections, especially in patients who are intolerant of penicillins. Cephalosporins such as cephalothin have little efficacy in treating enterococcal infections, especially enterococcal endocarditis, and should be avoided in most cases.

REFERENCES

Gardner P, Provine HT: Manual of Acute Bacterial Infections. Boston, Little, Brown and Co., 1975, pp 215-216

Root RK, Hierholzer WJ Jr: Infectious disease. In: Clinical Pharmacology, Basic Principles in Therapeutics. Second Edition. Melmon KL, Morrelli HF (Eds). New York, Macmillan Publishing Co. Inc., 1978, pp 752-753

Watanakunakorn C: Changing epidemiology and newer aspects of infective endocarditis. Adv Intern Med 1977; 22:21

RATIONALE 123-e

Bacterial endocarditis in elderly men with prostatism or women with genitourinary infections is often caused by the enterococcus (Streptococcus faecalis). The correct bacteriological diagnosis is crucial, as these organisms are frequently resistant to penicillin. The combination of penicillin and an aminoglycoside such as streptomycin, gentamicin, or tobramycin is synergistic. Penicillin G is administered in doses of 12-24 million units/day, and gentamicin in a dose of 3-5 mg/kg•day in divided doses. Therapy for at least 4 weeks is mandatory.

If bacteriological diagnosis is delayed for any reason, it is useful to begin an aminoglycoside with penicillin and consider discontinuing the aminoglycoside if the organism turns out to be Streptococcus viridans. Some authorities, however, believe use of an aminoglycoside enhances treatment of Streptococcus viridans with penicillin.

This combination is a good example of antimicrobial synergism. It results because each agent has a different mode of action. Penicillin decreases permeability of bacterial cell walls by interfering with synthesis of wall units; aminoglycosides apparently then enter bacterial cells more easily and are able to exert their lethal effect by interfering with protein synthesis.

REFERENCES

Cherubin CD, Neu HD: Infective endocarditis at the Presbyterian Hospital in New York City from 1938-1967. Am J Med 1971; 51:83

Moellering RC Jr, Watson BK, Kunz LJ: Endocarditis due to Group D streptococci: A comparison of disease caused by Streptococcus Bovis with that produced by the enterococci. Am J Med 1974; 57:239

NOSOCOMIAL INFECTION

RATIONALE 124-b

Bacteremias in patients with surgically implanted Hickman or Broviac catheters may be cured without removing the catheter. If blood cultures remain positive after 3-5 days of intensive antibiotics, if the tunnel is grossly infected, or if septic emboli develop, the catheter must be removed. Aminoglycosides might be avoided in the face of cis-platinum therapy but they are not contraindicated. A recent study demonstrated no increased risk of nephrotoxicity when aminoglycosides were used in the cis-platinum treated patient. The rash associated with use of ampicillin does not usually represent a true allergy to penicillin and, therefore, it is generally safe to use cephalosporins in this setting.

REFERENCES

Haas A, Anderson L, Lad T: The influence of aminoglycosides on the nephrotoxicity of cis-Diamminedichloroplatinum in cancer patients. J Infect Dis 1983; 147:363

Kucers A, Bennett N: The use of antibiotics. London, William Heinemann Medical Books Ltd., 1977

Maki DG: Infections associated with intravascular lines. In: Current Clinical Topics in Infectious Diseases. Remington JS, Swartz MN (Eds). New York, McGraw-Hill Book Company, 1982

RATIONALE 125-c

Nosocomial infection is a major cause of morbidity and mortality in the critically ill. The more severe the underlying illness, the higher the incidence of nosocomial infection. Although the urinary tract is the most common site of hospital acquired infection, lower respiratory tract infection is associated with a higher mortality. Handwashing is considered the single most important procedure in preventing infection in the ICU. Colonization of the respiratory tract by gram-negative organisms is a frequent occurrence in the critically ill and plays a major role in the pathogenesis of nosocomial respiratory infection. Antibiotics may predispose to colonization and are not recommended unless definite infection is present.

REFERENCES

Albert RK, Condie F: Handwashing patterns in medical intensive care units. N Engl J Med 1981; 304:1465

Britt MR, Schleupner CJ, Matsumiya S: Severity of underlying disease as a predictor of nosocomial infection. Utility in the control of nosocomial infection. JAMA 1978; 239:1047

Donowitz LG, Wenzel RP, Hoyt JW: High risk of hospital-acquired infection in the ICU patient. Crit Care Med 1982; 10:355

Gross PA, Neu HC: Deaths from nosocomial infections: Experience in a university hospital and a community hospital. Am J Med 1980; 68:219

Johanson WG, Pierce AK: Nosocomial respiratory infections with gram-negative bacilli. Ann Intern Med 1972; 77:701

Wenzel RP, Thompson RL, Landry SM, et al: Hospital-acquired infections in intensive care unit patients: An overview with emphasis on epidemics. Infect Control 1983; 4:471

EDITORIAL COMMENT

Catheter contamination sleeves are widely used with pulmonary artery catheters. Theoretically, the sleeves enable repositioning while the catheter remains sterile. Initial studies reported no growth inside the contamination sleeves. Recent studies, however, indicate that the sleeves may not be as protective as previously thought. Baele reported a 12% incidence of valve contamination when the sleeve was used with a valved introducer.

ADDITIONAL REFERENCES

Baele P, Pedemonte O, Zech F, et al: Clinical use and bacteriological studies of catheter contamination sleeves. Intensive Care Med 1984; 10:297

Gamey F, Spagna PE, Lemole G: Improved techniques in using Swan-Ganz catheters. Ann Thorac Surg 1979; 27:468

Kopman EA, Sandza JG: Manipulation of the pulmonary artery catheter after placement: Maintenance of sterility. Anesthesiology 1978; 48:373

PEDIATRIC INFECTION

RATIONALE 126-c 127-a 128-b 129-d 130-a

Infection is the most common cause of death in sickle-cell anemia. The increased susceptibility is due in large part to the loss of splenic function. During the first 5 years of life, Streptococcus pneumoniae is the major offending organism. Osteomyelitis occurs with increased frequency in sickle-cell anemia and Salmonella is the most common organism.

Toxic epidermal necrolysis or scalded skin syndrome is a disease of infants and children under 10 years of age. It is caused by a group 2 phage type Staphylococcus aureus which elaborates an exotoxin. The toxin is responsible for the formation of fluid filled bullae which subsequently pull away leaving denuded areas. Excessive fluid loss, electrolyte imbalance, faulty temperature control, pneumonia and sepsis increase morbidity. Systemic therapy with a penicillinase-resistant penicillin is the treatment of choice.

Reye syndrome is heralded by a nonspecific viral prodrome followed by persistent vomiting, hepatic dysfunction, altered mental status and coma. There is an association with the influenza and varicella viruses.

Croup or laryngotracheobronchitis is caused by numerous respiratory viruses. Epiglottitis is an explosive, life-threatening bacterial infection of the epiglottis. The most common organism is Hemophilus influenzae - Type-B.

REFERENCES

Barrett-Conner E: Bacterial infection and sickle cell anemia. Medicine 1971; 50:97

Bass JW, et al: Acute epiglottitis: A surgical emergency. JAMA 1974; 229:671

Burgoon CF: The skin. In: Nelson Textbook of Pediatrics. Vaughan VC, McKay J, Nelson W (Eds). Philadelphia, WB Saunders Co.

Gorfinkel HJ, Brown R, Kabins SA: Acute infectious epiglottitis in adults. Ann Intern Med 1969; 70:289

Lukens JN: Sickle cell disease. DM 1981; 27:1

Schubert W, Bobo RC, Partin JC, et al: Reye's syndrome. DM 1975; December, pp 1-30

ROCKY MOUNTAIN SPOTTED FEVER

RATIONALE 131-b

Rocky Mountain Spotted Fever (RMSF) is an acute tick-borne febrile illness caused by Rickettsia rickettsii. It is characterized by the sudden onset of fever and headache. A characteristic rash beginning on the fourth febrile day is the most helpful diagnostic sign. The rash begins on the extremities (wrists, ankles, palms, soles, forearms) and spreads to the trunk. The first lesions are macular. After two to three days they become maculopapular, and about the fourth day the rash becomes petechial. Commonly these hemorrhagic lesions coalesce to form large ecchymotic areas especially over bony prominences. Ulcerations may form and eventually slough. Before the onset of the rash, differentiation from other acute infections may be difficult. Even after the rash develops, this disease may be confused with meningococcemia rubeola, murine typhus, Brill-Zinsser disease and Rickettsialpox. Careful attention to the details of the rash, however, will often make the diagnosis.

A nonproductive cough may occur in up to one-third of patients with RMSF. Altered pulmonary capillary permeability and increased lung water is thought to be responsible for the impaired gas exchange in most patients. The disease may have a fulminant course leading to death. The overall mortality rate is now 6%-7%. Treatment with chloramphenicol or tetracycline within the first 6 days of the illness almost uniformly leads to cure.

REFERENCES

Donohue JF: Lower respiratory tract involvement in Rocky Mountain spotted fever. Arch Intern Med 1980; 140:223

Hattwick MAW, O'Brien RJ, Hanson BF: Rocky Mountain spotted fever: Epidemiology of an increasing problem. Ann Intern Med 1976; 84:732

MacCaughelty TC: Rocky Mountain spotted fever from St. Louis County: Implications for early diagnosis and treatment. Crit Care Med 1982; 10:124

Medearis DN, Gang DL: Fever, rash, and circulatory collapse in a four-year-old boy. N Engl J Med 1978; 298:1071

EDITORIAL COMMENT

Other antimicrobial agents such as penicillins, cephalosporins, aminoglycosides, and trimethoprim-sulfamethoxazole have no effect on the course of the illness at clinically permissible doses.

ADDITIONAL REFERENCES

Harrell GT: Rocky Mountain spotted fever. Medicine 1949; 28:333

Walker DH: Rickettsial infection of the pulmonary microcirculation: The basis for interstitial pneumonitis in Rocky Mountain spotted fever. Hum Pathol 1980; 11:263

SPLENECTOMY

RATIONALE 132-d

Splenectomy is associated with an increase in the incidence of infections with pneumococci (Streptococcus pneumoniae), including pneumococcal peritonitis. The increased susceptibility to pneumococcal infections is greatest in children.

REFERENCES

Bisno AL: Hyposplenism and overwhelming pneumococcal infection: A reappraisal. Am J Med Sci 1971; 262:101

Eraklis AJ, Kevy SV, Diamond LK, et al: Hazard of overwhelming infection after splenectomy in childhood. N Engl J Med 1967; 276:1225

EDITORIAL COMMENT

Children are at high risk for pyogenic infection (particularly with Streptococcus pneumoniae and H. influenzae) following splenectomy for any cause. The use of prophylactic antibiotics (penicillin 250 mg p.o BID) has been recommended for at least two years following surgery. The necessity of lifelong prophylaxis is not clear. Polyvalent pneumococcal polysaccharide vaccine should be given to all patients undergoing splenectomy. The duration of immunity following vaccination is unknown. Booster doses should not be given.

ADDITIONAL REFERENCES

Dickerman JD: Bacterial infection and the asplenic host: A review. J Trauma 1976; 16:662

Gopal V, Bisno AL: Fulminant pneumococcal infections in "normal" asplenic hosts. Arch Intern Med 1977; 137:1526

Immunization Practices Advisory Committee, Centers for Disease Control: General recommendations on immunization. Ann Intern Med 1983; 98:615

O'Neal BJ, McDonald JC: The risk of sepsis in the asplenic adult. Ann Surg 1981; 194:775

TETANUS

RATIONALE 133-b

Wound debridement should be carried out after the administration of tetanus immune globulin. All but the mildest cases of tetanus will require neuromuscular blockade and appropriate ventilatory support. Morphine may help to control the sympathetic overactivity leading to myocardial irritability. Penicillin G or tetracycline are the antibiotics of choice. Thiacetazone is an antituberculous drug and is, therefore, NOT indicated in this setting.

REFERENCES

Edmonson RS, Flowers MW: Intensive care in tetanus: Management complications and mortality in 100 cases. Br Med J 1979; 1:1401

Rothstein RJ, Baker FJ: Tetanus: Prevention and treatment. JAMA 1978; 240:675

EDITORIAL COMMENT

Tetanus is a rare disease in the United States and other developed countries. In 1982 only 75 cases of tetanus were reported to the Centers for Disease Control. Most cases come from the rural southeast and south central states. The case fatality rate is still approximately 50%.

James and Mason recently reported their experience with magnesium sulfate infusions in 10 patients with tetanus. These patients had persistent autonomic dysfunction and myocardial irritability. They noted a significant reduction in heart rate, a decline in systemic vascular resistance, and an increase in stroke volume. Labetalol has also been used successfully in this setting.

ADDITIONAL REFERENCES

Dundee JW, Morrow WFK: Labetalol in severe tetanus. Br Med J 1979; 1:1121

Immunization Practices Advisory Committee: Diptheria, tetanus and pertussis. NY State J Med 1982; 82:1563

James MFM, Mason EDM: The use of magnesium sulphate infusions in the management of very severe tetanus. Intensive Care Med 1985; 11:5

Kerr JH: Current topics in tetanus. Intensive Care Med 1979; 5:105

Wellhoner H: Tetanus neurotoxin. Rev Physiol Biochem Pharmacol 1982; 93:1

TOXIC SHOCK

RATIONALE 134-a

Toxic shock syndrome (TSS) is a disease occurring (3/100,000) in young menstruating women. The disease, more common if tampons are used, begins within the first 5 days of menses. Women develop fever, rash, diarrhea, and vomiting initially. Marked hypotension may occur as early as 4 hours after onset of symptoms. Almost all patients exhibit altered mentation.

There is generally evidence of multisystem involvement: musculoskeletal - myalgias; mucous membrane - erythema; renal - elevated creatinine and BUN; hematologic - thrombocytopenia; CNS - disorientation and agitation, hepatic - elevated transaminases.

TSS is caused by a toxin produced by Staphylococcus aureus. This organism has been cultured in 98% of patients with the disease, but has only been isolated from the blood in a very few patients.

Therapy includes supportive measures to maintain adequate cardiopulmonary function. Large volumes of fluid may be needed to combat hypotension. Patients should be started on a penicillinase resistant penicillin although no studies have shown that antibiotics affect the natural history of the acute disease. Antibiotics do, however, decrease the incidence of recurrence.

REFERENCES

David J, et al: Toxic shock syndrome. N Engl J Med 1980; 303:1429

Fisher R, et al: Toxic shock syndrome in menstruating women. Ann Intern Med 1981; 94:157

Shands K, et al: Toxic shock syndrome in menstruating women. N Engl J Med 1980; 303:1436

Tofte R, et al: Toxic shock syndrome. Ann Intern Med 1981; 94:149

EDITORIAL COMMENT

Lysogenic bacteriophages incorporate genetic information into the host bacterium's DNA. Recent evidence suggests that S. aureus associated with TSS contain lysogenic bacteriophages that may be related to toxin production. The release of toxin(s) is thought to be responsible for the clinical manifestations of this disease. Removal of tampon or drainage of infected area as appropriate is indicated.

ADDITIONAL REFERENCES

Paris AL, Herwaldt LA, Blum D, et al: Pathologic findings in twelve fatal cases of toxic shock syndrome. Ann Intern Med 1982; 96:852

Schultzer SE, Fischetti VA, Zabriskie JB: Toxic shock syndrome and lysogeny in Staphylococcus aureus. Science 1983; 220:316

Section 9

135. The LEAST appropriate therapy of severe metabolic alkalosis is:

a. Trishydroxymethylaminomethane (Tromethamine)
b. Acetazolamide (Diamox)
c. Potassium chloride
d. Sodium chloride
e. Intravenous hydrogen chloride

136. A patient is found to have arterial PCO_2 = 20 mm Hg and pH = 7.1. The plasma bicarbonate concentration is about:

a. 1 mmol/L
b. 3 mmol/L
c. 6 mmol/L
d. 9 mmol/L
e. 12 mmol/L

137. In the patient with an arterial PCO_2 = 20 mm Hg and pH = 7.1, sudden hypoventilation increasing the PCO_2 to 80 mm Hg will result in a blood pH of about:

a. 6.5
b. 6.7
c. 6.8
d. 6.9
e. 7.0

138. Hyperventilation is associated with an INCREASED concentration in blood of:

a. Carbonic acid
b. Hydrogen ions
c. Potassium ions
d. Bicarbonate ions
e. Lactate ions

139. A patient with spontaneous hypothermia has a core temperature of 27°C. The blood gas laboratory assumes the patient to have a core temperature of 37°C when an arterial blood sample is analyzed.

Which of the following reports is most compatible with normal ventilation (i.e., actual patient PCO_2 = 40 mm Hg) and normal acid-base balance (i.e., actual patient pH = 7.40)?

a. PCO_2 = 24 mm Hg and pH = 7.25
b. PCO_2 = 24 mm Hg and pH = 7.55
c. PCO_2 = 24 mm Hg and pH = 7.40
d. PCO_2 = 56 mm Hg and pH = 7.25
e. PCO_2 = 56 mm Hg and pH = 7.55

Questions 140-144 refer to the following patient: A 20-year-old garage mechanic, weighing 60 kg, is admitted to your service when he is brought to the hospital by a friend who found him stuporous in his garage at midnight after he did not return home after work. The patient has been in good health, but has been despondent after his girlfriend recently deserted him. On examination, you find his BP = 140/90, P = 110, T = 37°C, and he is breathing deeply at a rate of 20 breaths/min with a "solvent" odor on his breath. He moans when hurt but does not answer questions. His pupils are dilated slightly and do not react to light though they rove conjugately to left and right. His neck is somewhat stiff, as is his abdomen, with moderate direct but no rebound tenderness. His admission hematological studies are normal, skull and chest roentgenograms are normal, and urinalysis is normal. Initial blood chemistry values are: Na = 140 mEq/L, K = 5 mEq/L, Cl = 90 mEq/L, HCO_3^- 10 mmol/L glucose = 90 mg/dl, urea nitrogen = 56 mg/dl, osmolality = 355 mOsm/kg, acetone and acetoacetate = normal, lactate = 1 mEq/L.

140. Which ONE of the following is the MOST likely cause of this condition?

a. Aspirin poisoning
b. Methanol poisoning
c. Ethylene glycol poisoning
d. Paraldehyde poisoning
e. Isopropyl alcohol poisoning

141. What is the concentration of occult anions ("anion gap") in this patient?

a. 10 mEq/L
b. 20 mEq/L
c. 30 mEq/L
d. 40 mEq/L
e. 50 mEq/L

142. What is the concentration of occult osmoles in this patient?

a. 10 mOsm/kg
b. 20 mOsm/kg
c. 30 mOsm/kg
d. 40 mOsm/kg
e. 50 mOsm/kg

143. If all of the occult osmoles are due to presence of the likely poison, and if it is present at equal concentrations throughout the whole body water, how much of the likely poison is present in this patient's body at this time?

a. 0.058 g
b. 0.58 g
c. 5.8 g
d. 58 g
e. 580 g

144. The patient is treated in part by giving ethanol intravenously. The sterile parenteral ethanol solution is labeled as containing 100% ethanol (molecular weight 46) at a specific gravity of 0.7893. How many ml of this ethanol solution should be added to 1000 ml of distilled water (to be given intravenously) to increase the patient's ethanol concentration in whole body water to 1.5 g/L?

a. 4.3 ml
b. 6.8 ml
c. 43 ml
d. 68 ml
e. 430 ml

145. In a patient with plasma protein concentration = 72 g/L, hematocrit = 40%, arterial pH = 7.40, PCO_2 = 40 torr, and PaO_2 = 100 torr at a temperature of 37°C, the whole blood buffer base is about 47 mEq/L.

Which ONE of the following factors contributes the GREATEST fraction of total buffering capacity under these circumstances?

a. Blood (plasma + erythrocyte) bicarbonate
b. Blood (plasma + erythrocyte) phosphate
c. Hemoglobin anions
d. Plasma protein anions
e. Carbamino anions

146. A 60-year-old female with a history of analgesic abuse is admitted to the ICU after emergency surgery for a perforated gastric ulcer with peritonitis. Over the next few hours she develops multiple episodes of hypotension responsive to volume infusions. You are asked to see the patient because of an electrolyte disturbance.

Temperature - 38°C (100.4°F)	Pulse - 95
Respiratory rate - 25	BP - 100/70

Examination reveals: Clear lung fields, normal cardiac exam, mildly tender abdomen, warm extremities, and peripheral and sacral edema.

Arterial blood gases and serum electrolytes are given below:

pH 7.30	$PaCO_2$ 30 mm Hg	PaO_2 89 mm Hg
Na^+ 140 mEq/L	Cl^- 115 mEq/L	
HCO_3^- 15 mEq/L	K^+ 4.8 mEq/L	

The etiology of this patient's problem is MOST likely secondary to which of the following:

a. Salicylate intoxication
b. Acute renal failure
c. Warm septic shock with an elevated lactic acid
d. Resuscitation with 0.9% saline
e. Respiratory alkalosis with metabolic compensation

147. A 19-year-old comatose male is admitted to a hospital. He is thought to have ingested a large quantity of phenobarbital in a suicide attempt. His physical examination reveals a rectal temperature of 35°C (96°F), a heart rate of 110, a respiratory rate of 7, and a blood pressure of 86/60. Breathing is shallow and precludes adequate chest examination. Except for the tachycardia, his heart examination is normal. Arterial blood gases obtained while the patient is breathing room air reveal:

pH 7.13	$PaCO_2$ 74 mm Hg	PaO_2 49 mm Hg

Which ONE of the following statements is TRUE?

a. Small tidal volumes have caused significant atelectasis and hypoxemia.
b. Hypoventilation explains the acidosis and hypoxemia.
c. Aspiration of gastric contents is a likely cause of the hypoxemia.
d. The acidosis is caused in part by generalized hypoperfusion.
e. The hypoxemia is secondary to noncardiogenic pulmonary edema with attendant pulmonary ventilation-perfusion mismatching.

148. A 33-year-old man recently complained of weakness and fatigue and lost 17 pounds in the past 3 months. He denies ingestion of prescription medication or other drugs. He is admitted to the ICU with a supine blood pressure of 70/40 and a heart rate of 130. Sitting, he becomes faint, his systolic blood pressure falls to 55 and his heart rate increases to 155. His rectal temperature is 97°F. He is noted to have increased pigmentation of the elbows, knees, and buccal mucosa. The following returns from the laboratory:

Na^+	119 mEq/L
K^+	6 mEq/L
Cl^-	105 mEq/L
HCO_3^-	21 mEq/L
Glucose	50 mg/dl

Which ONE of the following statements regarding this patient is TRUE?

a. The patient's ACTH level is probably elevated.
b. The most likely diagnosis is insulinoma.
c. The patient's plasma cortisol is probably elevated.
d. Glucose infusion is the most important clinical treatment.

149. Besides hepatic and uremic encephalopathy, asterixis may be found in the metabolic encephalopathies associated with which of the following?

a. Pulmonary insufficiency
b. Sedative overdose
c. Hypomagnesemia
d. Hypoglycemia
e. All of the above

150. In severe diabetic ketoacidosis with shock, which ONE of the following is LEAST likely to be true?

a. Acetoacetate concentration in blood is increased.
b. The ratio of acetoacetate to beta-hydroxybutyrate concentration in blood is increased.
c. The ratio of lactate to pyruvate concentration in blood is increased.
d. The ratio of $NADH^+$ to NAD in blood is increased.
e. Lactate concentration in blood is increased.

151. Which ONE of these statements is MOST correct about lactate?

a. Hyperventilation decreases blood lactate concentration.
b. Ethanol intoxication decreases blood lactate concentration.
c. An infusion of sodium lactate increasing blood lactate from 1-4 mmol/L decreases pH from 7.4 to about 7.1.
d. Accidental hypothermia leads to increased blood lactate concentration.
e. Pyruvate infusion decreases blood lactate concentration.

152. All the following statements about nutrition and the respiratory system are true EXCEPT:

a. Semi-starvation in normal man heightens the ventilatory response to hypoxia and hypercapnia.
b. Diaphragmatic mass is reduced in proportion to reduction in body weight in poorly nourished patients.
c. Vital capacity is progressively diminished in semi-starvation.
d. There is an increased level of CO_2 production in patients receiving total parenteral nutrition when glucose is used as the predominant source of nonprotein calories.
e. A fall in secretory IgA occurs in protein-calorie malnutrition.

153. Which statement concerning nutrition is TRUE?

a. Energy expenditure in patients with major burns may be increased up to two and one-half times the basal metabolic rate.
b. Abrupt discontinuation of parenteral solutions containing glucose and insulin may lead to hypoglycemia.
c. With proper care, a parenteral nutrition catheter may remain sterile for weeks to months and does not require routine changing every three to four days as does a pulmonary artery catheter.
d. In the absence of glucose, the brain metabolizes water soluble ketoacids such as acetoacetate, beta-hydroxybutyrate and acetone.
e. All of the above

154. The following parenteral nutrition fluids were given to an ICU patient in a 24-hour period:

2000 cc of a solution containing 25% hydrous dextrose and 4.25% crystalline amino acids, plus 500 cc of 20% lipid emulsion

Approximately how many Kcal did this fluid provide?

a. 3950
b. 3028
c. 2436
d. 1892
e. 1022

155. Which ONE of the following statements concerning metabolism and nutrition in severe hepatic failure is TRUE?

a. Ureagenesis is increased.
b. Metabolism of aromatic amino acids is increased.
c. Increase in the circulating concentration of branched-chain amino acids contributes to the development of encephalopathy.
d. Hypercaloric dextrose infusions which supply more Kcals than needed may potentiate hepatic dysfunction by causing fatty metamorphosis within the liver.

ANSWERS

135-a	136-c	137-a	138-e	139-d	140-b	141-d	142-e
143-d	144-d	145-a	146-d	147-b	148-a	149-e	150-b
151-d	152-a	153-e	154-b	155-d			

ACID BASE

RATIONALE 135-a

Metabolic alkalosis decreases the ventilatory drive and may complicate the weaning of patients from mechanical ventilators. It occurs commonly when potassium, sodium and chloride are depleted, as with excessive gastrointestinal or urinary electrolyte losses. Many patients respond to intravenous therapy with NaCl and KCl. Elimination of excessive bicarbonate may be hastened by oral or intravenous administration of acetazolamide that inhibits carbonic anhydrase, thereby limiting bicarbonate reabsorption in the kidney tubules. Rarely is it necessary to give HCL directly intravenously. Tromethamine (Tris, THAM) is an organic buffer that binds H^+ and some carbon dioxide directly. It alkalinizes urine in poisoning with salicylates or barbiturates or in hemoglobinuria and myoglobinuria. However, such an alkalinizing agent would be MOST inappropriate in metabolic alkalosis.

REFERENCES

Bleich HL, Schwartz WB: Tris Buffer (THAM): An appraisal of its physiologic effects and clinical usefulness. N Engl J Med 1966; 274:782

Makoff DL: Acid-base metabolism. In: Clinical Disorders of Fluid and Electrolyte Metabolism. Second Edition. Maxwell MH, Kleeman CK (Eds). New York, McGraw-Hill Book Company, 1972, pp 330-334

RATIONALE 136-c

The Henderson-Hasselbalch equation relates the ratio of the concentrations of base and acid (in this case bicarbonate and carbonic acid) to the solution pH. For carbonic acid there are two important constants to remember. The carbonic acid concentration in mEq/L is equal to the PCO_2 in mm Hg multiplied by the solubility factor of 0.03. The pH at which the concentrations of base and acid are equal (defined as pKa) is equal to 6.1. Both the carbon dioxide solubility and pKa change slightly with temperature, but for most purposes such changes can be neglected.

$$pH = pKa + \log_{10} \frac{[HCO_3^-]}{[CO_2]}$$

$$pH = 6.1 + \log_{10} \frac{[HCO_3^-]}{0.03 \times 20}$$

$$7.1 = 6.1 + \log_{10} \frac{[HCO_3^-]}{0.6}$$

$$1.0 = \log_{10} \frac{[HCO_3^-]}{0.6} = \log_{10} \frac{6}{0.6} = \log_{10}(10)$$

As a general rule, the bicarbonate concentration is halved when pH is decreased 0.3 units or when PCO_2 is halved with no change in pH. Thus, in this patient the pH has decreased from 7.4 to 7.1, and this would be expected to reduce bicarbonate from a normal value of 28 mEq/L to 14 mEq/L. The further reduction in PCO_2 from a normal 40 mm Hg to 20 mm Hg would be expected to reduce bicarbonate again to half, or from 14 to 7 mEq/L. The calculated concentration of 6 mEq/L is only 14% from the bicarbonate concentration estimated by this rule of thumb.

REFERENCES

Filey GF: Acid-Base and Blood Gas Regulation. Philadelphia, Lea & Febiger, 1971

Wilson RF: Principles and Techniques of Critical Care. Kalamazoo, MI, The Upjohn Co., 1978

RATIONALE 137-a

As in question 136, we may calculate the pH using the rule of thumb. If PCO_2 doubles from 20 to 40 mm Hg and then doubles again to 80 mm Hg, we would expect pH to decrease 0.3 units for each doubling of PCO_2. Thus, the pH would be expected to be about 6.5.

By Henderson-Hasselbalch:

$$pH = pKa + \log_{10} \frac{[HCO_3^-]}{[CO_2]}$$

$$7.1 = 6.1 + \log_{10} \frac{[HCO_3^-]}{0.03 \times 20}$$

$$1.0 = \log_{10} \frac{6}{0.6} = \log_{10}(10)$$

So the initial bicarbonate concentration is 6 mEq/L.

Then:

$$pH = 6.1 + \log_{10} \frac{[HCO_3^-]}{0.03 \times 80} = \log_{10} \frac{6}{2.4}$$

$$pH = 6.1 + \log_{10} (2.5) = 6.1 + 0.398 = 6.5$$

Patients who develop low bicarbonate concentrations but maintain viable blood pH values by hyperventilation need bicarbonate therapy. Such patients are in precarious balance. Momentary underventilation may increase PCO_2 to double or quadruple initial values, lowering pH by 0.3 to 0.6 units and causing fatal electrolyte shifts, cardiac dysrhythmias, etc. Such underventilation is common when patients have endotracheal suctioning, seizures, or are being repositioned especially for lumbar or other special procedure. Although the patient with a PCO_2 of 20 mm Hg is clearly not "underventilating," great care must be used to prevent even momentary elevations of carbon dioxide tensions that may cause permanent sequelae if bicarbonate concentrations and buffering capacity are quite low.

RATIONALE 138-e

Hyperventilation lowers carbon dioxide tensions, thereby reducing the concentrations of carbonic acid and hydrogen ions directly. Bicarbonate concentrations are reduced quickly as bicarbonate is converted to carbonic acid (that is exhaled as carbon dioxide) and over hours as bicarbonate excretion in urine is augmented. The alkalosis resulting from hyperventilation leads to a shift of potassium from extracellular fluids to within cells. Lactate concentrations are increased in hyperventilation, with lactate anions taking the place of lost bicarbonate anions. This lactate presumably arises in the mesenteric circulation and is generated together with pyruvate to maintain a normal lactate/pyruvate ratio and thus a normal oxidation potential in tissues. In shock, blood lactate concentrations greater than 2.7 mEq/L are associated with a mortality of more than 50%, but concentrations more than this (but at normal lactate/pyruvate ratios) may be associated with hyperventilation. As prolonged hyperventilation with progressive bicarbonate loss may cause profound metabolic (lactic) acidosis and death, severe hypocarbia should be prevented or treated properly with controlled ventilation, dead-space ventilation, or inhaled carbon dioxide.

REFERENCES

Cady LK, Weil MH, Afifi AA, et al: A quantitation of severity of critical illness with special reference to blood lactate. Crit Care Med 1973; 1:75

Eichenholz A, Mulhausen RO, Anderson WE, et al: Primary hypocapnia: A cause of metabolic acidosis. J Appl Physiol 1962; 17:283

Huckabee WE: Relationships of pyruvate and lactate during anaerobic metabolism: I. Effects of infusion of pyruvate or glucose and of hyperventilation. J Clin Invest 1958; 37:244

RATIONALE 139-d

Blood gas values are usually measured at 37°C, but the patient may have quite different core temperatures. Remember that warming gas increases its pressure and, if bicarbonate concentrations are not changed, warming blood will lower pH. Thus, in this hypothermic patient, a PCO_2 of 40 mm Hg in the patient will be read by the blood gas electrode at 37°C as 56 mm Hg (an increase of about 4% per °C). If the patient's pH is actually 7.40 at 27°C, the measuring electrode calibrated at 37°C will read it as 7.25 (a change of 0.0154 units/°C).

The hypothermic patient with blood gases measured at 37°C may be thought to have underventilation, respiratory acidosis, and adequate oxygen tensions. Actually, hypoxemia is common due to atelectasis and such patients should receive oxygen. Assisted ventilation, however, must be done very carefully because carbon dioxide production is reduced and overventilation with alkalosis may precipitate ventricular tachyarrhythmias. Thus, correct carefully the blood gas values for patient core temperature when this differs from 37°C.

REFERENCES

Grote J, Thiews G, Wuenscher WD: Nomograms for the interdependence of PO_2, SO_2, PCO_2, CCO_2 and pH in human blood at 28°C and 32°C. Respiration 1972; 29:193

Nunn JF, Bergman NA, Bumatyan A, et al: Temperature coefficients for PCO_2 of blood in vitro. J Appl Physics 1965; 20:23

RATIONALE 140-b 141-d 142-e 143-d 144-d

There are two important clues from usual laboratory tests that help establish the diagnosis of methanol poisoning in this young man. First, examine the concentration of occult anions: Na - Cl - CO_2 = 140 - 90 - 10 = 40 mmol/L. Usually the occult anions in healthy subjects are 8 to 12 mmol/L. There are both endogenous and exogenous causes of metabolic acidosis with excess occult anions.

Endogenous causes include uremia (not present here), lactic acidosis (not present here with normal lactate concentration), diabetic ketoacidosis, alcoholic ketoacidosis, and starvation. In each of these latter cases, the acidosis is associated with increased production of ketones; and you ordinarily expect the nitroprusside reaction (Acetest or Ketostix) for acetoacetate and acetone to be positive. However, the reduction-oxidation (redox) state is also changed in these three conditions, and an excess of $NADH^+$ and a relative deficiency of NAD is reflected in increased ratios of lactate/pyruvate and beta-hydroxybutyrate/acetoacetate. When there is severe reductosis, the increased concentrations of ketone bodies may be predominantly in the form of beta-hydroxybutyrate that is NOT detected by the nitroprusside reaction. During treatment of ketoacidosis, as the reductosis is corrected, the concentration of total ketones may decrease but the concentration of acetone may increase. Acetone is weakly reactive with nitroprusside; thus, an increase in nitroprusside reactivity during treatment may not indicate worsening of ketosis, but merely an appropriate correction of reductosis and concomitant normalization of the balance among the three ketone bodies. Do not conclude that diabetes is impossible in this patient, as hypoglycemic ketoacidosis is well recognized. In starvation, plasma bicarbonate rarely falls below 17 mEq/L. Alcoholic ketoacidosis is a real possibility and cannot be dismissed because of the lack of history of alcohol abuse, as such histories are elicited often only on repeated questioning of patient, friends, and relatives.

Exogenous causes of metabolic acidosis with increased occult anions include ingestions of: salicylates, methanol, ethylene glycol, and paraldehyde. Salicylates stimulate the respiratory center and the hyperventilation leads to loss of bicarbonate that is replaced with lactate. Later, the initial respiratory alkalosis becomes a metabolic acidosis. If the hypocarbia is prevented, by inhalation of carbon dioxide, the subsequent acidosis is abated. A useful screening test for salicylate intoxication is the ferric chloride reaction. Also, Phenistix (used to test for phenylketonuria) will become brownish-purple to gray when moistened with urine or serum containing as little as 200 mg/L of salicylate. The urine may be positive after therapeutic doses, but a positive reaction with serum may indicate salicylism, or poisoning with phenothiazines and other drugs that also change the color of this test strip.

Paraldehyde metabolic acidosis is unexplained, but it can be reproduced in animals given fresh paraldehyde in large doses. Paraldehyde acidosis is accompanied by "false" positive nitroprusside reactions for "ketones." Ethylene glycol is oxidized by alcohol dehydrogenase to glycoaldehyde, and then by aldehyde dehydrogenase to glycolate that causes the acidosis and most of the toxicity.

	ACIDOSIS	KETOSIS
Methanol	+	-
Ethanol	+ (alcoholic ketoacidosis)	+
Ethylene glycol	+	-
Isopropanol	-	+ (acetone)
Paraldehyde	+	+ (pseudoketosis)

The second important clue to the diagnosis here is the osmolality of the patient's blood serum. The osmolality is measured by freezing point depression as 355 mOsm/kg. The osmolality can also be estimated from the measured solute concentrations as: 2 x Na + glucose/18 + urea nitrogen/2.8 = 280 + 5 + 20 = 305 mOsm/kg. Thus, this patient has (355 - 305 =) 50 mOsm/kg of occult osmoles. This may be caused by accumulation of large amounts of small molecules. The alcohol poisons fit this description. They are impotent poisons, requiring high absolute concentrations for toxicity. With their low molecular weights, the alcohols when toxic have appreciable numbers of molecules in body water and, therefore, significant occult osmoles:

	ADULT LETHAL DOSE (ml)	LETHAL BLOOD CONCENTRATION (g/L)	(mmol/L or mOsm/kg)
Methanol	100	1.8	50
Ethanol	400	5.0	100
Ethylene glycol	100	3.0	50
Isopropanol	250	3.0	50
Paraldehyde	50	1.0	10

In this case, there are several clues to suggest methanol rather than ethylene glycol as the culprit. First, urinalysis is normal, and the absence of oxalate crystals and hematuria are important. Second, dilated pupils that are unreactive suggest the toxicity of methanol's metabolite, formate, on the eyes. Third, the stiff neck ("pseudomeningitis") and direct abdominal tenderness are characteristic of methanol intoxification. Usually after ingestion of methanol, in 1-48 hours, there are visual changes (blurred vision, flashes, snowstorm, "skin" over the eyes, or dim vision) with headache, dizziness, nausea, vomiting, epigastric pain, obstipation, and dyspnea. On examination, the patient may have hyperemia of the optic disc, retinal edema, especially about blood vessels, engorged retinal veins, enlarged blind spot, Kussmaul breathing, and diminished visual acuity. It is not so important to distinguish at this stage methanol from ethylene glycol, as both poisonings will be treated the same, but it is essential to suspect one or the other, because supportive therapy is not adequate and immediate specific interventions must be effected.

To understand the treatment, we must examine the pathophysiology of alcohol poisonings. Methanol, ethanol, ethylene glycol, and isopropanol are, themselves, about equally toxic and have similar tastes. Methanol is as colorless as gin, as pleasant in odor and taste as vodka, and until metabolized, as harmless as aquavit. The differences in toxicity are due to metabolites.

```
                           ALCOHOL                        ALDEHYDE
                        DEHYDROGENASE                  DEHYDROGENASE

Methanol -------------------> formaldehyde ------------> formate
Ethanol --------------------> acetaldehyde ------------> acetate
Ethylene glycol ------------> glycoaldehyde -----------> glycolate
Isopropanol ----------------> acetone
Paraldehyde ----------------> acetaldehyde ------------> acetate
```

Some of the acute and chronic effects of ethanol may be due to acetaldehyde, and the "ketosis" of isopropanol ingestion is due to acetone, but these metabolites are far less toxic than those of methanol and ethylene glycol. Virtually all of the acidosis and toxicity of methanol and ethylene glycol are due to formate and glycolate. When oxidation of methanol is inhibited with 4-methyl-pyrazole, methanol accumulates but acidosis and toxicity are prevented. The first metabolite of methanol is formaldehyde, but this ordinarily is oxidized rapidly to formate. The formate combines with tetrahydrofolate (from folic acid) and may become a substrate in variety of "one-carbon" reactions. Folate deficiency in rodents and monkeys slows formate metabolism and enhances toxicity of methanol. In monkeys, all of the acidosis and ocular toxicity of methanol can be reproduced by administration of comparable amounts of formate alone. How does formate cause ocular damage? Formate inhibits cytochrome oxidase (ki = 5-30 mmol/L) and white matter, with low levels of cytochrome oxidase, may be especially susceptible. Inhibition of cytochrome oxidase may impede axo-plasmic transport that normally carries proteins, mitochondria, and neurotubules from their sites of synthesis along the axon segments. Transport system stoppages may cause formation of vesicles. In the eye, a major cause of damage may be intracellular edema of the optic disc fibers and proximal optic nerve, possible related to swelling of astroglia and oligodendroglia.

There are three important aspects to treatment of methanol (or ethylene glycol) poisoning: "A A A."

ALKALINIZE the patient. A fatal dose of methanol of 3 g/kg may generate 6000 mEq of formic acid that will require aggressive treatment with bicarbonate (6 mol = 40 L of isosmolar $NaHCO_3$). Alkalinization may decrease ocular toxicity somewhat. Even though formic acid is highly ionized throughout the body (pKa = 3.75), it will tend to accumulate in more alkaline spaces. Systemic metabolic acidosis causes hyperventilation, lowering blood and brain PCO_2. With a slow diffusion of bicarbonate into brain, the brain may remain alkaline relative to blood, thereby theoretically increasing brain formate accumulation. Correction of the blood metabolic acidosis may promote formate diffusion out of brain.

ACCELERATION of elimination of methanol (and formate) by hemodialysis is essential. Normally about 2% of methanol is exhaled, 10% is excreted in urine, but hemodialysis can increase elimination substantially. Peritoneal dialysis is little more effective than diuresis.

ALCOHOL treatment may inhibit metabolism of methanol (or ethylene glycol) to formaldehyde (or glycoaldehyde). All three substrates are oxidized by alcohol dehydrogenase; in man this enzyme can be saturated at low ethanol concentration in blood. In healthy adults, the maximum rate of ethanol oxidation (Vmax) is about 0.157 ml/kg•h and the alcohol dehydrogenase is half-saturated with ethanol at blood ethanol concentrations of 0.175 ml/L (km). A blood concentration of 1.5 g/L ethanol is associated with intoxication, but not stupor or coma. As ethanol weighs 0.7893 g/ml, this concentration is equal to 1.5/0.7893 = 1.9 ml/L. Ethanol distributes in whole body water (that is about 60% of body weight), so the distribution volume in this 60-kg patient will be about 60 x 0.6 = 36 L. The initial dose of ethanol, therefore, should be 1.9 ml/L x 36 L = 68.4 ml of absolute ethanol. This could be given orally if the patient were alert and cooperative, but in the present case, intravenous therapy is more appropriate.

Maintenance doses of ethanol can be determined from the Michaelis-Menten equation:

$$\text{Drug Metabolism Rate} = \frac{\text{Vmax x concentration}}{\text{Km + concentration}}$$

$$= \frac{0.157 \times 1.9}{0.175 + 1.9} = 0.1 \text{ ml/kg}\bullet\text{h}$$

Thus in this 60-kg patient, one would give an initial dose of 68 ml ethanol and then give (60 x 0.14 =) 8.6 ml every hour to maintain a blood concentration of about 1.5 g/L. It is important to monitor the blood ethanol concentration by a specific assay, such as head-space gas-liquid chromatography, as the alcohol dehydrogenase activity may be altered. Remember that the molecular weight of ethanol is 46.07, so a concentration of 1.5 g/L = 32.6 mmol/L = 33 mOsm/kg.

During dialysis, ethanol as well as methanol may be removed. The easiest way to prevent dialysis from removing ethanol is to add ethanol to the dialysis fluid to a concentration of 1.5 g/L. To a hemodialysis bath of 100 L one can add 190 ml of absolute ethanol, 200 ml of 95% ethanol, a pint (473 ml) of 80-proof whiskey, or 8 "shots" (378 ml) of 100-proof whiskey.

An additional treatment of methanol poisoning may be administration of large doses of folic acid. In monkeys, 50 mg/kg of folate accelerates metabolism of formate to carbon dioxide by 50% when folate concentrations are 2000 times normal. Although there are no reports of efficacy of this treatment in humans, the toxicity of folic acid is minimal.

The burden of methanol in this patient can be calculated from its distribution volume, concentration (in Osm/kg), and molecular weight. For 50 mOsm/kg that are about 50 mmol/L in a distribution volume of 36 L, this = 1.8 moles. Methanol (CH_4O) has a molecular weight of 32.04 (12 + 4 + 16). So 1.8 moles = 1.8 x 32.04 = 57.67 g. The lethal dose of methanol in adults varies from 6 ml to more than 200 ml. In the present subject, the low bicarbonate concentration is a poor prognostic sign and intensive alkalinization, alcohol treatment, and hemodialysis are indicated.

REFERENCES

Baumback GL, Cancilla PA, Martin-Amat G, et al: Methyl alcohol poisoning. IV: Alterations of the morphological findings of the retina and optic nerve. Arch Ophthalmol 1977; 95:1859

Clay KL, Murphy RC: On the metabolic acidosis of ethylene glycol intoxication. Toxicol Appl Pharmacol 1977; 39:39

Cooperman MT, Davidoff F, Spark R, et al: Clinical studies of alcoholic ketoacidosis. Diabetes 1974; 23:433

Eichenholz A, Mulhausen RO, Anderson WE, et al: Primary hypocapnia: A cause of metabolic acidosis. J Appl Physiol 1962; 17:283

Emmet M, Narins RG: Clinical use of the anion gap. Medicine (Baltimore) 1977; 56:38

Hadden JW, Metzner RJ: Pseudoketosis and hyperacetaldehyde in acidosis. Am J Med 1969; 47:642

Hayreh MS, Hayreh SS, Baumback GL, et al: Methyl alcohol poisoning. III: Ocular toxicity. Arch Ophthalmol 1977; 95:1851

Johnson PK, Free HM, Free AH: A simplified urine and serum screening test for salicylate intoxication. J Pediatr 1963; 63:949

Keyvan-Larijarni H, Tannenberg AM: Methanol intoxication. Comparison of peritoneal dialysis and hemodialysis treatment. Intern Med 1974; 134:293

Makar AB, Tephyl TR: Methanol poisoning. VI. Role of folic acid in the production of methanol poisoning in the rat. J Toxicol Environ Health 1977; 2:1201

Martin-Amat G, McMartin KE, Makar AB, et al: The monkey as a model in methanol poisoning. In: Alcohol and Aldehyde Metabolizing Systems. Vol 2. Thurman RG, Williamson IR, Drott H, et al (Eds). New York, Academic Press, 1978

Martin-Amat G, Tephyl TR, McMartin KE, et al: Methyl alcohol poisoning. II. Development of a model for ocular toxicity in methanol poisoning using the rhesus monkey. Arch Ophthalmol 1977; 95:1847

Maxwell MH, Kleeman CR (Eds): Clinical Disorders of Fluid and Electrolyte Metabolism. Third Edition. New York, McGraw-Hill Book Company, 1980, pp 6-10, 205-213, 1348-1349

McMartin KE, Makar AB, Martin G, et al: Methanol poisoning. I. The role of formic acid in the development of metabolic acidosis in the monkey and the reversal by 4-methylpyrazole. Biochem Med 1975; 13:319

McMartin KE, Martin-Amat G, Makar AB, et al: Methanol poisoning. V. Role of formate metabolism in the monkey. J Pharmacol Exptl Ther 1977; 201:564

Sulway MJ, Malins IM: Acetone in diabetic ketoacidosis. Lancet 1970; 2:736

RATIONALE 145-a

Buffer base is defined as the sum of available buffer anions in 1 L of whole blood. This is represented by the sum of bicarbonate ion, hemoglobin anion, protein anion, hemoglobin carbamino anion, and a correction factor that must be applied if hemoglobin is not fully saturated. The latter correction factor relates to alterations in buffering capacity of deoxyhemoglobin compared to oxyhemoglobin.

Under normal conditions indicated in the question, carbamino anion concentration is 0.67 mEq/L. Hemoglobin anion concentration is 16.9 mEq/L (slightly less when partially saturated), and plasma protein anion concentration is 10.4 mEq/L. Total whole blood (plasma + red cell) bicarbonate concentration is 19.4 mEq/L. Hence, hemoglobin and bicarbonate represent major sources of buffering capacity.

The ionization constant for phosphate (HPO_4/H_2PO_4) is pK = 6.8, and the ionization constant for the bicarbonate system (HCO_3^-/H_2CO_3) is pK = 6.1. Thus, near the physiological pH (7.4), the phosphate system is the more efficient buffer. However, phosphate is present in only small concentrations in plasma and red cells, precluding its importance as a major source of buffering capacity. Moreover, the bicarbonate buffer system is altered by pulmonary carbon dioxide exchange, as well as renal bicarbonate excretion, thus providing additional mechanisms to moderate acid-base status.

Buffering capacity is a function of the ionization constant of the buffer, as well as the buffer concentration. In whole blood, red cell membrane permeability also plays a role as the red cell membrane is permeable to HCO_3^- and Cl but not to hemoglobin anion. Based on noncarbonic acid titration, bicarbonate in plasma and red blood cells contributes most to whole blood buffering capacity, followed by hemoglobin and plasma protein. The role of carbamino hemoglobin in the buffer value of blood is slight, although it does account for up to 30% of carbon dioxide transport.

Carbon dioxide transport between venous and arterial blood is equally divided between cells and plasma. Nearly all of the carbon dioxide transport in plasma is in the form of HCO_3^-. In the red cell, nearly two-thirds of the carbon dioxide is carried in the form of carbamino-CO_2 and the remainder as HCO_3^-.

The concept of buffer base and base excess provides a means to incorporate several factors related to acid-base balance into one derived parameter. Thus, nomograms computed by Singer and Hastings and Siggaard-Andersen allow description of acid-base status based upon measured quantitites of pH, PCO_2, bicarbonate, and hemoglobin concentration.

REFERENCES

Roughton FJ: Transport of oxygen and carbon dioxide. In: Handbook of Physiology. Section 3: Respiration. Vol 1. Fenn WD, Rahn M (Eds). Washington, American Physiological Society, 1964, pp 767-825

Ruch TC, Patton HD (Eds): Physiology and Biophysics. Circulation, Respiration and Fluid Balance. Vol 2. Philadelphia, WB Saunders Co., 1974

Siggaard-Andersen O: Titratable acid or base of body fluids. Ann NY Acad Sci 1966; 133:41

Simmons DH: Evaluation of acid-base status. Basics of respiratory disease. Am Thorac Soc 1974; 3:1

Singer RB, Hastings AB: An improved clinical method for the estimation of disturbances in acid-base balance of human blood. Medicine (Baltimore) 1948; 27:223

Thomas LJ: Algorithms for selected blood acid-base and blood gas calculations. Appl Physiol 1972; 33:154

RATIONALE 146-d

The patient has a metabolic acidosis with respiratory compensation. The metabolic acidoses are divided into two groups: those with increased anion gaps and those without. The anion gap $NA^+ - (Cl^- + HCO_3^-)$ is normally 12 mEq/L ± 2 mEq/L. An increased anion gap is caused by ingestion or production of organic or inorganic acids. Etiologies include renal failure, lactic acidosis, ketoacidosis, and ingestion of salicylates, ethylene glycol, methanol or paraldehyde.

The differential diagnosis of a normal anion gap (hyperchloremic) acidosis includes: diarrhea, pancreatic fistula, renal tubular acidosis, hyperparathyroidism, hyperalimentation and dilutional acidosis. This patient has a nonanion gap acidosis and has been receiving large volumes of an isotonic solution (0.9% NaCl). Rapid ECF volume expansion with fluids that do not contain HCO_3^- will lead to a temporary reduction in serum HCO_3^-. The condition is rapidly corrected by the kidneys.

REFERENCES

Narins RG, et al: Diagnostic strategies in disorders of fluid, electrolyte and acid base disorders. Am J Med 1982; 72:496

Narins RG, Goldberg M: Renal tubular acidosis: Pathophysiology, diagnosis and treatment. DM 1977; 23:1

Renal & Electrolyte Disorders. Second Edition. Schrier RW (Ed). Boston, Little, Brown and Co., 1980

RATIONALE 147-b

The patient has a normal alveolar-arterial oxygen gradient (8 mm Hg):

$$P_AO_2 = (P_B - P_{H_2O})\ FIO_2 - \frac{PaCO_2}{.8}$$

$$P_AO_2 = (760-47).21 - 74/.8$$

$$P_AO_2 = 57$$

$$PaO_2 \text{ (given)} = 49$$

$$57 - 49 = 8 \text{ mm Hg}$$

This patient's hypercapnia, acidosis and hypoxemia are all explained by hypoventilation. Aspiration pneumonitis, significant atelectasis and noncardiogenic pulmonary edema are generally associated with an abnormal alveolar-arterial oxygen gradient.

REFERENCE

West JB: Respiratory Physiology, The Essentials. Baltimore, Williams & Wilkins Co., 1979

==

ADRENAL INSUFFICIENCY

==

RATIONALE 148-a

Primary adrenal insufficiency is the most likely diagnosis to explain weight loss, increased pigmentation, hypotension, hyponatremia, hyperkalemia and hypoglycemia. Plasma levels of ACTH are increased and cortisol decreased in this condition. Insulinomas do not produce the above described pigmentary changes and do not usually produce hypotension in the absence of severe hypoglycemia.

Although infusion of glucose is indicated, it is not the most important first step in the treatment of adrenal crisis. Corticosteroids should be given immediately and every 4-6 hours during the first several days following the crisis (hydrocortisone hemisuccinate 100 mg iv as the initial bolus followed by 50 mg every 4-6 hours is usually adequate). Large volumes of saline-containing fluid may be needed to restore adequate circulatory function.

REFERENCES

Axelrod L: Glucocorticoid therapy. Medicine 1976; 55:39

Liddle GW, Melmon KL: The adrenals. In: Textbook of Endocrinology. Fifth Edition. Williams RH (Ed). Philadelphia, WB Saunders Co., 1974, p 233

Speckart PF, Nicoloff JT, Bethune JE: Screening for adrenocortical insufficiency with cosyntropine (synthetic ACTH). Arch Intern Med 1971; 128:761

==

ASTERIXIS

==

RATIONALE 149-e

Asterixis is a nonrhythmic asymmetric lapse in voluntary sustained posture of the extremities, head and trunk. It is usually best demonstrated as a sudden palmar flapping movement of the hands and wrists. This finding is often seen in awake but lethargic patients, but disappears with stupor or coma.

Asterixis is a CNS release phenomena that was first described in hepatic coma. It is a nonspecific finding, however, and may also be seen in uremia, ventilatory failure, drug intoxication, other forms of metabolic brain disease, and with several structural lesions.

REFERENCES

Adams RD, Foley JM: The neurological disorder associated with liver disease. Res Publ Assoc Res Nerv Ment Dis 1953; 32:198

LaMont JT, Koff RS, Isselbacher KJ: Cirrhosis. In: Principles of Internal Medicine. Tenth Edition. Petersdorf RG, et al (Eds). New York, McGraw-Hill Book Company, 1983, pp 1804-1816

Leavitt S, Tyler HR: Studies in asterixis. Arch Neurol 1964; 10:360

Plum F, Posner JB: The Diagnosis of Stupor and Coma. Contemporary Neurology. Vol 3. Philadelphia, FA Davis Co., 1980

Shahani BT, Young RR: Asterixis - A disorder of the neural mechanisms underlying sustained muscular contraction. In: The Motor System. Neurophysiology and Muscle Mechanisms. Shahani M (Ed). New York, Elsevier, North Holland, 1976, pp 301-306

DIABETIC KETOACIDOSIS

RATIONALE 150-b

Major pathways of fatty acid metabolism in the liver include oxidation to carbon dioxide and ketogenesis. With increased mobilization of fatty acids from adipose tissues in diabetes mellitus, the oxidative capacity of hepatic and extrahepatic tissue is overwhelmed and ketogenesis occurs. Ketones being strong acids, are buffered by bicarbonate causing an elevation in the calculated anion gap ($Na^+ + K^+ - Cl^- - HCO_3^-$).

The equilibrium between the two major forms of ketones, acetoacetate (AA), and beta-hydroxybutyric acid (BHB), is determined by the ratio of reduced and oxidized nicotinamide adenine dinucleotide. In patients with diabetic ketoacidosis with shock, hypotension and hypoxia, the level of reduced nicotinamide adenine dinucleotide ($NADH_2$) is increased and the reaction is driven to BHB reducing the previously elevated values of AA to low levels and yielding a weekly reactive "ketone test" by the nitroprusside method (Ketostix Acetest). The ratio of AA to BHB is, thus, reduced. However, in this setting severe depression of serum bicarbonate remains and is associated with a wide anion gap indicative of continuing life-threatening ketoacidosis.

As in other forms of shock, lactic acid levels are also elevated in response to hypoxia and hypotension. Whether there is a specific defect in lactate metabolism in diabetes is still debated. Well-controlled diabetics have normal lactate levels at rest and have a normal tolerance to a lactate load. In diabetic ketoacidosis there is a decrease in lactate tolerance and an increase in the lactate/pyruvate ratio. Whether this is related to metabolic factors or to the development of hypoperfusion is still in question.

REFERENCES

Cohen RD, Woods HF: Clinical and Biochemical Aspects of Lactic Acidosis. Oxford, Blackwell Scientific Publications, 1976

Emmett M, Narins RG: Clinical use of the anion gap. Medicine (Baltimore) 1977; 56:38

Foster DW, McGarry JD: The metabolic derangements and treatment of diabetic ketoacidosis. N Engl J Med 1983; 309:159

Kreisberg RA: Diabetic ketoacidosis: New concepts and trends in pathogenesis and treatment. Ann Intern Med 1978; 88:681

Oliva PB: Lactic acidosis. Am J Med 1970; 48:209

Smithline N, Gardner KD Jr: Gaps--anionic and osmolal. JAMA 1976; 236:1594

LACTATE

RATIONALE 151-d

All tissues have the ability to produce lactic acid. Blood lactic acid concentration reflects the quantity of lactic acid produced and the quantity metabolized, primarily by the liver and kidney. Tissue hypoxia due to circulatory, respiratory, and cellular dysfunction results in lactic acid overproduction while impaired hepatic perfusion results in under utilization. Most instances of lactic acidosis occur as a result of a combination of both processes. The most common cause of lactic acidosis is hypoperfusion due to cardiogenic shock, hypotension, hypothermia, or sepsis. Lactic acidosis occurs early in the shock syndrome, often preceding a fall in blood pressure or urine output and other signs of impaired perfusion. Prospective studies suggest that serum lactate levels of 4 mmol/L or greater are usually associated with a fatal outcome.

Lactic acid, the end product of anaerobic glucose metabolism, is formed by the reduction of pyruvic acid with reduced nicotinamide adenine dinucleotide ($NADH_2$) which forms lactic acid and nicotinamide adenine dinucleotide (NAD). The postulate that the lactate/pyruvate ratio measures the $NADH_2$/NAD ratio may not be entirely valid as additional pools of $NADH_2$/NAD exist within the cell.

Huckabee infused sodium lactate solution into human subjects and recorded a mild rise in pyruvate as well as lactate concentration during the period of infusion. This was associated with a normal ratio of lactate/pyruvate. The increase in pyruvate may be related to the alkalinizing effect of sodium lactate since similar elevations in lactate and pyruvate were recorded with bicarbonate infusion.

Ringer's lactate solution is frequently utilized for replacement of extracellular fluid. As prepared commercially, Ringer's lactate is composed of 28 mEq/L lactate (with nearly equal D and L forms). Because it is unbuffered, minimal neutralization is required to return the pH to 7.4 after intravenous infusion. Sodium lactate in Ringer's solution is not an acid and does not lower pH. Rather it has an alkalinizing effect after its metabolism.

Passive and voluntary hyperventilation in man and animals have consistently produced elevations in serum lactate levels ranging from 2-10 mmol/L. Breathing 5% carbon dioxide during hyperventilation abolishes this effect and reverses it if it has occurred. The elevated blood lactate levels have been attributed to intracellular hypocapnea and inhibition of pyruvate carboxylase, intracellular alkalosis, enhanced red cell glycolysis, and to a decreased hepatic uptake of lactate due to reduced hepatic perfusion.

Along with renal excretion of bicarbonate, lactate accumulation serves as a compensatory mechanism during the development of respiratory alkalosis.

Lactate production during ethanol ingestion occurs as a result of the effects of intermediate cellular metabolism. Alcohol is converted to acetaldehyde and acetic acid by alcohol dehydrogenase and nicotinamide adenine dinucleotide within the cytoplasm. The reduced nicotinamide adenine dinucleotide which is produced by this reaction is oxidized by the pyruvate lactate system resulting in an increase in lactate and a decrease in pyruvate concentrations. Ordinarily, the elevation in lactate levels are minor and the acidosis is not severe.

REFERENCES

Canizaro PC, Prager MD, Shires GT: The infusion of Ringer's lactate solution during shock changes in lactate, excess lactate and pH. Am J Surg 1971; 122:494

Emmett M, Narins RG: Clinical use of the anion gap. Medicine (Baltimore) 1977; 56:38

Gabow PA, Kaehny WD, Fennessey PV, et al: Diagnostic importance of an increased serum anion gap. N Engl J Med 1980; 303:854

Huckabee WE: Relationships of pyruvate and lactate during anaerobic metabolism. I: Effects of infusion of pyruvate or glucose and of hyperventilation. J Clin Invest 1958; 37:244

Kreisberg RA: Lactate homeostasis and lactic acidosis. Ann Intern Med 1980; 92:227

Kreisberg RA: Pathogenesis and management of lactic acidosis. Annu Rev Med 1984; 35:181

Oliva PB: Lactic acidosis. Am J Med 1970; 48:209

Olson RE: "Excess lactate" and anaerobiosis. Ann Intern Med 1963; 59:960

Weil MH, Afifi AA: Experimental and clinical studies on lactate and pyruvate as indicators of the severity of acute circulatory failure (shock). Circulation 1970; 41:989

NUTRITION

RATIONALE 152-a

The nutritional management of the critically ill patient is a topic of intense controversy. The optimum nutritional therapy for a patient with respiratory failure is unknown. Numerous studies, however, suggest that starvation and refeeding impact the respiratory system at many levels.

It has been shown that the normal ventilatory response to hypoxia and hypercapnia is diminished in humans semistarved for ten days. This response returns toward normal following refeeding. Fatigue of the muscles of respiration is thought to be an important contributor to respiratory discoordination and respiratory failure. Diaphragmatic mass has been shown to diminish in proportion to reduction of body weight in malnutrition. Vital capacity, likewise, diminishes in a progressive fashion in undernourished patients. The suggestion that surfactant production may be abnormal in starvation is supported by numerous animal studies. Pulmonary infection is often a complication of starvation. One possible contributor to this increased infection rate is a decreased level of secretory IgA in undernourished patients. Because of the high RQ (respiratory quotient) associated with carbohydrate feedings, CO_2 production is increased. In patients with ventilatory deficiency this increased CO_2 production may make weaning from ventilatory support more difficult. At this time the optimum carbohydrate/fat ratio has not been defined. It has been suggested, however, that under these circumstances fat make up 40%-50% of total nonprotein calories.

REFERENCES

Arora NS, Rochester DF: Effect of general nutritional and muscular states on the human diaphragm. Am Rev Respir Dis 1977; 115:84

Askanazi J, Weissman C, et al: Nutrition and the respiratory system. Crit Care Med 1982; 10:163

Doekel RC Jr, Zwillich CW, Scoggin CH, et al: Clinical semi-starvation. Depression of hypoxic ventilatory response. N Engl J Med 1976; 95:358

Keys A, Brozek J, Henschel A, et al: Biology of Human Starvation. Minneapolis, University of Minnesota Press, 1950

Macklem PT: Respiratory muscles: The vital pump. Chest 1980; 78:753

RATIONALE 153-e

Patients with extensive burns have energy requirements that may be increased up to two and one-half times the basal rate. Survival may be dependent upon meeting these requirements.

Increased oxygen consumption in critically ill patients reflects the metabolic demands of fever, increased glucose turnover, and increased serum levels of catecholamines, glucagon, and glucocorticoids. Catabolism continues unless appropriate calories are provided. Without proper care, TPN catheters may become a source of positive blood cultures, unexplained fever spikes, and phlebitis. With proper care, they may be left in place for weeks to months. Abruptly stopping glucose-insulin infusions can cause hypoglycemia, especially with high insulin dosages, as the effect of the insulin lasts longer than that of the glucose. Although most tissues are able to catabolize fat for energy, the brain consumes glucose or ketone bodies only. Free fatty acids do not cross the blood-brain barrier. The brain does metabolize water soluble ketoacids as a glucose alternative.

REFERENCES

Fisher JE: Nutritional support in the seriously ill patient. Curr Probl Surg 1980; 27:466

Mann S, Wentenskow DR, Houtchens BA: Measured and predicted caloric expenditures in the acutely ill. Crit Care Med 1985; 13:173

Parsa MH, Shoemaker WC: Nutritional failure. In: Textbook of Critical Care. Shoemaker WC, Thompson WL, Holbrook PR (Eds). Philadelphia, WB Saunders Co., 1984, pp 664-693

Saffel JR, Medina E, et al: Use of indirect calorimetry in nutritional management of burned patients. J Trauma 1985; 25:32

Sanders BA, Sheldon RF: Septic complications of total parenteral nutrition. Am J Surg 1976; 132:214

Turner WW, Ireton PS, Hunt JL, et al: Predicting energy expenditure in burned patients. J Trauma 1985; 25:11

RATIONALE 154-b

2000 cc of 25% hydrous dextrose contains 500 gm of hydrous dextrose

Hydrous dextrose = 3.4 Kcal/gm

500 gm x 3.4 Kcal/gm		1700 Kcal
2000 cc of 4.25% crystalline amino acids contain approximately 82 gm of protein equivalent		
Protein = 4 Kcal/gm		
82 gm x 4 Kcal/gm		328 Kcal
20% lipid emulsion contains approximately 2.0 Kcal/cc		
500 cc x 2 Kcal/cc		1000 Kcal
	TOTAL	3028 Kcal

REFERENCE

Grant JP: Handbook of Total Parenteral Nutrition. Philadelphia, WB Saunders Co., 1980

EDITORIAL COMMENT

The avoidance of underfeeding the critically ill patient has been appropriately emphasized. Overfeeding the patient is also detrimental and may be associated with excessive carbon dioxide production, hyperglycemia, hyperosmolarity, cholestasis, steatosis and volume overload. Traditional methods of predicting metabolic requirements (Harris-Benedict basal energy expenditure) often significantly overestimate the caloric needs of acutely ill patients. To avoid this problem it has been suggested by Mann and others that caloric needs should be measured by indirect calorimetry rather than estimated.

ADDITIONAL REFERENCES

Askanazi J, Rosenbaum S, Hyman AI, et al: Respiratory changes induced by the large glucose loads of total parenteral nutrition. JAMA 1980; 243:1444

Herve P, Simonneau G, Girard P, et al: Total parenteral nutrition induces hypercapnia in mechanically ventilated patients with chronic respiratory insufficiency. Am Rev Respir Dis 1983; 127:255

Laaban JP, Lemaire F, Baron JF: Influence of caloric intake on the respiratory mode during mandatory minute volume ventilation. Chest 1985; 87:67

Mann S, Westenskow DR, Houtchens BA: Measured and predicted caloric expenditure in the acutely ill. Crit Care Med 1985; 13:173

Sheldon GF, Peterson SR, Sanders R: Hepatic dysfunction during hyperalimentation. Arch Surg 1978; 113:504

RATIONALE 155-d

Increasing exogenous protein supply may precipitate encephalopathy in patients with severe liver disease. Ureagenesis, gluconeogenesis and other metabolic activities are curtailed. The liver's inability to metabolize aromatic amino acids and ammonia have been suggested as possible causes of hepatic encephalopathy. Branched-chain amino acids may provide protection from developing this complication. Carbohydrate calories administered in excess of need may result in fatty infiltration of the liver.

REFERENCES

Cerra FB: Metabolic monitoring: The key to the microcirculation and cellular metabolism. In: Critical Care: State of the Art. Vol 3. Shoemaker WC, Thompson WL (Eds). Fullerton, CA, Society of Critical Care Medicine, 1982, pp III(L):1-21

Fischer JE, Rosen HM, Ebeid AM, et al: The effect of normalization of plasma amino acids on hepatic encephalopathy in man. Surgery 1976; 80:77

Freund H, et al: Infusion of branched-chain enriched amino acid solution in patients with hepatic encephalopathy. Am J Surg 1982; 196:209

Jeejeehboy KN: Nutrition in critical illness. In: Critical Care: State of the Art. Vol 5. Shoemaker WC, Thompson WL (Eds). Fullerton, CA, Society of Critical Care Medicine, 1984, pp V(B):1-74

Section 10

156. In a patient with one isoelectric electroencephalogram, which of the following is LEAST likely to be associated with recovery of normal neurologic function?

a. Recent (> 10 minutes) cardiopulmonary resuscitation
b. Hypothermia
c. Hyperosmolality
d. Glutethimide overdose
e. Hypocapnia

157. Which ONE of the following conditions is LEAST likely to cause reversible electrical silence on EEG?

a. Phenobarbital overdose
b. Induced hypothermia
c. Hypoglycemia
d. Fresh water immersion
e. Brain stem herniation

158. Following a hypotensive hypoxic insult a patient fulfills criteria for certification of brain death. Which ONE of the following is NOT found in such a patient?

a. Absent eye movements to ice water caloric testing
b. Absence of intracranial blood flow on arteriography
c. Isoelectric EEG recorded at full gain
d. Tachycardia induced by 1 mg atropine intravenously

159. Increased intracranial pressure is decreased LEAST often by:

a. Glycerol
B. Furosemide
c. Mannitol
d. Nitroprusside sodium
e. Halothane

160. Cerebral blood flow is LEAST likely to be increased by:

a. Norepinephrine
b. Halothane
c. Thiopental
d. Mannitol
e. Hypercapnia

161. Which ONE of the following statements concerning the cerebral circulation is FALSE?

a. Cerebral perfusion pressure equals mean arterial pressure minus intracranial pressure.
b. Neuronal ischemic damage may occur in spite of an adequate cerebral perfusion pressure and a normal amount of cerebral blood flow.
c. Normally cerebral blood flow does not change as the mean arterial pressure rises from 70 to 120 mm Hg.
d. Sodium nitroprusside, nitroglycerin and trimethaphan are direct cerebral vasodilators and may elevate intracranial pressure.
e. A $PaCO_2$ below 40 mm Hg causes a progressive decrease in cerebral blood flow.

162. A young man is found on the street in deep coma, breathing slowly, and is admitted to your service. You find his left eye to have an old injury and the right pupil to be 6 mm in diameter and unreactive.

Which ONE of the following is LEAST likely to be the SOLE cause of this finding?

a. Glutethimide Poisoning
b. Scopolamine poisoning
c. Right-sided subdural hematoma
d. Left-sided subdural hematoma
e. Damage to the right sixth cranial nerve

163. You are treating a 40-year-old man found comatose in bed. His eyes do not move after irrigating each ear with 200 ml of ice water. When observing the edge of his iris with your ophthalmoscope, you observe the iris to constrict when you shine a very bright light directly into either eye.

Which ONE of the following conditions is the MOST likely cause of this finding?

a. Postanoxic brain damage
b. CNS syphilis
c. Sedative drug overdose
d. Subdural hematoma

164. Which ONE of the following disorders is LEAST likely to produce coma?

a. Anoxic damage to both cerebral hemispheres
b. Basilar artery thrombosis
c. Infarct of the lateral medulla
d. Pontine hemorrhage
e. Vitamin B_1 deficiency

165. The Glasgow Coma Scale is frequently used to standardize clinical assessments of comatose patients and to monitor these patients over time. This scale involves an assessment of each of the following EXCEPT:

a. Eye opening
b. Vestibular response
c. Best motor response
d. Best verbal response
e. Withdrawal from pain

166. Which ONE of the following statements concerning herpes simplex encephalitis is TRUE?

a. Brain biopsy is of no diagnostic value.
b. Therapy with acylovir decreases morbidity and mortality.
c. Diffuse cerebral involvement is commonly seen on brain scan or head CT scan.
d. Coma is associated with a poor prognosis.

167. Which ONE of the following is LEAST often found in a patient with classical Guillain-Barre' syndrome?

a. Lower extremities weaker than upper extremities
b. Paresthesias of toes
c. Postural hypotension
d. Spinal fluid contains many lymphocytes with normal globulin concentration.
e. Weakness progresses symmetrically up both lower extremities.

168. Which ONE of the following is NOT a primary concern in the ICU management of Guillain-Barre' syndrome?

a. Pulmonary embolism
b. Seizures
c. Nutrition
d. Pulmonary infections

169. Which ONE of the following statments concerning intracranial hemorrhage is FALSE?

a. The incidence of the progressive ischemic syndrome from cerebral vasospasm following subarachnoid hemorrhage is related to the quantity of blood found in the basal cisterns.
b. The most common cause of spontaneous intracranial hemorrhage is rupture of an intracranial aneurysm.
c. Rebleeding after subarachnoid hemorrhage occurs most frequently in the first 14 days and is a major source of morbidity and mortality.
d. The most common site of intracranial hemorrhage in hypertensive patients is the putamen.

170. Intracranial pressure is most likely to be reduced by:

a. Decreased arterial blood pH
c. Increased arterial blood norepinephrine concentration
c. Increased cardiac output
d. Decreased arterial blood carbonic acid concentration
e. Increased arterial blood lactic acid concentration

171. Which ONE of the following statements about the Wernicke-Korsakoff syndrome is FALSE?

a. Confabulation is a prominent feature of Korsakoff's psychosis.
b. Gaze palsies, nystagmus and ataxia are prominent features of Wernicke's encephalopathy.
c. The pathologic changes found in the brains of patients dying in the acute stages of Wernicke's encephalopathy are very similar to those of patients dying with chronic Korsakoff's psychosis.
d. Intravenous glucose should be administered prior to thiamine in alcoholic patients presenting with altered mental status.

172. You are monitoring intracranial pressure in a young patient resuscitated after prolonged immersion in a freshwater swimming pool. During the first hour of admission you observe the intracranial pressure to rise.

Which ONE of the following treatments is LEAST likely to minimize or reverse the rise of intracranial pressure?

a. Controlled ventilation lowering arterial carbon dioxide tension from 50 to 32 torr
b. Drainage of 50 ml of cerebrospinal fluid
c. Intravenous pentobarbital infusion in large doses
d. Diuresis lowering right atrial pressure from 15 to 5 mm Hg
e. Norepinephrine titrated to increase mean arterial pressure from 90 to 110 mm Hg

173. Which ONE of the following treatments is LEAST likely to decrease intracranial pressure in a patient with a glioma?

a. Glycerol orally
b. Mannitol intravenously
c. Furosemide intravenously
d. Methylprednisolone sodium succinate intravenously
e. Positive end-expiratory pressure

174. Which ONE of the following statements regarding a brain injured patient with a focal expanding mass lesion and midline shift on head CT scan is FALSE?

a. The ICP may be normal.
b. The amount of CSF within the cranium is decreased.
c. Iatrogenic hyperventilation is an aid in preventing secondary damage.
d. All fever should be treated with antipyretics.
e. Volatile inhalational anesthetics are preferable to intravenous narcotic anesthetics.

NEUROLOGIC

175. A 30-year-old, 70 kg accident victim arrives in the Emergency Department and on examination does not open his eyes to pain or respond verbally but does localize pain bilaterally. His pupils are unequal is size. He has a normal oculocephalic response. The patient maintains a clear airway and has a respiratory rate of 20/min. A head CT scan is ordered.

Which ONE of the following statements is CORRECT?

a. The patient should be intubated and hypoventilated.
b. Mannitol 200 gm should be administered prior to scanning.
c. Following removal of an intracranial hematoma, a sudden rise in ICP above 30 mm Hg (in the absence of neurologic deterioration) may indicate a need for reoperation.
d. The patient's initial Glasgow Coma Score (15 point scale) is 5.

176. Which of the following statements regarding controlled hyperventilation in patients with intracranial hypertension is TRUE?

a. The cerebral vasoconstrictive effects of hyperventilation usually diminish after 48 to 72 hours.
b. Improved survival has been clearly demonstrated in patients who have suffered hypoxic brain damage following cardiopulmonary resuscitation when controlled hyperventilation is used.
c. When hyperventilation is discontinued, the $PaCO_2$ may be rapidly returned to normal.
d. None of the above

177. Which of the following statements regarding controlled hyperventilation in patients with intracranial hypertension is FALSE?

a. Controlled hyperventilation decreases the incidence of cerebral vasospasm following subarachnoid hemorrhage.
b. When controlled hyperventilation is used, the $PaCO_2$ is usually lowered to 10-15 mm Hg.
c. Morbidity and mortality are sharply decreased following head trauma if controlled hyperventilation is utilized.
d. All of the above

178. Glucocorticoid therapy is MOST effective in treating cerebral edema associated with which ONE of the following?

a. Vasogenic edema associated with brain tumor
b. Edema from acute cerebral infarction
c. Edema from cerebral trauma
d. Hypo-osmolality edema
e. Hypoxic edema

179. The most logical reason for treating children with acute bacterial meningitis with ampicillin AND chloramphenicol is:

a. Hemophilus influenzae - Type B is a common causative organism and some strains are resistant to ampicillin.
b. Ampicillin and chloramphenicol have synergistic action against Neisseria meningitidis when tested in vitro.
c. Chloramphenicol toxicity is reduced by ampicillin.
d. Ampicillin penetration into bacteria is enhanced by chloramphenicol.
e. Streptococcus pneumoniae is not sensitive to the small amounts of ampicillin reaching the cerebrospinal fluid in meninigitis.

180. You are treating a patient with myasthenia gravis with pyridostigmine (Mestinon). She is getting weaker. Which ONE of the following is MOST likely to be present in a cholinergic crisis caused by excessive doses of pyridostigmine?

a. Decreased bowel sounds
b. Decreased sweating and dry skin
c. Increased heart rate
d. Urinary retention
e. Increased salivation

Questions 181-183 refer to the following case history: A 55-year-old, 60 kg female with myasthenia gravis had been well managed with pyridostigmine. One month prior to admission, she developed increasing muscle weakness and fatigue. The dose of pyridostigmine was increased and she was started on prednisone. One week later, she presented with fever, cough and worsening fatigue. She was admitted to the hospital and started on penicillin and gentamicin for a suspected aspiration pneumonia.

Arterial Blood Gases:	pH 7.45	PaO_2 70 mm Hg
	FIO_2 .21	PCO_2 35 mm Hg

Maximum Negative Inspiratory Pressure:	-18 cm H_2O
Forced Vital Capacity:	500 cc
Chest Radiograph:	Normal

181. Which ONE of the following statements describes the BEST management for this patient?

a. Intubation and mechanical ventilation
b. Increase the dose of pyridostigmine.
c. Discontinue the pyridostigmine and observe the patient in the ICU.
d. Perform a tensilon (edrophonium hydrochloride) test.
e. Perform a thymectomy.

182. All of the following can precipitate respiratory failure in patients with myasthenia gravis EXCEPT:

a. Aminoglycoside antibiotics
b. Postoperative myasthenic crisis
c. The initiation of corticosteriod therapy
d. Intercurrent infection
e. "Anticholinergic crisis"

183. Which ONE of the following is the BEST predictor of impending respiratory failure in the patient with myasthenia gravis?

a. Arterial blood gases
b. Chest radiograph
c. A negative tensilon test
d. Maximal inspiratory pressure

184. Which ONE of the following drugs is capable of altering pupillary eye signs?

a. Atropine
b. Morphine
c. Trimethaphan
d. Dopamine
e. All of the above

185. A 4-year-old boy presents to the emergency department with minimal response to painful stimuli. His mother relates a history of nausea and vomiting over the preceding day. Vital signs: pulse 100, respiratory rate 18, BP 110/60, temperature 37°C (98.6°F).

Admission laboratory work includes:

Hematocrit	-	40
WBC	-	14,000
Na^+	-	145 mEq/L
HCO_3^-	-	26 mEq/L
BUN	-	20 mEq/L
Glucose	-	50 mEq/L

Which ONE of the following statements about the disease process and its treatment is TRUE?

a. Hepatitis B surface antigen is frequently positive.
b. Serum transaminase and serum bilirubin levels are markedly elevated.
c. Accepted therapy for this patient includes controlled mechanical ventilation with paralysis, intracranial pressure monitoring and barbiturates titrated to control intracranial pressure.
d. Serum ammonia levels above 100 mcg/100 ml are associated with poor prognosis.

186. Which ONE if the following statements regarding the treatment of status epilepticus is INCORRECT?

a. Recurrent seizures are a potential problem with diazepam (Valium) treatment alone due to its short half-life.
b. Phenytoin is effective in controlling most seizures but is slower in action than diazepam.
c. Combining a barbiturate and diazepam in the treatment of seizure disorders has a significant risk of respiratory depression.
d. Phenytoin should only be given in dextrose containing solutions.

ANSWERS

156-e	157-e	158-d	159-e	160-c	161-d	162-e	163-c
164-c	165-b	166-d	167-d	168-b	169-b	170-d	171-d
172-e	173-e	174-e	175-c	176-a	177-d	178-a	179-a
180-e	181-a	182-e	183-d	184-e	185-c	186-d	

BRAIN DEATH

RATIONALE 156-e

The EEG may be isoelectric for at least 10 minutes after cardiopulmonary resuscitation and yet the patient may recover fully. Most brain-death criteria require at least 30 minutes between two isoelectric EEGs. Hypothermia, hyperosmolality and glutethimide may cause isoelectric EEGs in patients who subsequently recover normal brain function. Hypocapnea alone, however, does not make the EEG isoelectric and is not a component in most brain-death criteria.

After cardiopulmonary resuscitation some patients are hyperventilated ($PaCO_2 \cong$ 30 mm Hg) to minimize intracranial pressure. Such mild hyperventilation does not interfere with use of the electroencephalogram to evaluate brain function.

REFERENCES

Diagnosis of brain death. Conference of Royal Colleges and Faculties of the United Kingdom. Lancet 1976; 2:1069

Myers RR, Stockard JJ: Neurologic and electrocephalographic correlates in glutethimide intoxication. Clin Pharmacol Ther 1975; 17:212

Powner DJ, Snyder JV, Grenvik A: Brain death certification: A review. Crit Care Med 1977; 5:230

RATIONALE 157-e

High dose barbiturate therapy is often administered to patients with Reye syndrome, and induced hypothermia is frequently utilized in pediatric cardiac surgery. The lack of long-term neurological side effects of these therapeutic maneuvers is well documented. Likwise, barbiturate overdose does not necessarily produce lasting neurological dysfunction if maximal medical supportive therapy is employed. Bird and Plum reported a patient who remained in deep coma with an isoelectric EEG for 5 days after a barbiturate overdose, who was subsequently able to return to work. Induced hypothermia causes a rapid fall in CNS oxygen consumption, and is commonly thought to be protective during a simultaneous CNS anoxic-ischemic event. In primates, electrical silence on the EEG is achieved between 18 to 20°C, and monkeys have been reported to tolerate up to 2 hours of cardiac stand-still at 2°C. Recovery from drowning or near-drowning is frequently reported in children who have sustained an icy freshwater near-drowning. Kvittigen and Naess reported a 5-year-old child who survived immersion for 22 minutes in icy fresh water, and subsequent cardiopulmonary resuscitation for 2 hours, whose pupils remained fixed and dilated for 48 hours, yet who later achieved relatively normal neurological function. The suspected key to this and similar intervals is the induced hypothermia in such freshwater immersions.

Hypoglycemia in a relatively controlled situation has not been documented to produce complete electrical silence. Himwich and Hoegland studied serial EEGs in schizophrenic patients undergoing induced insulin shock and documented loss of alpha waves. Markedly abnormal delta rhythms and diffuse high-voltage slow waves were documented at blood sugars ranging from 0-22 mg/dl. The EEG change lagged behind the blood sugar change by approximately 30 to 45 minutes. In contrast, herniation of the brain stem with acute compression of the aqueduct of Sylvius is a terminal event from which the change of neurological resuscitation is remote.

REFERENCES

A definition of irreversible coma: Report of the Ad Hoc Committee of the Harvard Medical School to examine the definition of brain death. JAMA 1968; 205:337

Bird TD, Plum F: Recovery from barbiturate overdose coma with prolonged isoelectric electroencephalogram. Neurology 1968; 18:456

Himwich HE, Frostig JP, Fazekas JF, et al: Clinical, electroencephalographic, and biochemical changes during insulin hypoglycemia. Proc Soc Exptl Biol Med 1939; 40:401

Hoegland H, Rubin MH, Cameron DE: The electroencephalogram of schizophrenics during insulin hypogylcemia and recovery. Am J Physiol 1937; 120:559

Kvittingen TD, Naess A: Recovery from drowning in freshwater. Br Med J 1963; 1:1315

Lougheed WM: The central nervous system in hypothermia. Br Med Bull 1961; 17:61

RATIONALE 158-d

Brain death identifies a permanent loss of all integrated neuronal brain function. It is important to realize that "brain death" indicates death of the cerebrum, cerebellum and the entire brain stem. Specific criteria for determining brain death have originated from many different groups. In general, a patient fulfilling the criteria for brain death has no spontaneous muscular movement, no decorticate or decerebrate posturing, no cranial nerve reflexes, no evidence of blood flow above the foramen magnum and an isoelectric EEG. Atropine has no effect on heart rate in this setting. Spinal cord reflexes may be present in the brain dead patient. The President's Commission for the Study of Ethical Problems in Medicine recommends that a single EEG may be obtained but it is not required.

REFERENCES

Bernat JL, Culver CM, et al: On the definition and criterion of death. Ann Intern Med 1981; 94:389

Goodman JM, Miskin FS, Pyken M: Determination of brain death by isotope angiography. JAMA 1969; 209:1869

Grenvik AR, Powner DJ, Snyder JV, et al: Cessation of therapy in terminal illness and brain death. Crit Care Med 1978; 6:284

Jastremski MJ, Powner DJ, et al: Problems in brain death determination. Forensic Science 1978; 11:201

Posner JB: Coma and other states of consciousness: The differential diagnosis of brain death. Ann NY Acad Sciences 1978; 315:1

President's Commission for the Study of Ethical Problems in Medicine and Bio-medical and Behavioral Research: Deciding to forego life sustaining treatment. Washington, DC, US Government Printing Office, 1983, p 554

Walker AE: Cerebral Death. Second Edition. Urban and Schwarzemberg, 1981

CEREBRAL BLOOD FLOW

RATIONALE 159-e

Glycerol and mannitol establish an osmotic gradient between blood and brain promoting osmotic flow of water out of the brain and reducing intracranial pressure. Furosemide inhibits chloride reabsorption in the ascending limb of the loop of Henle in the kidney, promoting loss of salt and water from the body and thereby reducing increased intracranial pressue. Nitroprusside sodium may lower intracranial pressure if systemic venous and arterial pressures are reduced by its direct vasodilating action on systemic vascular smooth muscle. In some animal models, however, nitroprusside causes a transient initial increase in cerebral blood flow and intracranial pressure. Halothane, however, causes cerebral vasodilatation and increased intracranial pressure in animals and patients.

Many critically-ill patients have increased intracranial pressures. Treatments should be chosen carefully to avoid further elevations of pressure.

REFERENCES

Christensen MS, Hoedt-Rasmussen K, Lassen NA: Cerebral vasodilation by halothane anesthesia in man and its potentiation by hypotentsion and hypercapnia. Br J Anaesth 1967; 39:927

Fishman RA: Brain edema. N Engl J Med 1975; 293:706

Tabaddor K, Tavares A, Marmarou A, et al: Intracranial pressure and cerebral compliance during hypotension induced by sodium nitroprusside. Acta Neurol Scand [Suppl] 1977; 56:310

RATIONALE 160-c

Thiopental in anesthetic doses has been observed to reduce cerebral blood flow as much as 48% in contrast to halothane which is a cerebral vasodilator. Hypercania is a potent stimulus to cerebral vasodilatation and mannitol, by increasing intravascular volume, would tend to increase cerebral blood flow. Norepinephrine has little direct effect on cerebral vascular resistance, but by increasing mean aortic pressure tends to increase cerebral blood flow.

REFERENCES

Betz E: Cerebral blood flow: Its measurement and regulation. Physiol Rev 1972; 52:595

Christensen MS, Hoedt-Rasmussen K, Lassen NA: Cerebral vasodilatation by halothane anesthesia in man and its potentiation by hypotension and hypercapnia. Br J Anaesth 1967; 39:927

Marshall LF, Shapiro HM, Rauscher A, et al: Pentobarbital therapy for intracranial hypertension in metabolic coma. Crit Care Med 1978; 6:1

Pierce EC Jr, Lambertsen CJ, Deutsch S, et al: Cerebral circulation and m etabolism during thiopental anesthesia and hyperventilation in man. J Clin Invest 1962; 41:1664

RATIONALE 161-d

Cerebral perfusion pressure (CPP) equals the mean arterial pressure (MAP) minus the intracranial pressure (ICP). Cerebral blood flow (CBF) is determined by the CPP and the cerebral vascular resistance (CVR). Autoregulation is that property of the cerebral vasculature which maintains a constant CBF as CPP changes. Normally, CBF is constant between a MAP of 60 to 150 torr. Below 60 torr, CBF falls and above 150 torr, CBF rises. These parameters describe overall perfusion and may be normal in spite of significant regional hypoperfusion and ischemia. Nitroprusside and nitroglycerin dilate cerebral arterioles and veins but also increase cerebral blood volume. In a noncompliant brain, this may result in a dangerous rise in the ICP. Trimethaphan, a ganglionic-blocking agent, does not directly dilate cerebral vessels. The partial pressure of CO_2 is a potent regulator of cerebral vasodilation/vasoconstriction. As $PaCO_2$ declines, cerebral vessels constrict and CBF decreases in a linear fashion.

REFERENCES

Marsh ML, et al: Changes in neurologic status and ICP associated with sodium nitroprusside. Anesthesiology 1979; 51:336

Safar P, Grenvik A (Eds): Brain failure and resusciation. New York, Churchill Livingstone, 1981

Shapiro H: Physiologic and pharmacologic regulation of cerebral blood flow. ASA Annual Refresher Course, 1977

COMA

RATIONALE 162-e

We are faced with a comatose patient with a fixed dilated right pupil and we have no idea about the condition of the left pupil. Damage to the right sixth cranial nerve by itself does not explain the coma. However, as trauma or infection are frequently the cause for a sixth nerve paresis, the level of consciousness may be consistent. The parasympathetic pupiloconstrictor fibers travel in the third cranial nerve. The pupil dilates because of involvement of this nerve, either directly or indirectly, when uncal herniation compresses the nerve against the posterior cerebral artery or tentorium. Involvement of the sixth cranial nerve affects the ability to abduct the right eye (paralysis of right lateral gaze) but does not affect the pupil.

Several drugs are known to cause dilated and fixed pupils. Atropine and scopolamine may do this when taken in doses large enough to cause delirium or stupor. Glutethimide (Doriden) characteristically produces midposition or moderately dilated (4-8 mm) pupils. These may be unequal and can be fixed to light for several hours after ingestion of enough drug to cause coma. Fixed and dilated pupils do not necessarily signify a poor prognosis.

Subdural hematomas have been classified as acute, subacute and chronic. The acute and subacute varieties most often present with alterations in the level of consciousness, whereas headache is the more common presentation in the chronic group. Pupillary inequality is common in acute bleeds. McKissock found that the dilated pupil was on the side of the lesion in 79% of patients with subdural hematomas. Eight percent of the cases presented with pupil dilation contralateral to the subdural hematoma.

A right sided subdural is consistent with this patient's course and findings although a left sided subdural is possible.

REFERENCES

McKissock W, Richardson A, Bloom WH: Subdural hematoma: A review of 389 cases. Lancet 1960; 1:1365

Plum F, Posner JB: The Diagnosis of Stupor and Coma. Third Edition. Philadelphia, FA Davis Co., 1980

RATIONALE 163-c

The concurrence of diverse signs that reflect convergence of neurons in one contiguous area of damage suggests structural rather than metabolic lesions. A pattern of damage that progresses systematically from rostral to caudal is particularly suggestive of progressive structural damage often associated with increased intracranial pressure.

Absence of pupillary light reflexes is more commonly associated with structural than metabolic lesions. The Argyll Robertson pupil is usually small, irregular, unequal to its fellow pupil, fails to react to light directly or consensually, and reacts poorly to pain or mydriatics, though it may constrict on accommodation. Such pupils are common in tabes dorsalis, but are also found in other types of neurosyphilis as well as diabetes, alcoholism, multiple sclerosis, tumors of the midbrain, and encephalitis.

Irrigation of the right ear with the head flexed forward 30° from the horizontal position stimulates the lateral semicircular canal that is then vertical. Cooling this canal causes downward currents, away from the ampulla. After cerumen has been removed and the tympanic membrane shown to be intact, the ear may be irrigated with 200 ml of iced water using a soft plastic tube. The usual response is tonic deviation of the eyes toward the irrigated ear for 2 or 3 minutes. This indicates intact brain stem function, at least between cranial nerves 3 and 8. In addition, there may be nystagmus with the rapid component directed away from the irrigated ear; that indicates intact connections with the cerebral cortex. After 5 minutes, if there is no response, the contralateral ear may be tested. Caloric responses are often present in patients who show no eye movement to head rotation and, therefore, are valuable signs to elicit.

Most structural lesions that eliminate the caloric responses of the eyes also cause unreactive pupils. To observe light reflexes, one should observe the edge of the iris with a +20 to +40 diopter lens, possibly with a green filter, from the side in a dark room, and then shine a bright light directly into the eye. If the eyes do not move to proper caloric testing, but the pupils do react to light, metabolic cause of coma is suggested rather than a structural lesion.

REFERENCES

Bannister R: Brain's Clinical Neurology. Fourth Edition. London, Oxford University Press, 1973

Bass E: Cardiopulmonary arrest: Pathophysiology and neurologic complications. Ann Intern Med 1985; 103:920

Merritt HH: A Textbook of Neurology. Fifth Edition. Philadelphia, Lea & Febiger, 1973, pp 119-122

Plum F, Posner JB: The Diagnosis of Stupor and Coma. Third Edition. Philadelphia, FA Davis Co., 1980

RATIONALE 164-c

Anoxic damage to both cerebral hemispheres, such as that sustained during a cardiopulmonary arrest, frequently produces coma if the anoxic ischemia persists for longer than 4 to 6 minutes. Willoughby and Leach examined 48 patients after 53 episodes of cardic arrest. Eighteen patients at 1 hour after the arrest demonstrated deep coma, which was a negative prognostic sign.

Basilar artery thrombosis presents with stupor or coma, flaccid quadriplegia, bulbar paralysis, and is rapidly fatal. Pontine hemorrhage, representing approximately 10% of all primary hemorrhages in the CNS, presents an acute event, with or without prodromal symptoms, with deep coma and quadriplegia. Seventy-five percent of patients die within the first 24 hours.

Vitamin B_1 (thiamine) deficiency has been thought to be causally related to a number of disorders, including nutritional polyneuropathies, retrobulbar neuropathies, cerebellar degeneration, and degeneration of the corpus callosum, Wernicke's encephalopathy, and Korsakoff's psychosis. In Wernicke's encephalopathy, mental symptoms occur in 90% of the cases, primarily as a quiet global confusional state. Stupor and coma are an uncommon initial feature of the illness, although Victor et al. reported 9 stuporous patients and 2 deeply comatose patients in a series of 239 such patients.

Infarction of the lateral medulla is related to disease in the inferior, superior, or middle arteries of the medulla, the posterior inferior cerebellar artery, or the vertebral artery. The presentation of this striking and unusual syndrome depends upon the size and precise anatomic location of the lesion. Patients usually present with vertigo and dizziness, facial dysesthesias, hiccuping, vomiting, dysphagia, nystagmus, and hypotonia of the ipsilateral limbs. Consciousness is rarely disturbed in such patients.

REFERENCES

Haymaker W, Kuhlenbeck W: Disorders of the brainstem and its cranial nerves. In: Clinical Neurology. Baker AB, Baker LH (Eds). Hagerstown, MD, Harper and Row, 1976

Victor M: Alcoholism. In: Clinical Neurology. Baker AB, Baker LH (Eds). Hagerstown, MD, Harper and Row, 1977

Victor M, Adams RD, Collins GH: The Wernicke-Korsakoff Syndrome. Philadephia, FA Davis Co., 1971

Willoughby JO, Leach BG: Relation of neurological findings after cardiac arrest to outcome. Br Med J 1974; 3:437

RATIONALE 165-b

The Glasgow Coma Scale is widely used as a means of quantitating and monitoring the level of consciousness. Scores are given as follows:

FUNCTION	SCORE
Eye Opening:	
Spontaneous	4
To speech	3
To pain	2
Nil	1
Best Motor Response:	
Obeys	6
Localizes	5
Withdraws	4
Abnormal flexion	3
Extension	2
Nil	1
Best Verbal Response:	
Oriented	5
Confused conversation	4
Inappropriate words	3
Incomprehensible sounds	2
Nil	1

The maximum score is 15; scores less than 7 are defined as coma.

REFERENCES

Jennett B, Teasdale G: Aspects of coma after severe head injury. Lancet 1977; 1:878

Jennett B, Teasdale G, Braakman R: Predicting outcome in individual patients after severe head trauma. Lancet 1976; 1:1031

EDITORIAL COMMENT

Although this score is convenient and reproducible, it does not replace a standard neurologic evaluation. The Glasgow Coma Scale accurately describes patients with near normal states of consciousness and those who are deeply comatose, however, it quantitates poorly those patients with moderate cerebral impairment.

ADDITIONAL REFERENCES

Tabaddor K: Emergency care: Initial evaluation. In: Head Injury. Cooper PR (Ed). Baltimore, Williams & Wilkins Co., 1982, pp 15-26

Teasdale G, Jennett B: Assessment of coma and impaired consciousness. A practical scale. Lancet 1974; 2:81

ENCEPHALITIS

RATIONALE 166-d

Herpes simplex virus infection of the CNS is the most common cause of fatal sporadic encephalitis. It occurs in all sexes, races and ages throughout the year. Cerebral infection with herpes simplex tends to localize in the temporal lobes. The most common symptoms are personality change, disorientation and hallucinations, frequently leading to a misdiagnosis of psychiatric disturbance. The disease progresses through changes of consciousness to coma which has a poor prognosis. The exact role of brain biopsy remains controversial. It is, however, the only means currently available to make a definitive diagnosis. In the early stages, therapy with adenine arabinoside improves morbidity and mortality.

REFERENCES

Barza M, Pauker SG: The decision to biopsy, treat or wait in suspected herpes encephalitis. Ann Intern Med 1980; 92:641

Caplan LR: Brain biopsy in herpes simplex encephalitis. N Engl J Med 1980; 303:700

Nahmias AJ, Whitley RJ, Visintine AN, et al: Herpes simplex virus encephalitis: Laboratory evaluations and their clinical significance. J Infect Dis 1982; 145:829

Streuli RA, Ultmann JE: Herpes simplex encephalitis: A great clinical challenge. Ann Intern Med 1980; 93:696

Whitley RJ: Diagnosis and treatment of herpes simplex encephalitis. Annu Rev Med 1981; 32:335

Whitley RJ, Soong SJ, et al: Herpes simplex encephalitis. N Engl J Med 1981; 304:313

GUILLAIN-BARRE'

RATIONALE 167-d

Guillain-Barre' syndrome (GBS) is an insidiously progressive demyelination of segmental spinal nerve roots and proximal nerve segments, occurring following a nonspecific infectious illness, trauma, or pregnancy. Usually, maximal neurological deficit has been achieved within 3 weeks of the onset of the illness. The pattern of neurological dysfunction is usually symmetrical and ascending. Muscle weakness tends to be more severe in the proximal than the distal musculature. Fifty-five percent of patients initially present with paresthesias or pain. Lichtenfeld noted postural hypotension in 43% of patients in his series of 25 consecutive patients with GBS, perhaps related to sporadic chromatolysis of the preganglionic neurons of the sympathetic nervous system in the intermediolateral cell column as suggested by Birchfield and Shaw. Other autonomic nervous system derangements are seen frequently. Lichtenfeld observed a 61% incidence of hypertension, 25% incidences of persistent facial flushing, 21% incidence of bradycardias, and a 30% incidence of urinary retention. The CSF is abnormal, with protein values ranging up to 1300 mg/dl, although the first CSF sample on initial presentation may be normal. Minimal lymphocytic pleocytosis in the range of 2 to 3 lymphocytes per ml may be noted. The observation of pronounced lymphocytic pleocytosis in the presence of a normal protein concentration in the CSF suggests that the initial diagnosis of GBS was in error.

REFERENCES

Birchfield RI, Shaw CM: Postural hypotension in the Guillain-Barre' syndrome. Arch Neurol 1964; 10:149

Eisen A, Humphreys P: The Guillain-Barre' syndrome: A clinical and electrodiagnostic study of 25 cases. Arch Neurol 1974; 30:438

Lichtenfeld PL Autonomic dysfunction in the Guillain-Barre' syndrome. Am J Med 1971; 20:772

McFarland HR, Heller GL: Guillain-Barre' disease complex: A statement of diagnostic criteria and analysis of 100 cases. Arch Neurol 1966; 14:196

RATIONALE 168-b

Guillain-Barre' syndrome presents as flaccid, symmetric, ascending motor paralysis. There are usually minimal sensory findings. Seizures are not a part of the classic complex. The primary neurological concern is paralysis of the muscles of respiration with resultant hypoxemia and hypoventilation. Prolonged bedrest places the patient at high risk for thromboembolic complications. Ineffective cough increases the chance of pneumonia, which is often recurrent. Staphylococcus aureus, Klebsiella pneumoniae, and Pseudomonas aeruginosa are the predominant offending organisms. Forty percent of patients with Guillain-Barre' syndrome require ventilator support. The incidence of pneumonia in this group of mechanically ventilated patients is exceptionally high. General malaise and difficulty in swallowing lead to early nutritional deficits. The preferred method of feeding is by the enteral route.

REFERENCES

Jackson DL: Critical care neurology. In: Textbook of Critical Care. Shoemaker WC, Thompson WL, Holbrook PR (Eds). Philadelphia, WB Saunders Co., 1984, p 95

Kennedy RH, Danielson MA, Mulder DW, et al: Guillain-Barre' syndrome: A 42-year-old epidemiological and clinical study. Mayo Clin Proc 1978; 53:93

Moore PM, James D: Guillain-Barre' syndrome: Incidence, management and outcome of major complications. Crit Care Med 1981; 9:549

Raman TK, Blake JA, Harris TM: Pulmonary embolism in Landry-Guillain-Barre' Strohl syndrome. Chest 1971; 60:555

EDITORIAL COMMENT

The Guillain-Barre' Study Group recently reported experience with plasmapheresis vs. conventional therapy in 245 patients with the Guillain-Barre' Syndrome. The plasmapheresis treated group demonstrated clinical improvement at 4 weeks, decreased time to independent walking and improved outcome at 6 months. Plasmapheresis was not beneficial for all patients but those who received treatment within 7 days of onset and those who required mechanical ventilation seemed to benefit.

ADDITIONAL REFERENCE

Guillain-Barre' Syndrome Study Group: Plasmapheresis and acute Guillain-Barre' syndrome. Neurology 1985; 35:1096

INTRACRANIAL BLEED

RATIONALE 169-b

The third most common cause of stroke following atherosclerosis and embolism is intracranial hemorrhage. Although there are over a dozen causes of intracranial hemorrhage, the most common are hypertensive intracerebral hemorrhage, ruptured saccular aneurysm and hemorrhage associated with bleeding disorders (in that order). The most common site of intracranial hemorrhage is the putamen. Fifty-five to sixty percent of all hypertensive intracranial hemorrhages occur at this site. Saccular aneurysms that rupture into the subarachnoid space are most frequently found on the anterior half of the Circle of Willis. Following the initial bleed the most dreaded complications result from rebleeding or vasospasm. Both complications have the highest frequency in the first 14 days. CT scanning indicates that the amount of blood in the basal cisterns is prognostically associated with subsequent vasospasm and ischemic symptoms. At this time there is no widely accepted effective therapy to prevent or reverse vasospasm, however, recent studies with the calcium channel blocking agent Nimodipine are encouraging.

REFERENCES

Adams HP: Currrent status of antifibrinolytic therapy for treatment of patients with aneurysmal subarachnoid hemorrhage. Stroke 1982; 13:256

Allen GS, et al: Cerebral vasospasm - A controlled trial of Nimodipine in patients with subarachnoid hemorrhage. N Engl J Med 1983; 308:619

Drake CG: Management of cerebral aneurysm. Stroke 1981; 12:273

Jackson DL: Selected topics in critical care neurology. In: Critical Care: State of the Art. Vol 1. Shoemaker WC, Thompson WL (Eds). Fullerton, CA, Society of Critical Care Medicine, 1980, pp I(M):1-47

Peerless SJ: Pre and postoperative management of cerebral aneurysms. Clin Neurosurg 1979; 26:209

Sundt TM, et al: Subarachnoid hemorrhage from intracranial aneurysms. N Engl J Med 1977; 299:116

INTRACRANIAL PRESSURE

RATIONALE 170-d

A major determinant in control of cerebrovascular tone is the pH of cerebrospinal fluid. Hyperventilation quickly lowers carbonic acid concentration both in blood and cerebrospinal fluid, causing cerebral vasoconstriction and reducing intracranial pressure. If metabolic acidosis develops suddenly, the compensatory hyperventilation may for a brief time lead to a "paradoxical" increase in cerebrospinal fluid pH due to the slow diffusion of bicarbonate from CSF. Increased arterial pressure (from norepinephrine) increases intracranial pressure, and the same may result if increased cardiac output is accompanied by an increase in arterial pressure.

REFERENCES

Betz E: Cerebral blood flow: Its measurement and regulation. Physiol Rev 1972; 52:595

Safar PL Cerebral edema. In: Critical Care Medicine Handbook. Weil MH, Shubin H (Eds). New York, John N Kolen, 1974, pp 264-272

RATIONALE 171-d

Wernicke's encephalopathy consists of gaze palsies, nystagmus and ataxia. Korsakoff's psychosis is an amnestic-confabulatory disorder in which memory is impaired out of proportion to other mental function. The disorders occur in alcoholic patients, however, the exact role played by alcohol has not been established. They have been united under the name Wernicke-Korsakoff syndrome (WKS) because of similarities in brain pathology. Brain autopsy findings in patients dying of chronic Korsakoff's psychosis are virtually identical to those dying with acute Wernicke's encephalopathy. Patients with WKS have an abnormal thiamine-requiring transketolase. Thiamine (100 mg iv) usually reverses the symptoms of acute Wernicke's encephalopathy, and significant improvement may be expected in up to 50% of patients with Korsakoff's psychosis. Administration of glucose to a withdrawing alcoholic who has yet to receive thiamine can precipitate acute Wernicke's encephalopathy. Thiamine, therefore, should always be given prior to glucose infusion in this setting.

REFERENCES

Blass JP, Gibson GE: Abnormality of a thiamine-requiring enzyme in patients with Wernicke-Korsakoff syndrome. N Engl J Med 1977; 297:1367

Victor M, Adams RD, Collins GH: The Wernicke-Korsakoff Syndrome: A Clinical and Pathological Study of 245 Patients with Post-Morten Examinations. Philadelphia, FA Davis Co., 1971

RATIONALE 172-e

With an insult as described, autoregulation may be compromised and cerebral blood flow may vary directly with arterial pressure. Thus, an increase in blood pressure may augment intracranial blood volume and enhance cerebral edema formation further elevating intracranial pressure (ICP). The end result may be a decrease in cerebral perfusion pressure.

Cerebral blood flow and hence ICP vary directly with $PaCO_2$. Cerebral blood flow is most sensitive to CO_2 within physiological ranges of carbon dioxide tension. The vasoconstrictive effect of hypocapnia lowers ICP by lowering intravascular blood volume. Hypercapnia significantly increases cerebral blood volume, blood flow and ICP.

Drainage of cerebrospinal fluid via a ventricular catheter decreases intracranial volume. This is another rapid form of treatment for increased intracranial pressure. Placement of the intraventricular catheter is often difficult technically in the postanoxic patient who may have significant cerebral edema with small ventricles. Removing a large volume of CSF via lumbar puncture places the patient with increased intracranial pressure at risk for brain herniation.

Intravenous pentobarbital has been used to treat increased ICP from various causes. A level of 25-50 mg/L of pentobarbital in plasma has been used for acute reduction in ICP. Such therapy has been given for 3-5 days. In a patient with severe hypoxia, one must consider the cardiovascular depressant effects of barbiturates. The utility of barbiturate therapy remains questionable.

Diuretic therapy may be beneficial in this case for several reasons. By lowering right atrial pressure, diuretics facilitate jugular venous drainage and therefore lower ICP. Additionally, diuretics may directly decrease intracellular sodium and water transport in the brain which also significantly lowers ICP.

REFERENCES

Bruce DA, Gennarelli TA, Langfitt TW: Resuscitation from coma due to head injury. Crit Care Med 1978; 6:254

Buhrley LE, Reed DJ: The effect of furosemide on sodium-22 uptake into cerebrospinal fluid and brain. Exptl Brain Res 1972; 14:503

Cottrell JE, Robustelli A, Post K, et al: Furosemide- and mannitol-induced changes in intracranial pressure and serum osmolality and electrolytes. Anesthesiology 1977; 47:28

Marshall LF, Shapiro HM, Rauscher A, et al: Pentobarbital therapy for intracranial hypertension in metabolic coma. Crit Care Med 1987; 6:1

Shapiro HM: Intracranial hypertension: Therapeutic and anesthetic considerations. Anesthesiology 1974; 43:445

Shapiro HM, Wyte SR, Loeser J: Barbiturate-augmented hypothermia for reduction of persistent intracranial hypertension. J Neurosurg 1974; 40:90

RATIONALE 173-e

Hyperosmolar agents, such as intravenous mannitol (in acute situations) and oral glycerol (that has been successful in long-term use) have proven very effective in lowering intracranial pressure (ICP). Furosemide lowers ICP in patients undergoing craniotomy for aneurysm surgery, repair of an arteriovenous malformation, or resection of a tumor.

The beneficial effects of steroids in patients with cerebral edema due to primary or metastatic brain tumors and pseudotumor are established. However, they does not cause rapid reduction of ICP.

Th use of positive end-expiratory pressure (PEEP) may increase ICP. PEEP could adversely affect this patient by decreasing cardiac output and arterial pressure (thereby decreasing cerebral perfusion pressure) or by impeding cerebral venous return (thereby increasing cerebral venous pressure and ICP). An increase in cerebral elastance (as tested by volume-pressure response) often predicted the patients most likely to be adversely affected by PEEP.

When PEEP is used in a patient with increased ICP, therapy must be individualized and continuous monitoring of ICP, intracranial compliance, arterial pressure and neurological status is important to permit optimal titration of therapy.

REFERENCES

Aidmis SJ, Lafferty J, Shaprio HM: Intracranial responses to PEEP. Anesthesiology 1976; 45:275

Apuzzo ML, Weiss MH, Petersons V, et al: Effect of positive end-expiratory pressure ventilation on intracranial pressure in man. J Neurosurg 1977; 46:227

Cottrell JE, Robustelli A, Post K, et al: Furosemide- and mannitol-induced changes in intracranial pressure and serum osmolality and electrolytes. Anesthesiology 1977; 47:28

Shapiro HM: Intracranial hypertension: Therapeutic and anesthethic considerations. Anesthesiology 1975; 43:445

Shapiro HM, Marshall LF: Intracranial pressure responses to PEEP in head injured patients. J Trauma 1978; 18:254

RATIONALE 174-e

Initial compensatory mechanisms (e.g., a reduction in the volume of CSF within the cranium) may keep intracranial pressure (ICP) low in spite of significant compression of brain matter. There is no consistent relationship between midline shift and ICP. Hyperventilation causes vasoconstriction, decreased blood flow, and decreased intracranial blood volume which may prevent secondary ischemic damage. Fever, inhalational anesthetics and sodium nitroprusside all cause cerebral vasodilatation which compromises an already compressed brain. Narcotics reduce cerebral metabolism and do not directly cause vasodilatation.

REFERENCES

Jennett B, Teasdale G: Management of Head Injuries. Contemporary Neurology Series 20, 1981

Koht A, Cerullo L: Management of patients with elevated intracranial pressure. In: Critical Care for Surgical Patients. Beal J (Ed). New York, Macmillan Publishing Co. Inc., 1982

Safar P, Grenvik A (Eds): Brain Failure & Resusciation. New York, Churchill Livingstone, 1981

RATIONALE 175-c

On admission, the Glasgow Coma Score is seven. The patient has focal findings and a CT scan is ordered. The airway should be protected and ventilation supplied in case deterioration continues during scanning. Osmotic agents and hyperventilation are recognized methods of delaying secondary brain damage in the face of an expanding mass lesion. The dosage of mannitol is .25-1 gm/kg. The utility of intracranial (ICP) monitoring after head injury is controversial but in the face of recent surgery a rising ICP may indicate the reaccumulation of a mass lesion.

REFERENCES

Jennett B, Teasdale G: Management of Head Injuries. Contemporary Neurology Series 20, 1981

Marshall L, Smith R, Rauscher LA, et al: Mannitol dose requirements in brain-injured patients. J Neurosurg 1978; 48:169

Safar P, Grenvik A (Eds): Brain Failure & Resusciation. New York, Churchill Livingstone, 1981

RATIONALE 176-a 177-d

Increased intracranial pressure (ICP) often complicates the course of patients with intracranial pathology and may be a major determinant of morbidity and mortality. One means to lower ICP in this population is by controlled hyperventilation.

An arterial PCO_2 acutely lowered to 25-30 mm Hg by hyperventilation causes an intense constriction of normal cerebral resistor vessels by increasing the local pH. This increase in cerebral vascular resistance lowers cerebral blood flow and cerebral blood volume which, in turn, lowers ICP. Within 48-72 hours of initiation of controlled hyperventilation, renal secretion of bicarbonate compensates for the lowered $PaCO_2$. Cerebral pH thus returns toward normal and cerebral blood flow increases towards baseline. Exactly how long hypocapnia will benefit a given patient is unknown. It is clear, however, that a sudden reversal of hypocapnia may cause an abrupt and dramatic rise in ICP even after several days. It is recommended, therefore, that when controlled hyperventilation is discontinued, the $PaCO_2$ should be brought back to baseline gradually.

Elevated ICP can be lowered by hyperventilation in patients who have sustained head trauma. Unfortunately there is little evidence that this maneuver has decreased morbidity or mortality in this group of patients. Similarly, no convincing evidence exists showing benefit from hyperventilation in patients with hypoxic cerebral edema.

There is no therapy available at this time to consistently prevent or reverse the cerebral vasospasm associated with subarachnoid hemorrhage. One could postulate a detrimental effect of hyperventilation induced cerebral vasoconstriction superimposed upon cerebral vasospasm.

REFERENCES

Alexander SG, Lassen NA: Hyperventilation in head injury. Anesthesiology 1970; 32:60

Bell JA, Hodgson HJ: Coma after cardiac arrest. Brain 1974; 97:361

Heffner JE, Sahn SA; Controlled hyperventilation in patients with intracranial hypertension: Application and management. Arch Intern Med 1983; 143:765

Kassel NF, Peerless SJ, Reilly PL: Intracranial pressure, aneurysms, and subarachnoid hemorrhage. In: Intracranial Pressure III. Beks JWF, et al (Eds). New York, Springer-Verlag, 1976

Trubuhovich RV: A note on cerebrovascular accidents. In: Management of Acute Intracranial Disasters. Boston, Little, Brown and Co., 1979

RATIONALE 178-a

High dose dexamethasone therapy has been shown to dramatically and rapidly reduce the focal and general signs of brain tumor. The effect is probably related both to decreasing peri-tumor edema, and to a transient reduction in size of the tumor. Although often used for the other causes of cerebral edema, no scientific evidence as yet supports the use of steroids.

REFERENCES

Cooper R, Moody S, Clark WK, et al: Dexamethasone and severe head injury: A prospective double-blind study. J Neurosurg 1979; 51:307

Fishman RA: Brain edema. N Engl J Med 1975; 293:706

Manz HF: The pathology of cerebral edema. Hum Pathol 1974; 5:291

Ward JD, Becker DP: Head trauma. In: Textbook of Critical Care. Shoemaker WC, Thompson WL, Holbrook PR (Eds). Philadelphia, WB Saunders Co., 1984, pp 926-928

MENINGITIS

RATIONALE 179-a

Beta-lactam antibiotics (penicillins and cephalosporins) inhibit bacterial cell wall synthesis and are most active in vitro when bacterial growth is not slowed by in inhibitor of protein synthesis such as chloramphenicol. Penicillins enhance penetration of aminoglycoside antibiotics into enterococci, but chloramphenicol does not have this effect. Although small amounts of beta-lactam antibiotics penetrate into normal brain and spinal fluid, meningitis enhances antibiotic penetration and adequate ampicillin concentrations for treatment of pneumococcal meningitis can be achieved. However, Hemophilus influenzae - Type B is a common cause of meningitis in infants (and increasingly in the older adult with chronic lung disease). Some strains are resistant to ampicillin and are best treated with chloramphenicol.

REFERENCES

Schiffer MS, MacLowry J, Schneerson R, et al: Clinical, bacteriological, and immunological characterisation of ampicillin-resistant Haemophilus influenzae type B. Lancet 1974; 2:257

Tomeh MO, Starr SE, McGowan JE Jr, et al: Ampicillin-resistant Haemophilus influenzae type B infection. JAMA 1974; 229:295

MYASTHENIA GRAVIS

RATIONALE 180-e

Increased salivation occurs as a response to cholinesterase inhibition. If swallowing is compromised by the myasthenia gravis, the patient may dribble and appear to be salivating more. A diagnostic dilemma thus exists in a myasthenic patient treated with a cholinesterase inhibitor who appears to have increased salivation. Overdosage with anticholinesterase drugs leads to increased gastrointestinal activity, with increased salivation, hyperactive bowel sounds, colic, and diarrhea. There may be muscle fasciculation, and the edrophonium (Tensilon) test is negative; it may even produce a nicotinic paralysis lasting up to 48 hours. Although atropine may ameliorate the salivation, it is considered a dangerous policy to use it routinely with pyridostigmine, as it may mask the early signs of a cholinergic crisis. Atropine should be used with neostigmine, as the muscarinic actions of neostigmine are more prominent that pyridostigmine, particularly bradycardia or cardiac arrest. Bradycardia is uncommon with pyridostigmine. Urinary retention may occur, but is a less constant feature. The skin is usually moist.

REFERENCES

Osserman KE, Foldes FF, Genkins G: Myasthenia gravis. In: International Encyclopedia of Pharmacology and Therapeutics. Section 14, Vol 2. New York, Pergamon Press, 1972, pp 561-618.

Seybold ME: Myasthenia gravis: A clinical and basic science review. JAMA 1983; 250:2516

RATIONALE 181-a 182-e 183-d

Myasthenia gravis results from an autoimmune attack on the nicotonic acetylcholine receptor in skeletal muscle. Although antibodies to the acetylcholine receptor are present in the serum of 80%-90% of patients with myasthenia gravis, their concentration does not correlate with disease activity. The cause of the immune response is unknown. Thymic abnormalities are present in 80% of persons with myasthenia gravis and may contribute to the pathogenesis of this disorder.

Respiratory failure is common in patients with myasthenia gravis. In a Mayo Clinic review, 7.6% of 288 patients with myasthenia gravis required mechanical ventilation for respiratory failure. Postoperative myasthenia crisis, especially after thymectomy, was the most common cause of respiratory failure. Cholinergic crisis (resulting from overdosage of anticholinesterase drugs) was the least common. Aminoglycosides, emotional stress, the initiation of steroid therapy, and infection are other causes.

Patients with myasthenia gravis frequently develop signs of respiratory insufficiency before blood gas abnormalities. The best predictor of impending failure seems to be the maximal inspiratory pressure. Commonly accepted criteria for intubation are alveolar-arterial oxygen gradient > 300 mm Hg (FIO_2 of 1.0), $PaCO_2$ > 45 mm Hg, pH < 7.35, maximum negative inspiratory pressures of < -30 cm H_2O, and an FVC < 10-15 cc/kg.

Intubation is necessary for most patients who develop abnormalities in one or more of these parameters.

REFERENCES

Bergufsky EH: Respiratory insufficiency in mechanical and neurological disorders of the thorax. In: Pulmonary Diseases and Disorders. Fishman AP (Ed). New York, McGraw-Hill Book Company, 1980, pp 156-166

Black LF, Hyatt RE: Maximal static respiratory pressures in generalized neuromuscular disease. Am Rev Respir Dis 1971; 103:641

Douglas JG, Ferguson RJ, Crompton GK, et al: Artificial ventilation for neurological disease: Retrospective analysis. Br Med J 1983; 286:1972

Ferguson HT, Murphy RP, Lascelles TG: Ventilatory failure in myasthenia gravis. J Neurol Neurosurg Psychiatry 1982; 45:217

Gracey DR, Divertie MB, Howard FM: Mechanical ventilation for respiratory failure in myasthenia gravis. Mayo Clin Proc 1983; 58:597

PUPILS

RATIONALE 184-e

Atropine is an antimuscarinic agent which blocks the responses of the sphincter muscle of the iris and the ciliary muscle of the lens to cholinergic stimulation; thus, it dilates the pupil (mydriasis) and paralyzes accommodation (cycloplegia). Trimethaphan (Arfonad) causes ciliary ganglionic blockade resulting in incomplete mydriasis and partial loss of accommodation. Morphine, like other narcotics, causes pupillary constriction (miosis) in man due to a central action on the Edinger-Westphal nucleus of the oculomotor nerve. Dopamine has also been reported to cause pupillary dilation (mydriasis) and fixation in patients treated with doses over 30 μg/kg•min.

REFERENCES

Goodman LS, Gilman A (Eds): The Pharmacologic Basis of Therapeutics. Fifth Edition. New York, Macmillan Publishing Co. Inc., 1979, pp 250, 514-518, 572

Guyton AC: Textbook of Medical Physiology. Philadelphia, WB Saunders Co., 1976, pp 822-825

Ong GL, Bruning HA: Dilated pupils due to administration of high doses of dopamine hydrochloride. Crit Care Med 1981; 9:658

REYE SYNDROME

RATIONALE 185-c

The patient has Reye syndrome (RS). Classically, RS begins with a nonspecific viral prodrome, followed by persistent vomiting progressing to altered mental status and coma. In addition to the neurologic symptoms, RS is characterized by severe hepatic dysfunction with elevation of serum transaminases, and prolongation of the prothrombin time. Hepatitis antigens are not positive in RS. The serum ammonia is always elevated but is only an index of poor prognosis when levels approach 500 mcg/100 ml. Serum bilirubin rarely rises above 3.0 to 4.0 mg/100 ml. Blood glucose is frequently below 50 mg/100 ml requiring intravenous dextrose infusions to prevent additional CNS damage. Over the last decade, improved recognition of the disease, early referral and aggressive intensive care have markedly reduced the mordibity and mortality of RS. Generally acknowledged methods of treatment for those patients with severe disease include controlled mechanical hyperventilation, ICP monitoring and treatment of elevated intracranial pressure.

REFERENCES

Boutros A: Reye Syndrome: A predictably curable disease. Pediatric Clinics 1980; 27:59

Schubert W, et al: Reye Syndrome. DM 1975; December, pp 1-30

Shaywitz BA, Rothsein P, Venes JL: Monitoring and management of increased ICP in Reye Syndrome. Pediatrics 1980; 66:198

STATUS EPILEPTICUS

RATIONALE 186-d

The therapy of status epilepticus is controversial but several conventional approaches are recognized. The maintenance of an open airway and adequate ventilation is paramount. All patients should receive a large intravenous catheter. Diazepam is effective in terminating status epilepticus in approximately 60%-80% of patients. The short half-life of intravenous diazepam (approximately 15 minutes) accounts for the frequent occurrence of breakthrough seizures. Many prefer to treat status with intravenous phenytoin which, when used properly, is generally safe and effective although slower in action than diazepam. The major hazard of phenytoin, when given intravenously, is hypotension and dysrhythmias which are directly related to the rate of administration. When the infusion rate is less than 50 mg/min this is rarely a problem.

The combination of diazepam and barbiturates is particularly likely to cause respiratory depression and should generally be avoided unless adequate artificial ventilation can be administered.

Phenytoin should be administered into a tubing filled with freely running normal saline, since the drug precipitates in dextrose-containing solutions.

REFERENCES

Beal F: Status epilepticus. In: Manual of Intensive Care Medicine. Rippe JM, Csete ME (Eds). Boston, Little, Brown and Co., 1983, pp 388-389

Celesia GG: Modern concepts of status epilepticus. JAMA 1976; 235

Cranford RE, Leppik IE, Patrick B, et al: Intravenous phenytoin in acute treatment of seizures. Neurology 1979; 29:1474

Delgado-Escueta V, Treiman DM, Walgh GD: The treatable epilepsies. N Engl J Med 1983; 308:1508

Penry JK, Newmark ME: The use of antiepileptic drugs. Ann Intern Med 1979; 90:207

EDITORIAL COMMENT

Reye syndrome is a self-limited disease of the hepatic mitochondria. Brain and muscle involvement may occur. The syndrome most commonly follows influenzae A, influenzae B and herpes varicella-zoster infections. Many other viral illnesses have been implicated but at lower frequency. Reye syndrome predominantly affects school age children, occasionally infants and rarely adults. The precise etiology and pathogenesis remain obscure. Salicylates may increase the risk of Reye syndrome in children with varicella or influenzae and, therefore, should be avoided. Partin found significantly higher serum salicylate levels on presentation of Reye syndrome in patients with a poor outcome as compared to those with a good outcome. The mortality in the United States has declined from 80% to 20%.

ADDITIONAL REFERENCES

Check WA: Reye's syndrome - aspirin link: A bit stronger. JAMA 1982; 247:1534

Edwards KM, Bennett SR, Garner WL, et al: Reye's syndrome associated with adenovirus infections in infants. ADJC 1985; 139:343

Mowat AP: Reye's syndrome: Twenty years on. Br Med J 1983; 286:1999

Partin JS, Partin JC, Schubert WK, et al: Serum salicylate concentrations in Reye's disease: Study of 130 biopsy-proved cases. Lancet 1982; 1:191

Section 11

187. You are managing a young woman in her 34th week of pregnancy who develops severe hypertension, proteinuria, confusion, and retinal hemorrhages. You begin an intravenous infusion of magnesium sulfate.

Which ONE of the following observations is the MOST serious contraindication to continued administration of magnesium sulfate?

a. Fetal heart rate decreases from 160 to 140/min.
b. Maternal serum magnesium concentration equals 3.0 mEq/L.
c. Maternal respiratory rate decreases from 24 to 16/min.
d. Maternal patellar reflexes change from 4+ to absent.
e. Maternal ECG shortening of PR and QRS interval durations

188. A young woman with an uncomplicated pregnancy begins spontaneous labor after 32 weeks of gestation.

Which ONE of the following tests would be MOST useful in predicting lung maturity of the fetus?

a. Estriol excretion in the mother's urine
b. Amniotic fluid estriol concentration
c. Alpha-antitrypsin concentration in the amniotic fluid
d. Ultrasonographic measurement of fetal chest dimensions
e. Amniotic fluid sphingomyelin and lecithin concentrations

189. A young healthy woman has the onset of spontaneous labor after 32 weeks of gestation. The fetal lungs are immature.

Which ONE of the following classes of drugs is MOST likely to be effective in delaying birth?

a. α-adrenergic agonist
b. β-adrenergic agonist
c. Histamine (H-2) receptor antagonist
d. Acetylcholine muscarinic receptor antagonist
e. Serotonin (5-HT) receptor antagonist

ANSWERS

187-d **188-e** **189-b**

ECLAMPSIA

RATIONALE 187-d

Preeclampsia and eclampsia have also been called "toxemia," but the toxin is not identified. Recent theories focus on an excess of thromboxane that causes platelet aggregation and vasoconstriction, and a deficit of prostacyclin, that inhibits platelet aggregation and promotes vasodilation. Whatever the pathophysiology, women with these syndromes have relative ischemia of the uterus, decreased sodium and water excretion, edema, hypertension, neuromuscular irritability, and convulsions.

Magnesium sulfate is commonly given in treatment, as it decreases neuromuscular irritability, decreases the incidence of seizures, ameliorates hypertension, promotes uterine relaxation and vasodilation, and may, therefore, treat some of the causes and effects of preeclampsia and eclampsia.

About 1300 mmol of magnesium are in the body, but only 13 mmol are in the extracellular fluid. Of the total of 0.84 mmol/L in plasma (1.68 mEq/L = 2 mg/dl), 60% is free, 25% is protein-bound, and 15% is complexed with bicarbonate, phosphate, and citrate. About 10% of the total body magnesium exchanges readily with injected magnesium. Magnesium is eliminated from the body primarily by the kidney. Little magnesium appears in urine at plasma concentrations less than normal, but at concentrations greater than 1.0-1.5 mmol/L renal tubular reabsorption maxima are exceeded, and excess magnesium appears in urine in direct proportion to the concentration in plasma and the glomerular filtration rate. The pregnant woman given magnesium may be especially at risk for magnesium toxicity if her renal perfusion and glomerular filtration decrease, permitting magnesium to accumulate in the blood.

Magnesium is generally given as magnesium sulfate, 50% (500 g/L), that provides in each 2-ml ampule 4 mmol of magnesium. Injected intramuscularly, this solution hurts. Intravenously, doses of 0.02 mmol/kg•hours are given for 1 day in treating severe magnesium deficiency. In a healthy 70-kg patient this provides, in 24 hours, 34 mmol of magnesium or about 2.6 times the total amount present in extracellular fluid and one-fourth of the total rapidly exchangeable magnesium in the healthy body. In severe magnesium deficiency, with blood concentrations less than 0.5 mmol/L, there often is peaking of the T wave, prolongation of the QRS complexes, and supraventricular and ventricular tachyarrhythmias, especially in patients receiving digitalis glycosides. Magnesium deficiency also causes anorexia, nausea, coarse tremor, muscle fibrillation, asterixis, choreiform twitches, myoclonic jerks, and focal and generalized major motor seizures. In addition, magnesium depletion leads to hypocalcemia in most patients, except those with primary reduction in tubular magnesium reabsorption and in the familial disorder associated with hypokalemia. The hypocalcemia is due to reduced secretion of parathormone, reduced responsiveness of target cells to parathormone, and abnormal responsiveness of bone calcium reserves to hypocalcemia.

Aggressive treatment of magnesium deficient patients is relatively safe in the presence of normal renal function, because excessive magnesium that elevates plasma concentrations are excreted promptly in the urine. However, women with eclampsia are treated with magnesium sulfate intravenously in doses as great as 0.07 mmol/kg•hours that provide, in 24 hours, 7.5 times the total amount of magnesium present normally in extracellular fluid. The target serum concentration is 3-4 mmol/L, but at the time of delivery women have had concentrations of 1.2-7 mmol/L. Fetal blood concentrations are similar to those in the mother, especially if magnesium has been given for 24 hours or more. As plasma magnesium concentrations rise to 5 mmol/L, there may be feeling of warmth, from superficial vasodilation, as well as nausea, vomiting, lethargy, confusion, hypotension, bradycardia, junctional rhythms, and neuromuscular blockade. Magnesium inhibits acetylcholine release and at plasma concentrations of 7-8 mmol/L, there may be complete paralysis of all muscles except the diaphragm, vocal cord abductors, and facial muscles. Levels only slightly greater lead to death from hypopnea and asystole. Thus, the most dangerous sign of magnesium intoxication in a patient is the loss of deep tendon reflexes that occurs at magnesium levels close to those associated with death.

Magnesium poisoning is not restricted to intramuscular or intravenous administration. The highest magnesium concentration ever recorded, 17.9 mmol/L, was noted in a patient who took by mouth about 1 mol of magnesium. Magnesium containing antacids or cathartics are especially dangerous in patients with acute or chronic renal failure. Even rectal administration may be dangerous, as one death resulted from enemas with magnesium sulfate to cleanse the bowel and decrease increased intracranial pressure.

Life-threatening hypermagnesemia may be treated in three ways. Calcium antagonizes most or all the effects of magnesium excess, and calcium 2.5-5.0 mmol, should be given intravenously. Remember that 1 g in 10 ml of calcium gluconate contains 2.2 mmol calcium, and the same mass of calcium chloride contains 9 mmol. The chloride salt is always preferred, as the gluconate complex is removed slowly and variably by the liver and is less reliable in increasing free calcium concentrations. Glucose and insulin promote intracellular incorporation of magnesium. Magnesium may also be removed by hemodialysis exchange transfusion.

REFERENCES

Dennis EJ III, Hester LL Jr: The preeclampsia-eclampsia syndrome. In: Obstetrics and Gynecology. Third Edition. Danforth DN (Ed). New York, Harper and Row, 1977, pp 391-409

Ditzler JW: Epsom-salts poisoning and a review of magnesium-ion physiology. Anesthesiology 1970; 32:378

Katz AI, Davision IM, Hayslett JP, et al: Pregnancy in women with kidney disease. Kidney Int 1980; 18:192

Lipsitz PJ: The clinical and biochemical effects of excess magnesium in the newborn. Pediatrics 1971; 47:501

Parfitt AM, Kleerekoper M: Clinical disorders of calcium, phosphorous, and magnesium metabolisn. In: Clinical Disorders of Fluid and Electrolyte Metabolism. Third Edition. Maxwell MH, Kleeman CR (Eds). New York, McGraw-Hill Book Company, 1980, pp 947-1151

Parfitt AM, Kleerekoper M: The divalent ion homeostatic system--physiology and metabolism of calcium phosphorous, magnesium, and bone. In: Fluid and Electrolyte Metabolism. Third Edition. Maxwell MH, Kleeman CR (Eds). New York, McGraw-Hill Book Company, 1980, pp 269-398

Pritchard JA: Management of preeclampsia and eclampsia. Kidney Int 1980; 18:259

Stevens AR Jr, Wolff HG: Magnesium intoxication: Absorption from the intact gastrointestinal tract. Arch Neurol Psychiatry 1950; 63:759

White RD, Goldsmith RS, Rodriguez R, et al: Plasma ionic calcium levels following injection of chloride, gluconate, and gluceptate salts of calcium. J Thorac Cardiovasc Surg 1976; 71:609

PREMATURE LABOR

RATIONALE 188-e

Amniotic fluid lecithin and sphingomyelin ratio (L/S ratio) has been shown to consistently reflect lung maturity of the growing fetus. Lecithin and sphingomyelin are phospholipids synthesized in the alveolar lining of the lungs. The site of production is the type II cells. These phospholipids are released into the fetal lung fluid, which freely contributes to amniotic fluid formation. Hence, the ingenious method developed by Gluck et al. provides an easy method of assessing fetal lung maturity by measuring L/S ratio in amniotic fluid obtained from amniocentesis. The phospholipids extracted from amniotic fluid are separated by thin layer chromatography and the individual phospholipids are quantitated. In a study of serial amniotic fluid measurements, lecithin and sphingomyelin concentrations remain low up to 35 weeks of gestation, but lecithin increases suddenly at 35 weeks. When expressed in L/S ratio, it reaches a level of > 2 at 35 weeks. Clinically, it has been shown that L/S ratios of 1 are associated with severe hyaline membrane disease; ratios of 1.0 to 1.5 mean moderately severe disease and 1.5 to 2.0 indicates mild disease. Thus, L/S ratio, a semiquantitative estimation of lung surfactants, is a most useful test in predictng lung maturity of the fetus.

Estriol excretion in the maternal urine predicts the state of fetal health. Urinary estriols in the mother are derived from fetal adrenal steroids which are converted by the placenta to estriols. These estriols enter into maternal circulation and are excreted. There is a wide variation of estriol excretion in the mother. Estriol excretions are, thus, dependent on the fetal, placental, and uterine status. Although urinary estriols increase with gestational age, low estriols are associated with uteroplacenta insufficiency and fetal distress and not fetal lung maturity.

Amniotic fluid α-antitrypsin has not been found to be a good predictor of lung maturity. In one study, it was shown to have no correlation to amniotic fluid phospholipid concentration. Whereas ultrasonographic measurement of biparietal diameter of fetal head is a useful tool to assess fetal growth, ultrasonographic measurement of fetal chest dimensions does not provide any information regarding fetal lung maturity.

REFERENCES

Campbell S: The assessment of fetal development by diagnostic ultrasound. Clin Perinatal 1974; 1:507

Gluck L, Kulovich MV, Borer RC Jr, et al: Diagnosis of the respiratory distress syndrome by amniocentesis. Am J Gynecol 1971; 109:440

Greene JW Jr, Touchstone JC: Urinary estriol as an index of placental function: A study of 279 cases. Am J Obstet Gynecol 1963; 85:1

Pritchard JA, MacDonald PC: Techniques to evaluate fetal health. Williams Obstetrics. Fifteenth Edition. New York, Appleton-Century-Crofts, 1976, pp 265-293

RATIONALE 189-b

The physiology of human labor is not yet fully understood. The process is complex and involves several endocrine changes in both the fetus and mother. The primary signal at term probably comes from the fetal central nervous system. A series of changes involving the fetal hypothalamic-pituitary-adrenal axis occurs with release of oxytocin. Similar changes in the same axis occur in the mother. It is thought that a decrease in progesterone stimulates labor, though this has not been proven unequivocally in the human. Prostaglandin levels are elevated during labor though their precise role also remains to be elucidated. The final common pathway in labor, however, is stimulation of the α-receptors in the myometrium and resultant contraction.

Therapeutic efforts to slow or halt premature labor have focused on four areas. The progesterone decrease has been treated with progesterone infusions. This has been largely unsuccessful. Blockade of the increase in prostaglandins with anti-inflammatory agents (e.g., aspirin or indomethacin) that inhibit prostaglandin synthesis have been criticized because of potential harmful effects on the fetus (e.g., closure of the ductus arteriosus).

Inhibition of oxytocin release from the pituitary by ethanol has been widely used and appears to produce statistically significant reduction in premature births. Criticisms of this therapy are based on lack of efficacy, difficulty in patient selection, and possible effects on the fetus.

Recently, data have been accumulating showing the efficacy of β-agonists in the treatment of premature labor. β-2 receptors are found in the myometrium and their stimulation causes uterine relaxation. Several β-2 agonists have been tested and, in the United States, ritodrine has been shown to stop premature labor more effectively than ethanol. Effects of ritodrine on the maternal cardiovascular system have not been alarming and significant effects on the fetus have not been noted, though few studies have yet been conducted. The β-adrenergic agonists and ethanol appear to work at different levels in the labor process and, thus, combined therapy may be possible.

Neither histamine nor serotonin (5-hydroxytryptamine) have significant effect on the human uterus. Similarly, muscarinic blockers such as atropine or scopolamine have little effect on uterine contractions.

REFERENCES

Fuchs F: Prevention of prematurity. Am J Obstet Gynecol 1976; 126:809

Fuchs F: Treatment of threatened premature labor with alcohol. Br J Obstet Gynaecol 1965; 72:1011

Landesman R, Wilson KH, Coutinho EM, et al: The relaxant action of ritodrine, a sympathomimetic amine, on the uterus during term labor. Am J Obstet Gynecol 1971; 110:111

Lauersen NH, Merkatz IR, Tejani N, et al: Inhibition of premature labor: A multicenter comparison of ritodrine and ethanol. Am J Obstet Gynecol 1977; 127:837

Zlatnik F, Fuchs F: A controlled study of ethanol in threatened premature labor. Am J Obstet Gynecol 1972; 112:610

Section 12

190. The MOST common cause of acute respiratory failure in the premature newborn is:

a. Heart failure from congenital heart disease
b. Diaphragmatic hernia
c. Neonatal sepsis and pneumonia
d. Hyaline membrane disease
e. Meconium aspiration syndrome

191. Which ONE of the following statements regarding circulatory causes of respiratory distress in the newborn is CORRECT?

a. Cardiac failure due to ventricular septal defect (VSD) usually occurs within the first six days after birth.
b. Cardiac murmurs are a reliable sign of functional heart problems in the newborn.
c. A patent ductus arteriosus is suggested by a higher PaO_2 in blood sampled from the umbilical artery compared with the PaO_2 drawn from the radial artery.
d. Cardiac failure occurring within several days of birth is compatible with hypoplastic left heart syndrome.

192. Which ONE of the following statements regarding renal function and fluid requirements in the pediatric patient is correct?

a. Total body water in the newborn is the same in relative proportion to total weight as in the five-year-old child.
b. Even the immature kidney in the neonate is able to avidly preserve sodium.
c. Rapid rehydration of the infant with hypertonic dehydration is beneficial in re-establishing the extracellular volume and poses no significant danger to the infant.
d. Even with severe dehydration the neonate is unable to concentrate urine more than 700 to 800 mOsm/L.

Questions 193-194 refer to the following patient: A 6-month-old infant is admitted to the ICU with a history of diarrhea. The child is very irritable. On physical examination, the infant has a pulse of 180/min and a blood pressure of 50/0. Laboratory results are shown below.

Serum Na^+	170 mEq/L
Serum K^+	5.5 mEq/L
Serum Cl^-	140 mEq/L
Serum CO_2	12 mEq/L
Serum BUN	50 mg%
Serum Creatinine	3.0 mg%

193. Which ONE of the following statements is TRUE?

  a. This patient must be closely monitored for hypercalcemia during rehydration.
  b. A fluid bolus of 20 ml/kg of normal saline is contraindicated because of the sodium load.
  c. Hypertonicity is confined to the extracellular space.
  d. Seizures may be a complication of therapy.

194. After initial rehydration, the above infant has a urinary output of 50 ml in 24 hours. The urine Na is 10 mEq/L, the urinary creatinine is 100 mg/dl, and the serum creatinine is 2 mg/dl. The infant weighs 5 kg.

Which ONE of the following statements is TRUE?

  a. This infant has sustained severe ischemic damage to the kidney, resulting in cortical necrosis.
  b. The urine:plasma osmolality ratio is probably less than 1.5.
  c. The infant will benefit from a normal saline bolus of 20 ml/kg over 1 hour.
  d. Furosemide 1 mg/kg iv is the treatment of choice.

PEDIATRICS/NEONATAL

ANSWERS

190-d 191-d 192-d 193-d 194-c

RATIONALE 190-d

Hyaline membrane disease (HMD) continues to be one of the most common causes of neonatal morbidity and mortality. It is the major cause of respiratory failure. Respiratory failure is secondary to lung immaturity. The main underlying mechanism in HMD is surfactant deficiency, which leads to severe alveolar instability. Because of surfactant deficiency, the lung tends to collapse. Retention of alveolar air following the first breath determines the subsequent amount of pressure required to sustain air exchange without collapse of the lung. The capability of retention of air within the lung at the end of expiration is the single most important physiologic phenomenon. This property of the alveolar stability at the end of expiration is attributed to the air-liquid interface formed by the phospholipids at the alveolar surface. There is sufficient evidence to support the finding that surfactant is deficient in infants with HMD. These factors, i.e., alveolar collapse, lead to severe intrapulmonary shunting. Resultant hypoxia leads to metabolic and respiratory acidosis, and atelectasis to increased work of breathing. All these factors end in acute respiratory failure.

Although congenital heart disease may present as acute respiratory failure in the premature infant, it is not the most common cause. Further, these infants develop primary cyanosis with little or no CO_2 retention. Only when severely hypoxic do the infants develop hypercapnia. Most infants with congenital disease are born at term.

Diaphragmatic hernia usually causes respiratory distress at birth. These infants usually are term. Clinically, they present with the following: scaphoid abdomen, bowel sounds in the chest, and roentgenography shows evidence of bowel in the thorax.

Neonatal sepsis and pneumonia are associated with respiratory distress and may lead to respiratory failure. In these infants, associated findings include severe hypothermia, hypotension, and changes in hematologic indices including neutropenia and granulocyte immaturity. However, sepsis as a cause of respiratory failure ranks only after HMD.

Meconium aspiration syndrome is usually associated with term infants. The major pathophysiology in these infants is an obstructive phenomenon, an inflammatory phenomenon, and physiological changes that result in severe pulmonary vasoconstriction and left to right shunt with severe cyanosis.

REFERENCES

Avery ME: Respiratory distress syndrome: State-of-the-art. In: Respiratory Distress Syndrome. Villee CA, Villee DB, Zuckerman J (Eds). New York, Academic Press, 1973, pp 1-6

Farrell PM, Avery ME: Hyaline membrane disease. Am Rev Respir Dis 1975; 111:657

RATIONALE 191-d

Early onset of heart failure with acyanotic respiratory disease suggests hypoplastic left heart syndrome, interrupted aortic arch, or other severe myocardial disorders. Cardiac failure due to coarctation of the aorta or large left-to-right shunts usually does not occur until six days or more after birth, as do septal defects, patent ductus arteriosus, endocardial cushion defects, anomalous pulmonary venous drainage without obstruction, and arteriovenous fistulas (often detected by auscultating the skull). Cardiac murmurs are not a reliable sign of abnormality in the first few days of life, since they are frequently functional and transient, and may be associated with ductal closure.

When history and physical examination fail to differentiate respiratory from circulatory disease, a variety of diagnostic techniques may be used. For example, a PDA is suggested by a lower arterial oxygen tension in arterial blood sampled from the aorta below the ductus (through the umbilical artery) compared with that obtained from preductal sampling (through right radial arteries).

REFERENCES

Bhat R, et al: Patent ductus arteriosus: Recent advances in diagnosis and management. Pediatr Clin North Am 1982; 29:1117

McNamara DB: Twenty-five years of progress in the medical treatment of pediatric and congenital heart disease. J Am Coll Cardiol 1983; 1:264

Swyer PR: Respiratory disturbances in the newborn other than the respiratory distress syndrome. In: Textbook of Critical Care. Shoemaker WC, Thompson WL, Holbrook PR (Eds). Philadelphia, WB Saunders Co., 1984, pp 286-301

RATIONALE 192-d

Newborns and small infants have a higher proportion of body water to total body weight primarily as extracellular fluid. As they mature, not only does the kidney become more able to preserve water and electrolytes through increasing concentrating ability, but the relative amount of fluid in the extracellular fluid space decreases in comparison to that in the intracellular fluid space. Maturation of the kidney during the first year of life gives the child about the same conserving and concentrating ability as the adult.

Infants with hypertonic dehydration pose a particular problem. The hypertonicity is shared by all body fluid compartments and rapid isotonic or hypotonic expansion of the extracellular space can lead to cellular swelling, causing, among other things, cerebral edema, seizures and even coma. Rehydration should be accomplished slowly and at such a rate that the serum sodium concentration drops by no more than 10 mEq/L per 24 hours.

REFERENCES

Edelmann C Jr: Fluid and electrolyte problems in the child. In: Critical Care: State of the Art. Vol 3. Shoemaker WC, Thompson WL (Eds). Fullerton, CA, Society of Critical Care Medicine, 1982, pp III(M):1-36

Finberg L: Hypernatremia (hypertonic) dehydration in infants. N Engl J Med 1973; 289:196

Tejani A, Dobias B, Mahadevan K: Osmolar relationships in infantile dehydration. Am J Dis Child 1981; 135:1000

RATIONALE 193-d 194-c

This infant has hypertonic dehydration and is in shock. Decreased blood pressure with hypertonic plasma implies severe volume depletion. A fluid bolus of 20 ml/kg of normal saline would be life-saving in this child and should be repeated if the initial dose does not restore the infant's perfusion. Hypertonicity is found in all compartments and, therefore, too rapid rehydration with hypotonic fluids may cause water to be drawn into the central nervous system with resultant cerebral edema and seizures. Hypocalcemia is occasionally seen with rehydration, particularly when the patient is hypertonic.

This infant is oliguric as defined by a urinary output of less than 15-20 ml/kg/24 hours. The urinary sodium is low and the urine Na/U:P creatinine ratio is less than 1 indicating intact tubular function. This implies functional oliguria rather than organic oliguria. Because the tubular system is intact, the urine:plasma osmolality ratio will probably be greater than 1.5. A normal saline bolus would be beneficial in this child. Furosemide is not indicated.

REFERENCES

Edelman C: Fluid and electrolyte problems in the child. In: Critical Care: State of the Art. Shoemaker WC, Thompson WL (Eds). Vol 3. Fullerton, CA, Society of Critical Care Medicine, 1982, pp III(M):15-17, 20-21

Feig PU, McCurdy DK: The hypertonic state. N Engl J Med 1977; 297:1444

Finberg L: Treatment of dehydration in infancy. Pediatrics in Review 1981; 3:113

Perkin R, et al: Shock in the pediatric patient. J Pediatr 1982; 101:163

Section 13

Questions 195-199: Match each drug below with the pattern in the table that MOST closely reflects its adrenergic receptor activity. Choices a-e can be used once, more than once, or not at all.

Table Code: 0 = No change
+ = Slight stimulation
++ = Moderate stimulation
+++ = Marked stimulation

195. Norepinephrine

196. Isoproterenol

197. Dobutamine

198. Dopamine

199. Phenylephrine

	Alpha (Peripheral)	Beta-1 (Cardiac)	Beta-2 (Peripheral)
a.	+	++	+
b.	+++	++	0
c.	++	++	+
d.	+++	0	0
e.	0	+++	+++

200. Each of the following drugs can be used as a vasopressor EXCEPT:

a. Dopamine
b. Dobutamine
c. Norepinephrine
d. Phenylephrine

201. Which ONE of the following statements concerning the effect of dopamine is CORRECT?

a. At infusion rates between 5-9 µg/kg•min, dopamine is predominantly a dopaminergic receptor stimulator (renal prophylaxis) with very little alpha- or beta-adrenergic action.
b. As a beta agent, dopamine is primarily an inotrope with minimal chronotropic effects.
c. The addition of dobutamine to dopamine therapy may allow a reduction in the dopamine infusion rate and maintenance of the same cardiac output with less alpha-adrenergic effect.
d. Any increase in urine output associated with institution of dopamine at 7 µg/kg•min is primarily due to its action as a diuretic.
e. Dopamine is most appropriately used in a peripheral vein.

202. Usual effects of digoxin on the heart include:

a. Increased resting membrane potential
b. Decreased rate of spontaneous (phase 4) diastolic depolarization
c. Decreased intracellular free calcium concentrations
d. Accelerated atrioventricular (AV) conduction velocity
e. None of the above

203. Which ONE of the following statements is LEAST correct about both dopamine and dobutamine?

a. Both increase heart force by an action antagonized by propranolol.
b. Both increase heart rate by an action antagonized by propranolol.
c. Both increase coronary blood flow if vessels are patent.
d. Both are normally present in the body.
e. Neither dilates bronchioles.

204. A 68-year old patient is admitted to the ICU in atrial fibrillation with a rapid ventricular response. Subsequent digitalization lowers the ventricular rate below 100 beats per minute. Because the arrhythmia persists, the patient is begun on quinidine sulfate 200 mg po every six hours.

Which of the following statements is true?

a. Concomitant use of digoxin and quinidine results in elevated quinidine levels and increased quinidine toxicity.
b. Quinidine impairs digoxin enhancement of transmembrane calcium flux.
c. Both digoxin and quinidine slow conduction through the AV node.
d. The dose of digoxin should be reduced.

205. Which ONE of the following statements concerning cephalosporins is LEAST correct?

a. Cefuroxime offers significantly greater CNS penetration when compared to other first and second generation cephalosporins.
b. Ceftriaxone offers adequate therapy for disseminated gonococcus if penicillin resistance is suspected.
c. Ceftazidime offers significant activity against pseudomonas as a single agent.
d. Ceftazidime offers considerable efficacy in the treatment of pulmonary infections in cystic fibrosis.
e. Ceftizoxime has high activity against pseudomonas meningitis but requires concomitant vitamin K therapy to avoid bleeding complications.

206. Which ONE of the following is NOT a sign of toxicity of gentamicin?

a. Increase in serum creatinine concentration
b. Tremors
c. Ataxia
d. Deafness
e. Respiratory insufficiency

207. Antimicrobial prophylaxis is effective in decreasing postoperative wound infection in each of the following EXCEPT:

a. Arterial reconstructive surgery of the abdominal aorta
b. Craniotomy for meningioma removal
c. Vaginal hysterectomy
d. Total hip replacement

208. Which ONE of the following drugs is primarily excreted via renal mechanisms?

a. Clindamycin
b. Chloramphenicol
c. Erythromycin
d. Cefoxitin

209. Which ONE of the following antibiotics LEAST effectively crosses the blood brain barrier?

a. Cefuroxime
b. Tobramycin
c. Chloramphenicol
d. Ampicillin
e. Ticarcillin

210. Which ONE of the following statements concerning third generation cephalosporins is TRUE?

a. Third generation cephalosporins offer an excellent single drug alternative for treatment of non-urinary tract pseudomonas infection.
b. Third generation cephalosporins are superior to first and second generation cephalosporins in surgical prophylaxis.
c. Third generation cephalosporins offer good coverage for Gram-negative bacillary meningitis.
d. Over 50% of healthy volunteers given high doses of moxalactum develop clotting factor abnormalities.

211. Which of the following statements is most correct about the mechanism of action of heparin as an anticoagulant?

a. Heparin augments the activity of a naturally occurring anti-coagulant.
b. Heparin inhibits hepatic synthesis of vitamin K-dependent coagulation proteins (II, VII, IX, X).
c. Heparin directly interferes with prothrombin conversion to thrombin.
d. Heparin inhibits activation of Hageman factor (XII).
e. None of the above

212. Quinidine, procainamide, propranolol, lidocaine and phenytoin (diphenylhydantoin) ALL share which common effect?

a. Increase effective refractory period relative to action potential duration
b. Increase rate of sodium influx through the fast channel
c. Decrease rate of sodium influx through the fast channel
d. Decrease RR interval in most patients
e. Decrease HV interval in most patients

Questions 213-215: For each numbered item, select the one lettered heading that is most closely associated with it. Each lettered heading may be used once, more than once, or not at all.

a. Verapamil
b. Nifedipine
c. Prazosin
d. Pindolol

213. Partial beta-1 agonist

214. Alpha-1 antagonist

215. Reflex tachycardia

216. Following acute myocardial infarction, which ONE of the following drugs is most likely to DECREASE the subsequent incidence of myocardial reinfarction?

a. Diltiazem
b. Verapamil
c. Pindolol
d. Timolol

Questions 217-221: For each numbered item, select the one lettered heading that is most closely associated with it. Each lettered heading may be used once, more than once, or not at all.

a. Minoxidil
b. Metoprolol
c. Captopril
d. Nadalol

217. Associated with increased renin and decreased aldosterone levels

218. Vasodilator

219. Hypertrichosis

220. Hyperkalemia

221. Beta-1 selective adrenergic blocker

222. Which ONE of the following statements concerning labetalol is FALSE?

a. Labetalol is a combined alpha- and beta-adrenoceptor blocking agent effective in the intravenous treatment of hypertensive emergencies.
b. Unlike conventional beta-adrenoceptor blocking drugs without intrinsic sympathomimetic activity, labetalol, when given acutely produces a decrease in peripheral vascular resistance and blood pressure with little alteration in heart rate or cardiac output.
c. Labetalol produces a significant reduction in cerebral blood flow and should be avoided in patients with cerebral vascular disease.
d. Labetalol should not be utilized in hypertensive emergencies in patients with active bronchospasm.
e. Decline in diastolic blood pressure following the initial dose of labetalol can be used to approximate the total intravenous dose required for hypertensive emergencies.

223. Which ONE of the following statements concerning aminophylline therapy is FALSE?

a. Aminophylline improves diaphragmatic contractility.
b. Aminophylline potentiates the effect of beta-agonist drugs.
c. Aminophylline has a positive chronotropic effect.
d. Erythromycin shortens the half-life of theophylline.

224. Which ONE of the following phrases about verapamil is TRUE?

a. Positive inotropic action
b. Increases AV nodal conduction
c. Positive chronotropic action
d. Vasodilator action

225. Which ONE of the following statements about the calcium channel antagonists diltiazem, nifedipine and verapamil is TRUE?

a. All three of these calcium antagonists have similar chemical structures.
b. All three are metabolized in the kidney.
c. All three slow AV conduction by increasing the HV time.
d. All three have limited usefulness in congestive heart failure.

226. Which ONE of the following corticosteroids has the MOST mineralocorticoid activity (i.e., tends to cause the most alkalosis)?

a. Hydrocortisone
b. Methylprednisolone
c. Prednisone
d. Dexamethasone

227. You are managing a patient who is comatose after severe head trauma. Your CT scanner is not functioning and because of rapidly progressive coma, you suspect a subdural hematoma and send the patient immediately for arteriography. Furosemide is given. Two hours after admission, a large subdural hematoma has been evacuated. Morphine was given preoperatively, vasopressin operatively, and the patient is now receiving dopamine at the rate of 2 μg/kg•min. At this time you observe the patient to have a urine output of 400 ml/h with a urinalysis of: clear, no observed sediment, pH = 6.5, specific gravity = 1.050, protein absent, glucose trace, acetone absent.

Which ONE of the following drugs is MOST likely to be the cause of this reaction?

a. Dopamine given at low doses
b. Vasopressin given during surgery
c. Morphine given preoperatively
d. Organic iodides given preoperatively
e. Furosemide given preoperatively

228. Hearing loss occurs LEAST frequently after large doses of:

a. Furosemide
b. Ethacrynic acid
c. Tobramycin
d. Vancomycin
e. Polymyxin B

229. Which ONE of the following drugs does not have its systemic clearance DECREASED by cimetidine?

a. Warfarin
b Propranolol
c. Theophylline
d. Tobramycin

230. When comparing intravenous ranitidine with intravenous cimetidine, which ONE of the following is the LEAST accurate?

a. Ranitidine has a longer duration of action than cimetidine.
b. Ranitidine is more likely to produce gynecomastia.
c. Cimetidine is associated with a higher incidence of central nervous system side effects.
d. Ranitidine exerts less interference with theophylline metabolism.

231. A patient is in the intensive care unit following abdominal surgery with narcotic/nitrous oxide anesthesia. He is mechanically ventilated with a ventilator rate set at 6 breaths/min and a tidal volume of 12 ml/kg. He is able to squeeze his hand lightly on command and lift his head from the bed on request. ABG's reveal PaO_2 120 mm Hg, $PaCO_2$ 48 mm Hg, pH 7.34. The patient is making no voluntary ventilatory effort.

Which statement below BEST explains the above findings?

a. Residual muscle relaxation from the anesthetic
b. Depressed ventilatory response to hypercapnia
c. Pain present during ventilation abolishes spontaneous respiratory effort.
d. Supernormal oxygenation decreases the need to breathe

Questions 232-233 refer to the following patient: A patient with a long history of chronic abdominal pain and multiple surgeries is in the intensive care unit and undergoes a right tube thoracostomy. The patient receives therapeutic doses of each of the following anesthetic agents: morphine for premedication, bupivacaine with 1/200,000 epinephrine for intercostal nerve block, xylocaine with 2/200,000 epinephrine for local incision block, and fentanyl citrate with droperidol. After the tube is placed, naloxone is administered, and the patient promptly develops tachycardia, restlessness, and generalized twitching.

232. Which ONE of the items below is the MOST probable diagnosis?

a. Bupivacaine toxicity
b. Xylocaine toxicity
c. Acquired tolerance to narcotic drugs
d. Vasovagal response

233. Which ONE of the following statements describes the MOST appropriate management for this condition?

a. Administration of oxygen and atropine
b. Administration of epinephrine
c. Administration of morphine intravenously
d. Close observation

234. Which ONE of the following drugs is LEAST likely to require a reduction in dose in a patient who develops anuric renal failure?

a. Gentamicin
b. Digoxin
c. Polymyxin B
d. Tetracycline
e. Chloramphenicol

235. Which ONE of the following drugs does not require a dose reduction in a patient who develops acute tubular necrosis?

a. Digitoxin
b. Gentamicin
c. Polymyxin B
d. Tobramycin
e. Trimethoprim-sulfamethoxazole

236. Which ONE of the following statements is MOST correct about the relative actions of intravenous nitroglycerin and nitroprusside in dilating venous and arterial vascular beds?

a. Both have about equal effects on venous and arterial beds.
b. Both dilate mostly venous beds.
c. Both dilate mostly arterial beds.
d. Nitroglycerin predominantly dilates venous beds and nitroprusside dilates both venous and arterial beds.
e. Nitroglycerin dilates arterial beds and nitroprusside both venous and arterial beds.

237. Which ONE of the following has NOT been used effectively to treat toxicity associated with sodium nitroprusside?

a. Thiosulfate
b. Hydroxocobalamin
c. Sodium nitrite
d. Cyanocobalamin

238. Which ONE of the following statements regarding the effects of nitroglycerin is LEAST correct?

a. Dilatation of venous capacitance vessels
b. Dilatation of collateral coronary blood vessels
c. A decrease in the left ventricular wall tension
d. No significant effect on intracranial pressure in patients with head trauma

ANSWERS

195-b	196-e	197-a	198-c	199-d	200-b	201-c	202-e
203-d	204-d	205-e	206-b	207-b	208-d	209-b	210-c
211-a	212-a	213-d	214-c	215-b	216-d	217-c	218-a
219-a	220-c	221-b	222-c	223-d	224-d	225-d	226-a
227-d	228-e	229-d	230-b	231-b	232-c	233-c	234-e
235-a	236-d	237-d	238-d				

ADRENERGIC AND INOTROPIC AGENTS

RATIONALE 195-b 196-e 197-a 198-c 199-d

The clinical effects of the sympathomimetic amines are predominantly determined by their adrenergic receptor activity which is indicated in the table below.

RELATIVE ADRENERGIC RECEPTOR ACTIVITY OF SYMPATHOMIMETIC AMINES

	Alpha (Peripheral)	Beta-1 (Cardiac)	Beta-2 (Peripheral)
Norepinephrine	+++	++	0
Isoproterenol	0	+++	+++
Dobutamine	+	++	+
Dopamine	++	++	+
Phenylephrine	+++	0	0

REFERENCES

Miller RD, Stoelting RK: Pharmacology of the autonomic nervous system. In: Anesthesia. Miller RD (Ed). New York, Churchill Livingstone, 1981, pp 539-562

Smith TW, Braunwald E: The management of heart failure. In: Heart Disease. Braunwald E (Ed). Philadelphia, WB Saunders Co., 1984, pp 503-559

Sonnenblick EH, Frishman WH, Le Jenitel TH: Dobutamine: A new synthetic cardioactive sympathetic amine. N Engl J Med 1979; 300:17

RATIONALE 200-b

Dopamine (at high infusion rates), norepinephrine and phenylephrine are all vasopressors which act directly or indirectly at alpha-adrenergic receptors to increase systemic vascular resistance. Dobutamine increases cardiac output and blood pressure by increasing cardiac contractility. It does not have alpha-adrenergic activity.

REFERENCES

Chernow B, Fletcher JR: Catecholamines, opioid peptides and prostaglandins. In: Critical Care: State of the Art. Vol 4. Shoemaker WC, Thompson WL (Eds). Fullerton, CA, Society of Critical Care Medicine, 1983, pp IV(E):1-53

Zaritsky A, Chernow B: Catecholamine and sympathomimetics. In: The Pharmacologic Approach to the Critically Ill Patient. Chernow B (Ed). Baltimore, William & Wilkins Co., 1983, pp 481-510

RATIONALE 201-c

At rates between 1-3 µg/kg•min, dopamine has little alpha- or beta-adrenergic effects and is predominantly a dopaminergic receptor stimulator, producing increased renal blood flow. Although dopamine has been shown to exert a diuretic effect, this is not proven to be of clinical efficacy. Dopamine's effect on increasing urine output is predominantly due to the increased cardiac output and not due to its known diuretic action. Dobutamine may be infused concurrently with dopamine in patients requiring both inotropic and peripheral vascular resistance support. In this capacity, it augments the inotropic action of dopamine with negligible direct effect on systemic vascular resistance, allowing dopamine dosage to be decreased. Thus, the same blood pressure may be maintained with less deleterious vasoconstricting effect. Infiltration of dopamine infusion in a peripheral vein may lead to significant tissue necrosis. Except in the arrest setting when no central line is available, it should be infused through a central line.

REFERENCES

Parker S, Carlon GC, Isaacs M, et al: Dopamine administration in oliguria and oliguric renal failure. Crit Care Med 1981; 9:360

Raiffer SI, Goldbert LI: Sympathomimetic amines in the treatment of shock. In: Textbook of Critical Care. Shoemaker WC, Thompson WL, Holbrook PR (Eds). Philadelphia, WB Saunders Co., 1984, pp 491-492

RATIONALE 202-e

Cardiac glycosides, such as digoxin, inhibit a myocardial Na^+/K^+ ATPase leading to a gradual reduction in intracellular potassium. As the resting membrane potential is related to the ratio of intra- to extracellular potassium, one of the direct effects of digoxin is to reduce the resting membrane potential. The inotropic effects of digoxin are probably caused by increased intracellular free calcium concentrations, possibly due to displacement of calcium from binding sites by higher concentrations of intracellular sodium. The rate of spontaneous (phase 4) diastolic depolarization is increased in digitalis intoxication, predisposing to ventricular tachyarrhythmias. Atrioventricular conduction is decreased by digitalis, both by enhanced vagal tone and by a direct effect.

REFERENCE

Nies AS: Heart failure. In: Clinical Pharmacology, Basic Principles in Therapeutics. Second Edition. Melmon KL, Morrelli HF (Eds). New York, Macmillan Publishing Co. Inc., 1978, pp 261-266

RATIONALE 203-d

Dopamine and dobutamine act directly upon beta-adrenergic receptors to increase heart rate and heart force. Their action is therefore antagonized by propranolol. Dopamine has a direct dose-dependent coronary vasodilating effect in special situations, but the predominant effect of both dopamine and dobutamine on myocardial blood flow is caused by their positive inotropic actions that increase oxygen demand. Increased heart work makes coronary blood flow increase, if the vessels are patent and capable of relaxation, if diastolic coronary perfusion pressure is maintained, if diastolic ventricular pressures are not increased, and if heart rates are sufficiently slow to permit coronary flow to occur during diastole. Of these factors, direct coronary vasodilation is probably the least important, especially in the seriously-ill, hypoperfused patient. All catecholamines may induce tachycardia, excessive myocardial oxygen demand, and myocardial ischemia and necrosis. Individual patient responses vary greatly in heart failure, shock and other hypoperfusion states. Neither dopamine nor dobutamine effectively dilate bronchioles.

Dobutamine is not a normal body product, but dopamine is decarboxylated L-dopa, an essential normal body constituent. Although dopamine is further beta-oxidized to norepinephrine, its hemodynamic effects are not dependent upon norepinephrine release or synthesis.

REFERENCES

Loeb HS, Khan M, Sandye A, et al: Acute hemodynamic effects of dobutamine and isoproterenol in patients with low output cardiac failure. Circ Shock 1976; 3:55

Maroko PR, Libby P, Covell JW, et al: Precordial ST segment mapping; an atraumatic method for assessing alterations in the extent of myocardial ischemia injury: The effects of pharmacologic and hemodynamic interventions. Am J Cardiol 1972; 29:233

Mueller HS: The heart and oxygen transport. In: The Organ in Shock. Thompson WL (Ed). New York, Informedia, 1977, pp 38-49

Robie NW, Goldberg LI: Comparative systemic and regional hemodynamic effects of dopamine and dobutamine. Am Heart J 1975; 90:340

Thompson WL: Drug therapy of shock. In: Recent Advances in Clinical Pharmacology. Vol 1. Turner P, Shand D (Eds). New York, Churchill Livingstone, 1978, pp 123-145

Toda N, Goldberg LI: Effects of dopamine on isolated canine coronary arteries. Cardiovasc Res 1975; 9:384

RATIONALE 204-d

Although the first published reports appeared less than seven years ago, the quinidine-digoxin interaction is a well-established clinical entity. Serum digoxin levels rise in 90% of patients who subsequently receive quinidine. Approximately half of these patients develop symptoms of nausea, vomiting, diarrhea and less frequently, cardiac arrhythmias. Since serum digoxin levels usually double, a reduction by one-half the daily dose is usually recommended.

Digoxin slows conduction through the AV node. Quinidine speeds conduction through the AV node and may increase the ventricular response if used for atrial tachycardias without prior digitalization.

REFERENCES

Doering W: Quinidine-digoxin interactions: Pharmacokinetics, underlying mechanism and clinical implications. N Engl J Med 1979; 301:400

Mungall DR, Robichaux RP, et al: Effects of quinidine on serum digoxin concentration. Ann Intern Med 1980; 93:689

EDITORIAL COMMENT

Studies continue to show a renal vasodilatory effect of low dose dopamine. This action persists despite infusions of strong vasopressors such as norepinephrine which decrease renal blood flow. Patients in shock maintained on potent vasopressors might, therefore, receive consideration for low dose dopamine therapy (2-3 μg/kg•min) even though absolute proof of clinical benefit is lacking.

The goal of shock treatment is improvement in delivery of oxygenated blood to peripheral tissues without jeopardizing the balance between myocardial oxygen supply and demand. When dopamine, dobutamine, and isoproterenol are compared as single agents in the treatment of shock after adequate intravascular volume expansion has been accomplished, the following has been shown: (1) Since dobutamine has less effect on increasing pulse, pulmonary artery occlusion pressure, and systemic vascular resistance when compared to isoproterenol and dopamine, it seems a reasonable first choice in the treatment of cardiogenic shock. (2) In patients with septic shock, in whom coronary perfusion reserve may exist when compared to cardiogenic shock, isoproterenol might offer an advantage since the increase in cardiac output, stroke volume, and LVSWI is greater than that observed with dobutamine.

Toxic shock syndrome with acute febrile multi-organ systemic illness can be associated with significant hypotension. Studies suggest a reversible toxic cardiomyopathy as the cause of cardiorespiratory failure in toxic shock syndrome. Inotropic support with dobutamine is beneficial in selective cases.

Acute right ventricular failure is a common cause of death in massive pulmonary embolism. Intravenous dobutamine was used in ten patients with massive pulmonary embolism and circulatory failure. Success was reported in nine out of ten patients. Dopamine infusion was associated with an increased cardiac index and stroke index, as well as reduced pulmonary vascular resistance. Patients required dobutamine support for a mean of 3.3 days after initiation. The patients received concurrent anticoagulant treatment as well.

Digitalis remains an important drug in the management of atrial tachyarrhythmias. Use in pre-excitation syndromes such as WPW may, however, be dangerous. Although mortality is unaffected by digitalis following myocardial infarction, the decrease in symptoms appears to justify its continued use in selected cases with severe cardiac failure in whom other inotropes seem less advantageous. Digoxin can exert favorable hemodynamic effects during acute myocardial infarction in patients with moderate left ventricular failure. This may well be due to a net decrease in myocardial oxygen requirements in spite of enhanced contractility. This is associated with reduced left ventricular volume and wall tension.

The serum digoxin concentration should be interpreted in light of the clinical setting. With the appropriate symptom complex, toxicity should be suspected even if levels are in the high therapeutic range. Some patients may, however, demonstrate beneficial arrhythmia control rather than toxicity with digoxin levels above the usual therapeutic range. This is particularly true when digoxin is being used to block AV conduction.

ADDITIONAL REFERENCES

Fisher CH, Horowitz BZ, Albertson TE: Cardiorespiratory failure in toxic shock syndrome: Effect of dobutamine. Crit Care Med 1985; 13:160

Jardin F, Genevray B, Brunney D, et al: Dobutamine: A hemodynamic evaluation in pulmonary embolism shock. Crit Care Med 1985; 13:1009

Marchionni N, Pini R, Vannucci A, et al: Hemodynamic effects of digoxin in acute myocardial infarction in man: A randomized controlled trial. Am Heart J 1985; 1:63

Schaer GL, Fink MP, Parrillo JE: Norepinephrine alone versus norepinephrine plus low-dose dopamine: Enhanced renal blood flow with combination pressor therapy. Crit Care Med 1985; 13:492

Stiles GL, Lefkowitz RJ: Cardiac adrenergic receptors. Annu Rev Med 1984; 35:149

Worthley LIG, Tyler P, Moran JL: A comparison of dopamine, dobutamine and isoproterenol in the treatment of shock. Intensive Care Med 1985; 11:13

ANTIBIOTICS

RATIONALE 205-e

Unlike any of the other first or second generation cephalosporins, cefuroxime has been demonstrated to produce therapeutic levels in cerebrospinal fluid (CSF). Cefuroxime is clinically and bacteriologically effective in treatment of meningitis. It has been shown to be very active against common pathogens causing purulent meningitis.

Ceftriaxone is effective against both penicillin-sensitive and penicillin resistant gonococcus. Therefore, in a patient with either uncomplicated or complicated gonococcus infection, if there is a question of penicillin resistance, ceftriaxone offers an adequate therapeutic option.

Ceftazidime is distinguished by its high activity against pseudomonas. Evidence is now accumulating that ceftazidime can be as effective as an aminoglycoside in some situations. Although the total numbers are still small, this drug has been used successfully as a single agent both in pseudomonas meningitis and in pseudomonas pulmonary infection in patients with cystic fibrosis. In this setting, ceftazidime is usually better tolerated than the alternative, an aminoglycoside.

Although not touted as single drug therapy for pseudomonas meningitis, ceftizoxime is a cephalosporin antibiotic that enters most body fluids including the CSF to produce therapeutic concentrations against clinically important bacteria. A bleeding diathesis has not been associated with its use.

REFERENCES

David TJ, Phillips BM, Connor PJ: Ceftazidime - A significant advance in the treatment of cystic fibrosis. J Antimicrob Chemother 1983; 12:337

del Rio M, Chrane DF, Shelton S, et al: Pharmacokinetics of cefuroxime in infants and children with bacterial meningitis. Antimicrob Agents Chemother 1982; 22:990

Elliott TSJ, Ispahani P, Choudhary BP: Successful treatment of pseudomonas aeruginosa meningitis with ceftazidime. J Infect 1983; 7:275

Harper PB: In vitro properties of ceftazidime, a highly active broad-spectrum cephalosporin with antipseudomonal activity. Clin Ther 1984; 6:411

Judson FN, Handsfield HH: Comparative study of ceftriaxone and spectinomycin in pharyngeal and anorectal gonorrhea. JAMA 1985; 253:10

Pfenninger J, Schaad UB, Lutschg J, et al: Cefuroxime in bacterial meningitis. Arch Dis Child 1982; 57:539

Waldvogel FA: Editorial comment: Third generation cephalosporins - A panacea for intensive care patients? Intensive Care Med 1985; 11:184

RATIONALE 206-b

All aminoglycoside antibiotics may cause kidney damage, hearing loss, vestibular damage, and neuromuscular blockade. Tremors are not an expected potential toxicity.

Aminoglycoside neuromuscular blockade is nondepolarizing, may be partially reversed by calcium, and is especially severe in patients given curariform muscle relaxants, patients with myasthenia gravis, or patients given drugs such as quinine, quinidine, or procainamide which inhibit neuromuscular transmission. It may therefore result in respiratory insufficiency.

Aminoglycosides kill the cochlea's outer hair cells beginning at the basilar turn, leading first to high-frequency hearing loss, often associated with tinnitus. Hearing loss is often permanent. Vestibular damage may lead to ataxic symptoms.

Aminoglycoside antibiotics are eliminated from the body almost entirely by glomerular filtration. Their most common side effect is reduction of glomerular filtration, causing aminoglycosides to accumulate in the body and thereby causing progressing damage to the kidney and ears.

In using aminoglycosides, it is important to frequently measure blood concentrations to prevent drug accumulation and to adjust upward to effective levels the dosage in patients with good renal function. In addition, the patient should be asked every day about tinnitus, hearing (especially at high frequencies), and steadiness of sitting or walking. As a minimum, creatinine clearance (not serum creatinine or urea concentration) should be monitored frequently during treatment if aminoglycoside assays are not available.

REFERENCES

Brummett RE, Fox KE, Bendrick TW, et al: Ototoxicity of tobramycin, gentamicin, amikacin and sisomicin in the guinea pig. J Antimicrob Chemother 1978; 4(Suppl A):73

Dukes MN (Ed): Meyler's Side Effects of Drugs. Vol 8. Amsterdam-Oxford, Excerpta Medica, 1975, pp 613-629

Dukes MN (Ed): Side Effects of Drugs Annual 3. Amsterdam, Excerpta Medica, 1979, pp 228-231

Reiner NE, Bloxham DD, Thompson WL: Nephrotoxicity of gentamicin and tobramycin given once daily or continuously in dogs. J Antimicrob Chemother 1978; 4(Suppl A):85

Smith CR, Lipsky JJ, Leitman PS: Relationship between aminoglycoside induced nephrotoxicity and auditory toxicity. Antimicrob Agents Chemother 1979; 15:780

Wade JC, Smith CR, Petty BG, et al: Cephalothin plus an aminoglycoside is more nephrotoxic than methicillin plus an aminoglycoside. Lancet 1978; 2:604

Warner WA, Sanders E: Neuromuscular blockage associated with gentamicin therapy. JAMA 1971; 215:1153

Waterman PM, Smith RB: Tobramycin-curare interaction. Anesth Analg (Cleve) 1977; 56:587

RATIONALE 207-b

Antimicrobial prophylaxis with a cephalosporin has been shown to decrease the incidence of postoperative wound infection after arterial reconstructive surgery of the abdominal aorta. Anti-staphylococcal drugs decrease the incidence of infection in prosthetic joints following total hip replacement. Antimicrobial prophylaxis (cefazolin) decreases morbidity after vaginal hysterectomy. The effectiveness of prophylactic antimicrobial agents in decreasing the incidence of infection has not been established in neurosurgery.

REFERENCES

Grossman JH, Greco TP, et al: Prophylactic antiobiotics in gynecologic surgery. Obstet Gynecol 1979; 53:537

Hill C, Flanrant R, et al: Prophylactic cefazolin versus placebo in total hip replacement. Lancet 1981; 1:795

Kaiser AB, Clayson KR, et al: Antibiotic prophylaxis in vascular surgery. Ann Surg 1978; 188:283

Sande MA, Mandell GL: Chemotherapy of microbial diseases. In: The Pharmacological Basis of Therapuetics. Sixth Edition. Gilman AG, Goodman LS (Eds). New York, Macmillan Publishing Co. Inc., 1980, pp 1080-1248

RATIONALE 208-d

The major excretion route for clindamycin, chloramphenicol and erythromycin is hepatic. The major excretion route for cefoxitin is renal.

REFERENCE

Kucers A, Bennett NM: The Use of Antibiotics: A Comprehensive Review with Clinical Emphasis. Third Edition. Philadelphia, JB Lippincott Co., 1980

RATIONALE 209-b

Antibiotics which cross the blood brain barrier even in the absence of meningeal inflammation include chloramphenicol, sulfonamides, metronidazole, ticarcillin, and the third generation cephalosporins. Agents that unreliably cross include most first and second generation cephalosporins, clindamycin and the aminoglycosides. One second generation cephalosporin, cefuroxime, does have excellent penetration into the central nervous system.

REFERENCES

Berk SL, McCabe WR: Meningitis caused by Gram-negative bacilli. Ann Intern Med 1980; 93:253

Buck LL, Douglas GW: Meningitis due to Hemophilus influenzae type e. J Clin Micro 1976; 4:381

Olson DA, Hoeprich PD, et al: Successful treatment of Gram-negative bacillary meningitis with moxalactum. Ann Intern Med 1981; 95:302-305

RATIONALE 210-c

The development of antibiotic resistance during therapy has been noted frequently with third generation cephalosporins. Mechanisms proposed include induction of beta-lactamase and alterations in binding sites on penicillin-binding proteins. This is most common with isolates of pseudomonas, enterobacter and serratia. Most feel that a third generation cephalosporin should not be used alone in the treatment of infections with pseudomonas and possibly not to treat serratia and enterobacter infections. An exception may be pseudomonas urinary tract infections.

Third generation cephalosporins are as effective as previous standard regimens for surgical prophylaxis. However, because the drugs are more expensive than standard regimens, their use is discouraged. Moreover, when these drugs are used alone, selection of highly resistant bacterial isolates exists as a distinct possibility. More work needs to be done to examine the efficacy of single preoperative doses of these drugs.

Probably the most important therapeutic use of the third-generation cephalosporins is in the treatment of meningitis, particularly Gram-negative bacillary meningitis (GNBM). Moxalactum, cefotaxime, and ceftazidime have 90% success rates in GNBM with rapid sterilization of the CSF.

Moxalactum and cefoperazone have been implicated in the development of hypoprothrombinemia and associated bleeding episodes. Although the mechanism is unclear, it may be related to the ability of thiomethyltetrazole side-chain found on the cephem nucleus to inhibit the vitamin K-dependent reaction system involved in the synthesis of prothrombin. Another possible mechanism involves eradication of anaerobic bacteria which are capable of producing vitamin K. No significant abnormalities in clotting factors have been seen in healthy volunteers given high doses of moxalactum. It thus appears that only those predisposed to this effect by poor nutrition or other underlying diseases develop the problem. Vitamin K usually prevents and/or reverses the hypoprothrombinemia.

REFERENCES

Bang NU, Tessler SS, Heindenreich RO, et al: Effects of moxalactum on blood coagulation and platelet function. Rev Infect Dis 1982; 4:S546

Barriere SL, Flaherty JF: Third-generation of cephalosporins: A critical evaluation. Clin Pharm 1984; 3:351

Cherubin CE, Corrado ML, Nair SR, et al: Treatment of Gram-negative bacillary meningitis: Role of the new cephalosporin antibiotics. Rev Infect Dis 1982; 4:S453

Gall SA, Hill G: Cefoperazone as a prophylactic agent in abdominal hysterectomy. Rev Infect Dis 1983; 5:S200

Landesman SH, Corrado ML, Shah PM, et al: Past and current roles for cephalosporin antibiotics in treatment of meningitis. Am J Med 1981; 71:693

Maki DG, Aughey DR: Comparative study of cefazolin, cefoxitin and ceftizoxime for prophylaxis in colorectal surgery. J Antimicrob Chemother 1982; 10:S281

Preheim LC, Penn RG, Sanders CC, et al: Emergence of resistance to beta-lactam and aminoglycoside antibiotics during moxalactum therapy of pseudomonas aeruginosa infections. Antimicrob Agents Chemother 1982; 22:1037

EDITORIAL COMMENT

Resistance may develop during treatment with third generation beta-lactam compounds. Most of the new third generation cephalosporins are not degraded by beta-lactamase producing bacteria and, therefore, are considered to be beta-lactamase stable. Recent investigations have shown, however, that full stability does not guarantee efficacy against beta-lactamase producing Gram-negative organisms. It is possible for Gram-negative organisms such as enterobacter, citrobacter and pseudomonas to become totally resistant to beta-lactamase resistant second and third generation cephalosporins.

Cefuroxime offers good coverage of meningitis due to susceptible strains of Hemophilus influenzae (including ampicillin-resistant strains), Streptococcus pneumonia, Neisseria meningitis, and Staphylococcus aureus. It is, therefore, an excellent choice for broad-spectrum coverage of outpatient acquired meningitis.

Using current recommended infusion dosages of tobramycin for treatment of septic shock, a significant percentage of patients have initial blood aminoglycoside concentrations below the recommended peak level of 5 mg/ml. An underestimation of the volume of distribution is thought to be the primary factor involved, and measurement of levels after the first rather than waiting until the third dose may be practical in selected patient populations.

A study analyzing the pharmacokinetics of tobramycin showed considerable variation in plasma levels among patients after initial loading dosages. It appears that a 1 hour 1 mg/kg infusion produces serum aminoglycoside levels below recommendations while a 2 mg/kg dose infused over the same period often leads to a peak concentration in the toxic zone. Therefore, the optimum dose may well be 1.5 mg/kg infused over one hour. In the non-neutropenic patient it is probably not necessary to have significant drug levels present at all times during the day. In the neutropenic patients it appears advantageous to have significant serum drug levels present continuously in the serum.

ADDITIONAL REFERENCES

Horrevorts AM, Degener JE, Dzoljic-Danilovic G: Pharmacokinetics of tobramycin in patients with cystic fibrosis. Chest 1985; 88:260

Lancon JP, Honnart D, Freysz M, et al: Serum aminoglycoside levels (Letter). Crit Care Med 1985; 13:995

Neu HC: The pharmacokinetics of new cephalosporins: Significance in clinical practice. Bull NY Acad Med 1984; 60:327

Neu HC: Ceftizoxime: A beta-lactamase-stable, broad-spectrum cephalosporin. Pharmacokinetics, adverse effects and clinical use. Pharmacotherapy 1984; 4:47

Summer WR, Michael JR, Lipsky JJ: Initial aminoglycoside levels in the critically ill. Crit Care Med 1983; 11:948

Waldvogel FA: Editorial comment: Third generation cephalosporins - A panacea for intensive care patients? Intensive Care Med 1985; 11:184

ANTICOAGULANTS

RATIONALE 211-a

Heparin is a negatively charged mucopolysaccharide that requires the presence of plasma co-factor antithrombin III (AT-III) for its anticoagulant activity. Anti-thrombin III is itself a naturally occurring anticoagulant whose activity is greatly enhanced by heparin.

REFERENCES

Deylsin D: The use of heparin. N Engl J Med 1967; 280:937

Rosenberg RD: Actions and interactions of antithrombin and heparin. N Engl J Med 1975; 292:146

EDITORIAL COMMENT

When various heparin preparations are compared for efficacy with coagulation assays they vary as much as 40%-50%.

Heparin's effectiveness in preventing thrombosis is related to heparin-induced restoration of the negative electrostatic charge of the endothelium. Heparin concentrations in the endothelium after administration are 1,000 times greater than the plasma concentration, indicating a highly specific uptake by endothelium.

Some of heparin's anticoagulation effect is secondary to its activation of plasma protein AT-III which has an antithrombin action. However, only one-third of commercial heparin combines with AT-III and combination itself does not ensure activation.

ADDITIONAL REFERENCE

Jacques LB: The new understanding of the drug heparin. Chest 1985; 88:751

ANTIDYSRHYTHMICS

RATIONALE 212-a

Quinidine and procainamide increase both the action potential duration and the effective refractory period. Lidocaine, phenytoin and propranolol decrease both action potential duration and effective refractory period. However, for all five antidysrhythmic drugs, the only common effect is that all increase the ratio of effective refractory period to action potential duration.

REFERENCES

Moe GK, Abildskov JA: Antiarrhythmic drugs. In: The Pharmacologic Basis of Therapeutics. Fifth Edition. Goodman LS, Gilman A (Eds). New York, Macmillan Publishing Co. Inc., 1975, pp 683-704

Nies AS: Arrhythmias. In: Clinical Pharmacology, Basic Principles in Therapeutics. Second Edition. Melmon KL, Morrelli HF (Eds). New York, Macmillan Publishing Co. Inc., 1978, pp 225, 258

EDITORIAL COMMENT

The antidysrhythmic drugs have been classified based on physiologic effects into the following four categories:

Class 1 drugs are membrane-stabilizing or local anesthetic agents which reduce conductivity, excitability and automaticity. Within Class 1 are drugs such as quinidine and procainamide which produce a moderate reduction in conductivity and prolong the action potential duration (1a); drugs such as lidocaine which exert little change on conductivity and shorten the action potential duration (1b); and drugs producing marked slowing of conduction with no change in action potential duration (1c).

Class 2 drugs include the beta-adrenergic blocking agents.

Class 3 drugs exert selective increase in action potential duration and refractory period and include bretylium.

Class 4 drugs include calcium-channel blockers.

Beta-adrenergic blockers are not first-line agents for the treatment of any specific dysrhythmia but may be drugs of choice when the dysrhythmia is found in a setting of elevated catecholamine levels such as occurs in hyperthyroidism or exercise. These drugs may also be effective when used as adjunctive therapy in combination with membrane stabilizing agents for a synergistic effect or in controlling the ventricular rate in atrial fibrillation and flutter even without converting the basic rhythm.

Mexiletine is a new 1b drug which has many properties in common with lidocaine. Except for rare isolated reports, it does not generally effect the PR, QS or QT intervals and has no effect on ventricular function. It is usually unnecessary to alter the dose in congestive heart failure or mild renal or hepatic insufficiency.

Lorcainide is a membrane active drug available for intravenous use. It is a 1c drug which may prolong the PR and QRS intervals. QT interval prolongation does not occur and there may be a transient mild depression of left ventricular contractility. It is metabolized by the liver with an elimination half-life of 7.6 hours.

Amiodarone has several unique pharmacologic effects. It is not placed in any of the routine classification categories. Its direct effect is prolongation of the action potential duration and refractory periods. It noncompetitively blocks both beta-adrenergic and alpha-adrenergic receptors and introduces blockade of calcium entry channels as well. Since it contains substantial amounts of iodine and interferes with the thyroxine metabolism, it may produce some antiarrhythmic activity through its interaction with thyroxine. Its primary electrophysiologic effect is a reduction in conduction through the atrioventricular node with prolongation of the refractory period. It produces significant EKG changes including PR and QT prolongation with the development of a prominent u wave. Sinus bradycardia is common as is vasodilatation in both peripheral and coronary arteries. It directly depresses left ventricular function, but the reduction in afterload generally counterbalances this maintaining cardiac output. Minor side effects occur in 70% of patients and serious side effects in 18% requiring drug discontinuation in approximately 8% of patients. One of the most serious side effects is pulmonary toxicity with 5% of the patients developing pulmonary infiltrates or fibrosis. Respiratory failure and death have been reported. Amiodarone has been reported by many investigators to be highly effective for preventing recurrent ventricular tachycardia and ventricular fibrillation although there are no studies showing uniform patient population or methods for evaluation of therapy.

ADDITIONAL REFERENCES

Podrid PJ: Antiarrhythmic Drug Therapy (Part 1) - Benefits and Hazards. Chest 1985; 88:452

Podrid PJ: Antiarrhythmic Drug Therapy (Part 2) - Benefits and Hazards. Chest 1985; 88:618

ANTIHYPERTENSIVE AGENTS AND CARDIOVASCULAR DRUGS/GENERAL

RATIONALE 213-d 214-c 215-b

Nifedipine may be associated with a reflex tachycardia due to peripheral vasodilatation. Prazosin, at one time thought to be a direct vascular smooth muscle dilator, actually is an alpha-1 antagonist. Pindolol is a beta-blocker with intrinsic cardiac sympathomimetic activity and thus has a partial beta-1 agonist effect.

REFERENCES

Frishman WH, Kostis J: The significance of intrinsic sympathomimetic activity in beta-adrenoceptor blocking drugs. Cardiovascular Reviews and Reports 1982; 3:503

Frishman WH: Pindolol: A new beta-adrenoceptor antagonist with partial agonist activity. N Engl J Med 1983; 308:940

Lefkowitz RJ: Pharmacologic principles related to the autonomic nervous system. In: Cecil Textbook of Medicine. Sixteenth Edition. Philadelphia, WB Saunders Co., 1985, pp 90-95

Zellis RF, Schroeder JS (Eds): Calcium, calcium antagonists and cardiovascular disease. Chest 1980; 78:121

RATIONALE 216-d

Controlled clinical studies of calcium channel antagonists such as diltiazem and verapamil have not yet been completed to assess their potential for protective effect from recurrent myocardial infarction. The Norwegian Multicenter Study Group conclusively showed that timolol had a protective effect against myocardial reinfarction and perhaps a lesser but significant protective effect on mortality. The beta-blocker heart attack trial produced equally convincing data using propranolol. Other beta-blockers such as metoprolol have this protective effect. Pindolol is a nonselective beta-adrenergic blocker which differs from timolol and propranolol in that it is a weak adrenergic agonist, thereby possessing some intrinsic sympathomimetic activity. No studies have shown that pindolol has a protective effect on myocardial reinfarction and many investigators feel that beta-blockers with partial beta-1 agonist activity will prove to be ineffective or less effective in the prevention of reinfarction when studies have been completed.

REFERENCES

Beta-Blocker Heart Attack Trial Research Group. A randomized trial of propranolol in patients with acute myocardial infarction. Morbidity results. JAMA 1983; 250:2814

Beta-blockers after myocardial infarction. The Medical Letter 1982; 24:43

Frishman WH, Furberg CD, Friedwald WT: Beta-adrenergic blockage for survivors of acute myocardial infarction. N Engl J Med 1984; 310:830

Lichstein E, Morganroth J, Harris R, et al: Effect of propranolol on ventricular arrhythmia: The beta-blocker heart attack trial experience. Circulation 1983; 67(Suppl I):5

Norwegian Multicenter Study Group. Timolol-induced reduction in mortality and reinfarction in patients surviving acute myocardial infarction. N Engl J Med 1981; 304:801

Pindolol. The Medical Letter 1983; 25:13

RATIONALE 217-c 218-a 219-a 220-c 221-b

In the last few years a number of new drugs have been approved by the FDA for use as oral antihypertensive agents.

Nadalol and metoprolol are beta-adrenergic blocking agents. Nadalol, like propranolol, is a non-selective beta-adrenergic blocker. Its long plasma half-life (24 hours) allows a once daily dose. Metoprolol is beta-1 selective and thus differs from nadalol and propranolol. This beta-1 selectivity makes metoprolol better tolerated in patients with bronchospastic disease. All beta-adrenergic blockers, however, including metoprolol should be used with caution in this setting.

Captopril is an angiotension converting enzyme (ACE) inhibitor. Because of ACE inhibition, renin levels are elevated while aldosterone levels are suppressed. It follows that during therapy patients may retain potassium. Thiazide-induced hypokalemia may often be corrected by the addition of captopril without need for potassium supplementation.

Minoxidil is a potent dilator of systemic arterioles. It is recommended for use in patients who cannot tolerate or who do not respond adequately to conventional three-drug antihypertensive therapy. Minoxidil causes retention of sodium and water and is therefore most often combined with a diuretic. A majority of female patients will develop hypertrichosis while taking this medication.

REFERENCES

Frishman WH: Beta-1 adrenoceptor antagonists: New drugs and new indications. N Engl J Med 1981; 305:500

Frishman WH: Nadolol: A new beta-adrenoceptor antagonist. N Engl J Med 1981; 350:678

Pettinger WA: Minoxidil and treatment of severe hypertension. N Engl J Med 1980; 303:922

Vidt DG, Bravo EL, Fouad FM: Captopril. N Engl J Med 1982; 306:214

EDITORIAL COMMENT

The combination alpha- and beta-blocker labetalol has found significant beneficial utilization in the treatment of severe hypertension. This drug produces a blood pressure lowering effect by reducing systemic vascular resistance and at the same time prevents reflex tachycardia. The beta blockade is non-selective and more potent than the alpha blockade with intravenous labetalol. The drug may also have direct vasodilator action as well as beta-2 agonist mediated vasodilation. Hemodynamic studies have shown that labetalol lowers systemic vascular resistance with minimal to no effect on cardiac output. Contraindications for utilization of the drug include greater than first degree heart block, decompensated primary congestive heart failure, bronchospasm, and pregnancy.

ADDITIONAL REFERENCES

Papademetriou V, Notargiacomo AV, Khatri IM, et al: Treatment of severe hypertension with intravenous labetalol. Clin Pharmacol Ther 1982; 32:431

Wilson DJ, Wallin JD, Vlachakis ND, et al: Intravenous labetalol in the treatment of severe hypertension and hypertensive emergencies. Am J Med 1983; 75:95

RATIONALE 222-c

Labetalol, a combination alpha- and beta-adrenoreceptor blocker, is considered by many to be the drug of choice for parenteral therapy of hypertensive emergencies in those patients in whom rapid blood pressure lowering is desired but in whom intravenous nitroprusside is impractical or dangerous because of an inadequate arterial pressure monitoring capability. Although bradycardia is a potential complication, most patients have little alteration in heart rate and no change in cardiac output. The drug offers several advantages over alternative parenteral antihypertensive agents since it permits controlled steady lowering of blood pressure without significant changes in heart rate or cardiac output. These properties enable the drug to be administered safely in patients with concomitant coronary artery disease. In addition, since intravenous labetalol produces no significant reduction in cerebral blood flow, it may be preferable for use in patients who also have cerebrovascular disease. After intravenous bolus administration of labetalol, the majority of patients show a blood pressure decrease that is usually maximized at 5 minutes. Subsequent doses of 40-80 mg are given at 10-minute intervals (blood pressure checked every 5 minutes). After the first significant decrease in diastolic pressure, the total amount needed to achieve a predetermined diastolic goal can be predicted based on the initial effect. For instance, if a cumulative dose of 80 mg of iv labetalol lowered diastolic pressures by 15 mm Hg, then a total dose of 240 mg would lower the diastolic pressure approximately 45 mm Hg. Bronchospastic disease greater than first degree heart block, primary decompensated congestive heart failure, and pregnancy are contraindications to its use. Maximum recommended dose is 300 mg of labetalol.

REFERENCES

Cressman MD, Vidt DG, Gifford RW, et al: Intravenous labetalol in the management of severe hypertension and hypertensive emergencies. Am Heart J 1984; 107:980

Lebel M, Langlois S, Belleau LJ, et al: Labetalol infusion in hypertensive emergencies. Clin Pharmacol Ther 1985; 37:615

MacCarthy EP, Bloomfield SS: Labetalol: A review of its pharmacology, pharmacokinetics, clinical uses and adverse effects. Pharmacotherapy 1983; 3:193

BRONCHODILATORS

RATIONALE 223-d

Aminophylline is a methylxanthine derivative used in the treatment of bronchospasm. It can act synergistically with sympathomimetic drugs to promote bronchodilation and it also potentiates the action of epinephrine.

Since the xanthines have fewer cardiac effects than ephedrine or isoproterenol, they should be used in preference to all but the newer beta-2 selective agents in patients with heart disease. However, xanthines do increase the rate and force of contraction of the heart, producing tachydysrhythmias and even ventricular fibrillation. This happens particularly with high plasma levels and usually occurs from too rapid an intravenous injection of aminophylline.

Recent studies by Viires, et al. have shown that aminophylline improves diaphragmatic contractility independent of changes in central nervous system output or lung mechanics. They have demonstrated that aminophylline in experimental animals is protective against diaphragmatic fatigue induced by shock or respiratory failure, even during persistent hypoxemia, and is therapeutic once diaphragmatic fatigue is established.

Important factors in planning theophylline therapy are: (1) the half-life varies widely between individuals; while plasma concentrations can assist in anticipating toxicity, they do not always predict toxicity; (2) the half-life is prolonged by heart failure, erythromycin, liver failure, obesity, fever, and pneumonia, and is reduced by barbiturates, smoking and young age.

REFERENCES

Koch-Weser J: Bronchodilator therapy. N Engl J Med 1977; 297:758

Park GD, et al: Use of hemoperfusion for treatment of theophylline intoxication. Am J Med 1983; 74:961

Viires N, Aubier M, Murciano D, et al: Effects of aminophylline on diaphragmatic fatigue during acute respiratory failure. Am Rev Respir Dis 1984; 129:396

EDITORIAL COMMENT

Although intravenous beta-agonist therapy has been reported in children, it is not recommended in adults due to the increased risk of myocardial ischemia and infarction.

For many years theophylline's action was believed to be related to phosphodiesterase inhibition. Although theophylline clearly inhibits phosphodiesterase at therapeutic concentrations, the degree of inhibition is minimal. Its primary effect may be instead a translocation of intracellular calcium, likely through adenosine antagonism.

The mechanism responsible for altered theophylline metabolism in congestive heart failure is unknown, but three explanations have been proposed: (1) passive congestion of the liver may alter extraction capability due to hepatocyte damage, (2) decreased blood flow to the liver likewise has been proposed as a reason for decreased clearance although the low hepatic extraction ratio of theophylline tends to make this explanation unlikely, and (3) liver hypoxia itself secondary to inadequate perfusion may also be a potential etiology.

Aminophylline, as well as doxapram, have been shown to decrease weaning time from mechanical ventilation in premature infants. Since aminophylline increases diaphragmatic contraction and is a central respiratory stimulant, the precise etiology of this beneficial effect is not known. The effect of aminophylline on the human diaphragm at therapeutic serum concentrations remains controversial.

Drugs commonly used in the intensive care unit that may increase theophylline levels include phenytoin and cimetidine. Rifampin and activated charcoal may decrease theophylline levels. A 1 mg/kg aminophylline loading dose roughly correlates with an increase in serum theophylline concentration of 2 μg/dl. Inhaled beta-2 selective adrenergic agonists remain the cornerstone of the treatment of acute and severe bronchospasm.

ADDITIONAL REFERENCES

Bauman JH, Lalonde RL, Self TH: Factors modifying serum theophylline concentrations: An update. Immunology & Allergy Practice 1985; 7:259

Bryant S, Edwards RHT, Faulkner JA, et al: Respiratory muscle failure: Fatigue or weakness - the role of theophylline. Chest 1986; 89:116

Bukowskyj M, Nakatsu K, Munt PW: Theophylline reassessed. Ann Intern Med 1984; 101:63

Eyal FG, Sagi EF, Alpan GAD, et al: Aminophylline versus doxapram in weaning premature infants from mechanical ventilation: Preliminary report. Crit Care Med 1985; 13:124

Jenne JW: Drug therapy of asthma (Part 1): Beta-adrenergic agonists and theophylline. Pulmonary Clinical Update. American College of Chest Physicians 1985; 1:1

Johnson AK, Spiro SG, Pidgeon J, et al: Intravenous infusion of salbutamol in severe asthma. Br Med J 1978; 1:1013

Moxham J, Miller J, Wiles CM, et al: Effect of aminophylline on the human diaphragm. Thorax 1985; 40:288

CALCIUM CHANNEL BLOCKERS

RATIONALE 224-d

Verapamil exerts its primary effect during phase 2 of the action potential. Like the other calcium channel blocking agents, verapamil interferes with the inward transmembrane flux of calcium through so-called "slow channels." These agents have a vasodilation action which accounts in part for their usefulness in atherosclerotic and vasospastic coronary artery disease. This vasodilation occurs both peripherally and in the coronary artery bed. They possess negative chronotropic, inotropic and dromotropic action.

REFERENCES

Antman EM, Stone PH, et al: Calcium channel blocking agents in the treatment of cardiovascular disorders. Part I. Basic and clinical electrophysiologic effects. Ann Intern Med 1980; 93:875

Stone PH, Antman EM, et al: Calcium channel blocking agents in the treatment of cardiovascular disorders. Part II. Hemodynamic effects and clinical applications. Ann Intern Med 1980; 93:886

RATIONALE 225-d

Despite the fact that these three calcium antagonists have similar pharmacokinetics, their chemical structures are strikingly different; yet they are all 80%-90% protein bound, metabolized in the liver and have a half-life elimination from 2-7 hours. Both verapamil and diltiazem slow AV conduction, but they do not increase the HV interval and, thus, are relatively safe in patients who have bundle branch block. Nifedipine has little effect on AV nodal conduction and can be used in patients who have second or third degree AV block. All three agents have a negative inotropic effect. This limits their utilization in congestive heart failure.

REFERENCES

Schwartz A (Ed): Symposium on cardiovascular disease and calcium antagonists. Am J Cardiol 1982; 49(Suppl):497

Zelis RF, Schroeder JS (Eds): Calcium, calcium antagonists and cardiovascular disease. Chest 1980; 78(Suppl 1):121

EDITORIAL COMMENT

An animal model has been used to investigate the effect of verapamil during beta-blockade. In these beta-blocked animals usual clinical doses of intravenous verapamil had no significant effect on cardiac output. Increases in stroke volume compensated for decreases in mean arterial pressure. With large pharmacologic doses in the dog, however, there was a decrease in left ventricular stroke work.

A combined overdose with a beta-adrenergic blocker and a calcium channel antagonist often leads to profound hypotension and bradycardia. Henry and associates reported two case studies that demonstrated an immediate and dramatic response to intravenous calcium chloride.

Dopamine's ability to augment cardiac output at a dose of 10 μg/kg per minute is not antagonized by 1.5 mg/kg of verapamil.

Like intravenous and oral verapamil, oral diltiazem has been shown to be effective for prophylaxis of paroxysmal supraventricular tachycardia.

Intravenously administered verapamil is effective in converting paroxysmal supraventricular tachycardia due to impulse reentry in the AV node. It is a drug of choice for this arrhythmia. Intravenous verapamil is useful in treatment of atrial fibrillation and flutter by slowing ventricular response rate. It may occasionally convert atrial flutter to atrial fibrillation.

Glucagon has been shown to reverse the hypotension and bradycardia of verapamil overdose alone in the rat model.

ADDITIONAL REFERENCES

Henry M, Kay MM, Viccellio P: Cardiogenic shock associated with calcium-channel and beta blockers: Reversal with intravenous calcium chloride. Am J Emerg Med 1985; 3:334

Iberti TJ, Weiner B, Stein JS, et al: Hemodynamic effects of verapamil in the beta-blocked dog. Crit Care Med 1985; 13:105

Sturm JT: The influence of verapamil on dopamine's ability to augment cardiac output. Ann Emerg Med 1985; 14;945

Yeh SJ, Fu M, Lin FC, et al: Serial electrophysiologic studies of the effects of oral diltiazem on paroxysmal supraventricular tachycardia. Chest 1985; 87:639

Zaloga GP, Malcolm D, Holaday J, et al: Glucagon reverses the hypotension and bradycardia of verapamil overdose in rats (Abstract). Crit Care Med 1985; 13:273

CORTICOSTEROIDS

RATIONALE 226-a

Mineralocorticoid activity is greatest in hydrocortisone and least in dexamethasone. Therefore, in asthmatics and other patients requiring steroids in the ICU, dexamethasone or methylprednisolone is preferable to hydrocortisone. Properties of commonly prescribed corticosteroids are shown in the table below.

Agent	Equivalent Dose (mg)	Mineralocorticoid Potency[1]	Glucocorticoid Potency[2]	Duration of Action
Dexamethasone	0.75	0.0	25.0	72 hrs.
Methylprednisolone	4.0	0.5	5.0	36 hrs.
Prednisolone	5.0	0.8	4.0	24 hrs.
Prednisone	5.0	0.8	4.0	24 hrs.
Cortisol	20.0	1.0	1.0	8 hrs.
Hydrocortisone	25.0	1.0	0.8	8 hrs.
Cortisone	25.0	1.0	0.8	8 hrs.

[1]The higher the number in this column, the more likely it is that the agent's use will cause metabolic alkalosis.

[2]The higher the number in this column, the more likely it is to cause suppression of hypothalmic CRF and pituitary ACTH.

REFERENCES

Chernow B: Hormonal and metabolic considerations in critical care medicine. In: Critical Care: State of the Art. Vol 3. Shoemaker WC, Thompson WL (Eds). Fullerton, CA, Society of Critical Care Medicine, 1982, pp III(J):1-52

Chernow B, Vernoski B, Zaloga GP, et al: Dexamethasone causes less steroid-induced alkalemia than methylprednisolone or hydrocortisone. Crit Care Med 1984; 12:384

DIURETICS

RATIONALE 227-d

Vasopressin has strong antidiuretic effects, and may increase the urine specific gravity and reduce urine volume. Furosemide is a potent diuretic, but it makes urine specific gravity resemble that of plasma and is, therefore, unlikely to result in a clinical pattern as described in this question. Dopamine enhances urine output and sodium excretion at low doses, but, again, a urine specific gravity of 1.050 is not likely to occur.

The effects of morphine on urine are more complex. Morphine vasodilates, and may increase renal blood flow and possibly enhance urine output. However, one would expect this to be accompanied by a decrease in urine specific gravity from a concentrated (≥ 1.023) to a more diluted (≤ 1.020) range, reflecting the increased renal blood flow. When vasodilation is extreme relative to intravascular volume, systemic arterial pressure and renal blood flow may decrease, resulting in a smaller volume of urine with higher specific gravity. Morphine also stimulates release of antidiuretic hormone, and this effect may result in a concentrated urine with high specific gravity, but low volume. Therefore, none of these actions of morphine could explain both high volume and high specific gravity.

Organic iodides in the contrast media used in roentgenography usually cause an osmotic diuresis because of their large osmotic load in the doses needed for visualization of large vessels. The diuresis is usually sustained, and care must be taken to replace the volume lost to avoid dehydration and renal failure. Infusion of organic iodides is also associated with a very high urine specific gravity, and is therefore the likeliest cause of the reaction described in this question.

REFERENCES

Streelen DHP, Moses AM, Miller M: Disorders of the neurohypophysis. In: Harrison's Principles of Internal Medicine. Eighth Edition. Thorn GW, Adams RD, Braunwald E, et al (Eds). New York, McGraw-Hill Book Company, 1977, pp 490-501

Walker WG: Clinical evaluation for renal function. In: The Principles and Practice of Medicine. Eighteenth Edition. Harvey AMcG, Johns RJ, Owens AH Jr, Ross RS (Eds). New York, Appleton-Century-Crofts, 1972, p 136

RATIONALE 228-e

Furosemide causes hearing loss that is more frequent and severe when it is injected rapidly intravenously. The hearing loss caused by ethacrynic acid is dose-dependent, more severe in renal failure, and may be permanent. All aminoglycosides, including tobramycin, cause hearing loss and vestibular damage. This is more common in patients with renal failure who accumulate high concentrations of these antibiotics. Vancomycin hearing loss may be preceded by tinnitus, although this is not a reliable warning sign, and is more common when patients with renal failure are given large doses for prolonged courses. Polymyxin B causes renal damage and neurotoxicity (circumoral and peripheral paresthesias and inhibition of neuromuscular transmission), but its penetration of the central nervous system is minimal and it does not cause ototoxicity.

REFERENCES

Breude A (Ed): Harmful reactions of antimicrobial drugs. In: Antimicrobial Drug Therapy. Philadelphia, WB Saunders Co., 1976, pp 100-147

Diamond C: Drug induced deafness. Adverse Drug Reactions Bulletin 1978; 69:244

Schuster CJ, Weil MH, Besso J, et al: Blood volume following diuresis induced by furosemide. Am J Med 1984; 76:585

EDITORIAL COMMENT

There is a common misconception by some clinicians that the intravascular volume in acute heart failure is by necessity increased. This perhaps relates to correlations of increased pulmonary capillary presure as being synonymous with increased intravascular volume. It has been demonstrated that patients may be in acute heart failure with a high pulmonary artery occlusion pressure byt yet with a low intravascular volume. These people may actually have hypotension responsive to volume (with decreased preload as defined by left ventricular end diastolic volume). Any volume replacement would exacerbate the pulmonary congestion although it may well improve cardiac output. The low intravascular volume is at least partially dependent on the increased gradient for movement of fluid across the capillary membrane due to the increased hydrostatic pressures.

It has been shown that furosemide therapy of acute pulmonary edema may increase intravascular volume and be associated with an increase in cardiac output and a decrease in afterload. The increase in intravascular volume may be related to the venous capacitance effects of furosemide with decreased venous resistance leading to lowering of the capillary hydrostatic pressure. In addition, there may be an increase in colloid osmotic pressure. Both mechanisms increase the effective oncotic hydrostatic pressure gradient, favoring reabsorption of extravascular (edema) fluid. It is probable that the beneficial effect of diuresis on the performance of the failing left ventricle comes not from preload reduction but from afterload reduction. Although debatable, it is unlikely that pure preload reduction will produce an increase in cardiac output. It may, however, decrease pulmonary congestion and improve oxygenation. Since most diuretics exert some effect on afterload and relieve pulmonary congestion, it is very difficult to isolate preload effect from other variables such as improved oxygenation and decreased afterload leading to decreased myocardial oxygen demand and increased myocardial delivery.

ADDITIONAL REFERENCES

Astiz M, Weil MH, Rackow E: Hypovolemia complicating acute heart failure. Practical Cardiology 1983; 7:250

Ross J Jr, Braunwald E: Studies on Starling's law of the heart. IX. The effects of impeding venous return on performance of the normal and failing human left ventricle. Circulation 1964; 30:719

Schuster CJ, Weil MH, Besso J, et al: Blood volume following diuresis induced by furosemide. Am J Med 1984; 76:585

Wilson JR, Reichek N, et al: Effect of diuresis on the performance of the failing left ventricle in man. Am J Med 1981; 70:234

H-2 RECEPTOR ANTAGONISTS

RATIONALE 229-d

Cimetidine inhibits microsomal drug metabolism in the liver and decreases hepatic blood flow. Commonly used drugs such as diazepam, warfarin, propranolol and theophylline are metabolized by the liver. When used concurrently with cimetidine, the systemic clearance of these drugs is reduced. Tobramycin is excreted in the urine by glomerular filtration. Its systemic clearance is not altered by cimetidine.

REFERENCE

Freston JW: Cimetidine II adverse reactions and patterns of use. Ann Intern Med 1982; 97:728

RATIONALE 230-b

Ranitidine has a significantly longer duration of action than cimetidine and less frequent intravenous dosing is required. Unlike cimetidine, ranitidine does not displace natural antrogens from their receptors and thus is devoid of antiandrogenic activity. There has been no clinical evidence of drug related gynecomastia with ranitidine.

Unlike cimetidine, the occurrence of mental confusion has not been significant with ranitidine. This is thought to be due to three reasons:

1. different structure
2. lower transfer to CSF
3. greater efficiency mole for mole and therefore a lower dose requirement

Most data indicates a nonsignificant effect of ranitidine on theophylline metabolism. This is in contrast to cimetidine. However, there have been isolated case reports inferring interference of ranitidine with kinetics of theophylline. Until further data is available, theophylline level should be followed closely in those patients who are treated with ranitidine.

REFERENCES

Bauman JH, Kimelblatt BJ: Cimetidine as an inhibitor of drug metabolism: Therapeutic implications and review of the literature. Drug Intell Clin Pharm 1982; 16:380

Bories P, Michel H, Duclos B, et al: Use of ranitidine, without mental confusion, in patient with renal failure. Lancet 1980; i:755

Breen KJ, et al: Effects of cimetidine and ranitidine on hepatic drug metabolism. Clin Pharmacol Ther 1982; 31:297

Cerra FB, et al: Mental status, the intensive care unit, and cimetidine. Ann Surg 1982; 196:565

Gardner ME, et al: Ranitidine and theophylline. Ann Intern Med 1985; 102:559

Kagevi I, et al: CSF concentrations of ranitidine. Lancet 1985; 1:164

Peden NR, et al: Effects of two histamine H-2 receptor blocking drugs on basal levels of gonadotrophins, prolactin, testosterone and estradiol - 17B during treatment of duodenal ulcer in male patients. Acta Endocrinol 1981; 96:564

Seggev JS, et al: Ranitidine does not ordinarily affect theophylline levels. Ann Allerg 1985; 55:402

Spence RW, et al: Gynecomastia associated with cimetidine. Gut 1979; 20:154

EDITORIAL COMMENT

In canine, cimetidine has been shown to blunt the hypoxia-induced increase in cerebral blood flow in all regions of the brain except the pons and the bulb. By blunting this increase in cerebral blood flow during hypoxia, oxygen supply to the brain might be reduced. Cimetidine has been suggested to acutely reduce liver blood flow in normal healthy subjects. The possibility that polytrauma patients might experience decreased hepatic blood flow during cimetidine therapy was tested by Ivatury and associates. No significant alteration in either hepatic blood flow or cardiovascular status was demonstrated in these critically ill patients.

Ranitidine and cimetidine administered preoperatively eliminate acid aspiration during anesthesia and elective surgery.

ADDITIONAL REFERENCES

Clozel JP, Philippe A, Saunier C, et al: Cimetidine inhibits the hypoxia-induced increase in cerebral blood flow in dogs. Crit Care Med 1985; 13:976

Ivatury RR, Khan MB, Nallathambi M, et al: Cimetidine and hepatic blood flow in polytrauma patients. Crit Care Med 1985; 13:436

Williams JG, Strunin L: Preoperative intramuscular ranitidine and cimetidine. Anaesthesia 1985; 40:242

NARCOTICS/ANESTHETICS

RATIONALE 231-b

All narcotics produce a dose-dependent depression of respiration, primarily through a direct action on the respiratory centers in the brain stem. Therefore, a higher $PaCO_2$ is tolerated without respiratory effort. Small doses of narcotics decrease respiratory rate without changing tidal volume. Tidal volume is occasionally increased. Carbon dioxide tension is usually elevated. Anesthetic doses of narcotics cause cessation of involuntary breathing. These patients may still respond to a verbal command and may initiate a normal tidal volume if requested. The apneic threshold is increased and the respiratory drive is absent if mechanical ventilation maintains the $PaCO_2$ below the new apneic threshold, frequently 45-50 mm Hg.

If residual muscle relaxation is present, weak, shallow, and rapid respirations are generally present. Pain counteracts the respiratory depressant effects of narcotics and itself is rarely a cause of apnea postoperatively.

REFERENCES

Eschenhoff JE: The effects of narcotics and antagonists upon respiration and circulation in man. Clin Pharmacol Ther 1960; 1:483

Kelsen SG, Fishman AP: Clinical assessment of the regulation of ventilation. In: Pulmonary Diseases and Disorders. Fishman AP (Ed). New York, McGraw-Hill Book Company, 1980

RATIONALE 232-c 233-c

Patients, for a variety of reasons, may receive narcotics for prolonged periods. If the critical care practitioner is not aware of this history, the use of a narcotic antagonist such a naloxone may precipitate the signs and symptoms of acute drug withdrawal. This fact may not be recognized and the patient may be mistreated. To avoid this complication, it is important to ascertain if patients have a history of prolonged use of narcotics. Toxic allergic reactions to topical anesthetics produce irritation to the central nervous system, followed by a respiratory and circulatory collapse. Since this patient developed a somewhat different symptom complex temporarily related to naloxone, this diagnosis is unlikely. A vasovagal response is generally associated with bradycardia and hypotension, neither of which were seen in this case.

The correct management of this patient involves intravenous administration of a narcotic agent. An obvious mistake would be to assume that this condition was a toxic reaction to the anesthetic agent used and to treat as such.

REFERENCES

Cousins MJ, Phillips GD: Sleep, pain, and sedation. In: Textbook of Critical Care. Shoemaker WC, Thompson WL, Holbrook PR (Eds). Philadephia, WB Saunders Co., 1984, p 793

Wylie WG, Churchill-Davidson HC: A Practice of Anesthesia. Third Edition. Chicago, Year Book Medical Publishers, Inc., 1972, pp 1068-1069

RENAL FAILURE

RATIONALE 234-e

Gentamicin and other aminoglycoside antibiotics are not metabolized and are excreted from the body almost entirely by glomerular filtration. In anuria the clearance of gentamicin is about 2 to 10 ml/min and the dose should be reduced 10-fold or more with careful monitoring of serum gentamicin concentrations. Polymyxin B and tetracycline are also excreted mostly by glomerular filtration and their doses should be reduced greatly. Digoxin in young healthy subjects is about 3/8 metabolized and about 5/8 excreted in urine. Anuria reduces clearance to about 3/8 of the usual dose. Chloramphenicol is largely metabolized with only 15%-20% appearing unchanged in urine. Some authorities suggest slight reduction in chloramphenicol dose in anuria, but its dose is adjusted much less than that of the other drugs listed.

REFERENCES

Anderson RJ, Gambertoglio JG, Schrier RW: Fate of drugs in renal failure. In: The Kidney. Brenner BM, Rector FC Jr (Eds). Philadelphia, WB Saunders Co., 1976, pp 1911-1948

Breude A (Ed): Pharmacological principles. In: Antimicrobial Drug Therapy. Philadelphia, WB Saunders Co., 1976, pp 67-99

Root RK, Hierholzer WJ Jr: Infectious disease. In: Clinical Pharmacology, Basic Principles in Therapeutics. Second Edition. Melmon KL, Morrelli HF (Eds). New York, Macmillan Publishing Co. Inc., 1978, pp 709-801

RATIONALE 235-a

Gentamicin, tobramycin, amikacin, neomycin, streptomycin, netilmicin, and other aminoglycoside antibiotics are eliminated from the body almost entirely by glomerular filtration. When renal function is minimal, there is almost no drug elimination. In anephric subjects, aminoglycoside antibiotic clearances are about 2 ml/min and doses of these drugs should be lowered significantly.

Polymyxin is excreted predominantly unchanged in urine. Both sulfamethoxazole and trimethoprim are excreted unchanged in urine to a large extent, but have alternate pathways of elimination. In severe renal failure, the doses of both of these drugs should be decreased.

Renal excretion of digitoxin is limited both by its binding to plasma proteins, preventing free diffusion through the glomerular pores, and by its lipid solubility that favors tubular reabsorption. Liver metabolism of digitoxin is also reduced by the high degree of protein binding. Thus, the plasma clearance of digitoxin is quite low, about 2.7 ml/min. In renal failure, as the acidic uremic products accumulate in blood, digitoxin binding to plasma proteins is reduced. This makes more free digitoxin available for metabolism and, in fact, its clearance is not changed at all in renal failure, even in anephric patients. Digitoxin, thus, has several advantages over digoxin. One tablet a day is sufficient because of the long half-life of about one week. Absorption is complete and elimination is relatively consistent with changing renal function.

Why not use digitoxin routinely? There are three disadvantages to digitoxin. First, its onset of action is about 40 minutes as compared with 20 minutes for digoxin. Second, the half-life in healthy patients is about 1.5 days for digoxin as compared with the 5-7 days of digitoxin. Third, digitoxin elimination theoretically may be altered in liver disease.

REFERENCES

Bennett WM, Porter GA, Bagby SP, et al: Drugs and Renal Disease. New York, Churchill Livingstone, 1978

Finkelstein FO, Goffinet JA, Hendler ED, et al: Pharmacokinetics of digoxin and digitoxin in patients undergoing hemodialysis. Am J Med 1975; 58:525

Nies AS: Cardiovascular disorders. In: Clinical Pharmacology, Basic Principles in Therapeutics. Second Edition. Melmon KL, Morrelli HF (Eds). New York, Macmillan Publishing Co. Inc., 1978, pp 709-801

Rasmussen K, Jervell J, Storstein L, et al: Digitoxin kinetics in patients with impaired renal function. Clin Pharmacol Ther 1972; 13:6

EDITORIAL COMMENT

Risk factors associated with aminoglycoside nephrotoxicity include pre-existing renal disease, previous therapy with an aminoglycoside, prolonged therapy, and concurrent administration of other nephrotoxic substances. Renal injury appears to be dose related and is more common in elderly debilitated patients, patients with a contracted intravascular volume, and those with pre-existing renal disease. It is usually mild and reversible, with onset after 5 to 7 days of therapy, but it may be clinically manifested after cessation of therapy. Predicting and monitoring toxicity in patients receiving aminoglycosides is best done by measurement of urinary cast excretion, which increases before the serum creatinine elevation. This is a more sensitive indicator of aminoglycoside effect on the proximal tubule than other tests of renal function. Nephrotoxicity is best correlated with trough concentrations consistently above 2 μg/ml for gentamicin or tobramycin or above 10 μg/ml for amikacin.

ADDITIONAL REFERENCE

Ristuccia AM: Aminoglycosides. In: Antimicrobial Therapy. Ristuccia AM, Cunha BA (Eds). New York, Raven Press, 1984, pp 305-328

VASODILATORS

RATIONALE 236-d

Intravenous nitroglycerin and nitroprusside dilate both arterial resistance and venous capacitance vessels, but their specificity for these vessels differs. With nitroprusside, there is balanced arterial and venous capacitance vessel dilation.

The indications for either dilator depend on the specific requirements and the condition of the patient. If a decrease in the systemic vascular resistance in patients without myocardial ischemia is desired, nitroprusside is usually the drug of choice. Nitroglycerin is particularly helpful if a decrease in left ventricular filling pressures by venodilation is preferred. In ischemic hearts, nitroprusside may aggravate ischemia by a coronary steal phenomenon, while nitroglycerin may alleviate it. Therefore, intravenous nitroglycerin is the inital drug of choice in patients with myocardial ischemia if lowering of systemic vascular resistance is desired.

Patients vary in response to nitroprusside and nitroglycerin. It is necessary to titrate each drug for desired effect and to change to alternate therapy when the desired effect is not manifest initially. The titration of nitroglycerin is readily accomplished by the use of an intravenous infusion, but sublingual tablets or topical ointments may be used.

REFERENCES

Chiariello M, Gold HK, Leinbach RC, et al: Comparison between the effects of nitroprusside and nitroglycerin on ischemic injury during acute myocardial infarction. Circulation 1976; 54:766

Cohn JN, Franciosa JA: Vasodilator therapy of cardiac failure. N Engl J Med 1977; 297:27

Helfant RH: Nitroglycerin: New concepts about an old drug. Am J Med 1976; 60:905

Kotter V, Von Leitner ER, Wunderlich J, et al: Comparison of haemodynamic effects of phentolamine, sodium nitroprusside and glyceryl trinitrate in acute myocardial infarction. Br Heart J 1977; 39:1196

Tinker JH, Michenfelder JD: Sodium nitroprusside: Pharmacology toxicology and therapeutics. Anesthesiology 1976; 45:340

RATIONALE 237-d

Sodium nitroprusside causes relaxation of arterial and venous smooth muscle. It has numerous clinical uses including acute hypertension, heart failure and controlled hypotension during surgery. Cyanide is liberated during the non-enzymatic degradation of sodium nitroprusside. The cyanide ion combines with cytochrome-c of the electron transport chain, interrupting aerobic metabolism. In the presence of a sulfur donor the cyanide is converted by the mitochondrial rhodanese system to thiocynate which is subsequently excreted by the kidneys. The first clinical effect of cyanide toxicity is usually an increase in ventilation because of the blockade of oxidative metabolism in the chemoreceptor cells. This is shortly followed by the complaints of headache, dizziness and nausea. Mild drowsiness may proceed quickly to obtundation and coma. Convulsions are common at this stage.

An infusion of thiosulfate provides the sulfur donor for the rhodanase system and facilitates the formation of the less toxic molecule thiocynate. Sodium nitrite causes the formation of methemoglobin which combines with the cyanide ion to form cyanomethemoglobin. Cyanide then gradually dissociates from cyanomethemoglobin. Hydroxocobalamin combines with cyanide to form the non-toxic molecule cyanocobalamin (vitamin B_{12}).

REFERENCES

Cohn JN, Burke LP: Nitroprusside. Ann Intern Med 1979; 91:752

Cottrell JE, Casthely P, et al: Prevention of nitroprusside-induced cyanide toxicity with hydroxocobalamin. N Engl J Med 1978; 298:808

Saunders JP, Himwich WA: Properties of the transsulfurase responsible for the conversion of cyanide to thiocyanate. Am J Physiol 1950; 163:404

Vesig CJ, Cole PV, et al: Some metabolic effects of sodium nitroprusside in man. Br Med J 1974; 2:140

RATIONALE 238-d

Nitroglycerin, like nitroprusside, exerts a vasodilatory effect on the cerebral vascular bed. Therefore, nitroglycerin may cause a significant increase in intracranial pressure in patients with intracranial pathology.

Another effect of nitroglycerin is a decrease in left ventricular wall tension (decreased myocardial ischemia) that may result in a decrease in myocardial oxygen consumption. Nitroglycerin also dilates collateral coronary vessels and venous capacitance vessels.

REFERENCES

Cohen MV, Downey JM, Sonnenblick EH: The effects of nitroglycerin on coronary collaterals and myocardial contractility. J Clin Invest 1973; 52:2836

Gagwan RL, Marsh ML: Intracranial hypertension caused by nitroglycerin. Anesthesiology 1979; 51:86

Hill NJ, Antman EN, Green LH, et al: Intravenous nitroglycerin. Chest 1981; 79:69

EDITORIAL COMMENT

Nitroprusside is the drug of choice for short-term control of hypertension when myocardial ischemia is not present. ST segment elevation has been observed in humans, as well as in animals during nitroprusside infusion and a coronary steal phenomenon has been described more likely occurring in patients with high filling pressures.

Cyanide toxicity may be a problem with nitroprusside infusion in patients with renal failure but is unlikely to occur in patients with normal hepatic and renal function receiving less than 1 µg/kg•min and a total dose less than 1.5-5 mg/kg over 24 hours.

It may be difficult to differentiate whether a nitroglycerin induced decrease in systemic vascular resistance is secondary to vasodilation or improved cardiac function in patients with myocardial ischemia. Patients with cardiac failure and profound elevations of systemic vascular resistance as a primary problem, particularly if unresponsive to initial nitroglycerin and/or beta-agonist therapy, should be considered for nitroprusside which has greater arterial bed vasodilating effects than nitroglycerin.

Phentolamine, an alpha-blocking agent, is capable of antagonizing or even reversing the vasoconstriction produced by catecholamines and in addition has a direct vasodilating effect on vascular smooth muscle. In cardiopulmonary bypass patients phentolamine has been shown to produce more uniform body rewarming and improved tissue perfusion. Phentolamine administration was also associated with lower blood lactate levels and less sodium bicarbonate requirements during rewarming.

In mechanically ventilated COPD patients with pulmonary artery hypertension, neither sodium nitroprusside nor hydralazine have been shown to exert significant influence on hemodynamic status.

Trimethaphan, a ganglionic blocking agent, decreases systemic vascular resistance without effect on cerebral blood flow, and may be useful in lowering blood pressure in head injury patients with cerebral edema. It does, however, cause dilated pupils, a disadvantage in this group.

ADDITIONAL REFERENCES

Bridges KG, Reichard GA, MacVaugh H, et al: Effect of phentolamine in controlling temperature and acidosis associated with cardiopulmonary bypass. Crit Care Med 1985; 13:72

Cerda E, Esteban A, De La Cal M, et al: Hemodynamic effects of vasodilators on pulmonary hypertension in decompensated chronic obstructive pulmonary disease. Crit Care Med 1985; 13:221

Kaplan JA, Finlayson DC, Woodward S: Vasodilator therapy after cardiac surgery: A review of the efficacy and toxicity of nitroglycerin and nitroprusside. Can Anaesth Soc J 1980; 27:254

Sarvotham SS, Patel C, Venus B, et al: Nitroglycerin vs. nitroprusside treatment of myocardial ischemia (Letter). Crit Care Med 1985; 13:212

Section 14

239. Signs of cyanide intoxication include all but which ONE of the following?

a. Metabolic acidosis
b. Decreased arterial blood PaO_2
c. Increased heart rate
d. Convulsions

240. Which ONE of the following electrolyte abnormalities causes an increased frequency of digoxin-induced tachyarrhythmias?

a. Hypocalcemia
b. Hyperkalemia
c. Hypermagnesemia
d. None of the above

241. Which ONE of the following drugs is MOST dangerous to administer to a patient with digitalis intoxication, sinus bradycardia, and recurrent ventricular tachycardia?

a. Atropine
b. Calcium chloride
c. Potassium chloride
d. Phenytoin
e. Propranolol

242. Which ONE of the following will likely remove the largest amount of glutethimide (Doriden) in an 18-year-old woman who is in deep coma one day after ingesting glutethimide?

a. Diuresis with alkaline urine
b. Peritoneal dialysis with saline
c. Hemodialysis with saline
d. Hemodialysis with oil
e. Hemoperfusion over resin

243. An 18-month-old male child is found by his mother in the garage sitting in a puddle of gasoline with the smell of gasoline on his breath. He is brought to the emergency room and is subsequently transferred to the ICU for management and observation.

Which ONE of the following statements regarding hydrocarbon aspiration or ingestion is CORRECT?

a. Danger from siphoning gasoline by mouth is present only if the liquid is ingested.
b. Cathartics have proven benefit in this setting.
c. Emesis and gastric lavage should never be attempted when hydrocarbons have been ingested.
d. Even when hydrocarbons are swallowed, the major pathology is pneumonitis.

244. Central nervous system manifestations of isoniazid (INH) overdose are most effectively managed with which ONE of the following agents?

a. Diazepam
b. Pyridoxine
c. Phenytoin
d. N-Acetylcysteine
e. Sodium bicarbonate

245. A 17-year-old man is admitted to your service after he was brought to the emergency department by two friends who found him comatose. He is a known heroin abuser. You find him to be cyanotic, breathing six times each minute with a pulse of 60/min and 4 mm diameter pupils. You give the appropriate antagonist intravenously.

Which ONE of the following reactions is LEAST likely?

a. Piloerection
b. Increased ventilation
c. Vomiting
d. Increased alertness
e. Constriction of pupils

246. Which of the following statements about phenobarbital is true?

a. Its major metabolite, the parahydroxyphenyl derivative, is inactive and is excreted in the urine.
b. Phenobarbital is 2%-5% bound to plasma proteins.
c. Acidification of the urine favors the poorly reabsorbed ionized form, thereby enhancing drug excretion.
d. The serum level of phenobarbital may be lowered by hemodialysis but not by charcoal hemoperfusion.
e. Phenobarbital is considered a short-acting barbiturate.

247. A previously healthy adult takes 100 Darvocet-N tablets (propoxyphene plus acetaminophen) and four hours later is seen in the critical care unit, mechanically ventilated with normal vital signs and arterial blood gases. The most important SINGLE drug to give is:

a. Naloxone
b. Nalorphine
c. Ipecac Syrup
d. Methylphenidate
e. Acetylcysteine

248. All of the following are appropriate in the management of the comatose patient who has taken a drug overdose EXCEPT:

a. Endotracheal intubation
b. Placement of an Ewald tube or equivalent for gastric lavage
c. Administration of syrup of ipecac through a gastric tube
d. Administration of charcoal through a gastric tube

249. Which of the following poisons (or medications taken in excess) is incorrectly matched with an antidote?

a. Acetaminophen - acetylcysteine
b. Cyanide - oxygen, sodium nitrite, hydroxocobalamin
c. Lead - naloxone, atropine
d. Propranolol - glucagon, pacing

Questions 250-252: You are treating a 30-year-old fireman who collapsed without apparent injury while inside a burning house. He is comatose but moves his arms and his legs when you pinch them. His pulse is 160, regular, and bounding, but his lips and skin are pale and blue. He breathes 30 times a minute, deeply, and he has no rales or wheezes. Although covered with soot, he has no external burns and his pharynx appears uninjured.

250. You draw an arterial blood sample for stat analysis while he is breathing room air. Which one of the following results is most likely to be WRONG (assuming other results to be correct)?

a. pH = 7.1
b. $PaCO_2$ = 20 mm Hg
c. HCO_3^- = 7 mEq/L
d. PaO_2 = 110 mm Hg
e. O_2 saturation = 97%

251. After vigorous appropriate treatment, over time the patient is alert and complains only of headache. The MOST important part of his treatment has been:

a. Intravenous sodium bicarbonate
b. Oxygen
c. Endotracheal intubation
d. Controlled mechanical ventilation
e. Positive end-expiratory pressure of 10 mm Hg

252. During the second and third days of hospitalization, he appears entirely healthy and you discharge him. Seven days after his initial admission, you reexamine him.

Which ONE of the following findings is MOST likely to be present?

a. Anemia (hematocrit = 20%)
b. Brain damage (confusion and ataxia)
c. Heart failure (edema, rales and dyspnea)
d. Jaundice (bilirubin = 10 mg/dl)
e. Uremia (serum creatinine = 5 mg/dl)

Questions 253-254: You are treating a 28-year-old woman who has been healthy until found comatose by her friends at 11 p.m. On admission, she is cyanotic with shallow ventilation. Her pulse is 140/min with a blood pressure of 100/70. Her rectal temperature is 35°C. She withdraws extremities to severe pain, but is otherwise unresponsive. Her eyes rove disconjugately and the pupils are 6 mm in diameter and react very slightly to light. Her muscle tone is increased, her deep tendon reflexes are increased, her plantar responses are extensor, and she has frequent myoclonic jerks. Her bowel sounds are absent. On EKG she has long PR, QRS, and QT intervals despite the rapid heart rate, and she is having premature ventricular systoles at a frequency of about 10/min.

253. The MOST likely cause of this presumed drug overdose is:

a. Acetaminophen
b. Aspirin
c. Amitriptyline
d. Diazepam
e. Heroin

254. The drug MOST likely to antagonize the probable cause of this syndrome is:

a. Atropine
b. Chlorpromazine
c. Epinephrine
d. Naloxone
e. Physostigmine

255. Ten days after injury you are asked to see a 5-year-old male in the burn unit because of cyanosis. The child had received 60% body surface area 2nd and 3rd degree flame burns to the chest, back, arms, neck and face during a house fire. The initial examination (one hour after injury) had revealed:

Temperature - 35°C (96°F)	Pulse - 130
Respiratory rate - 22	BP - 118/82

No cyanosis was noted.

The nasal hairs were singed but there was no carbonaceous material in the nose or mouth. There was no hoarseness or stridor. With the exception of tachypnea and tachycardia, the examination of the lungs and heart was normal.

Laboratory (on admission):		ABGs obtained on room air:	
Hgb	16.7	pH	7.50
Hct	48.5	$PaCO_2$	30 mm Hg
Carboxyhemoglobin	18%	PaO_2	110 mm Hg

Since admission, the patient had been treated with aqueous penicillin G 300,000 units iv q 6 hours, 0.5% silver nitrate solution to the burn wounds and hypertonic lactated saline (Na^+ 250 mEq/L, lactate 100 mEq/L, Cl 150 mEq/L). The patient had not required supplemental oxygen or mechanical ventilation until just prior to your arrival. Your examination now reveals:

Temperature - 38°C (101°F)	Pulse - 150
Respiratory rate - 30	BP - 140/90

Diffuse cyanosis is noted.

No hoarseness or stridor is observed. The lung fields are clear. The heart examination now reveals a hyperdynamic precordium with a II/VI systolic ejection murmur at the apex. Arterial blood gases drawn just before your arrival, while the patient was breathing room air, were noted to be "very dark" and revealed a pH of 7.48, a $PaCO_2$ of 31 mm Hg, and a PaO_2 of 108 mm Hg.

Repeat blood gases on a 40% Venturi mask were again noted to be "dark" and revealed a pH of 7.47, a $PaCO_2$ of 32 mm Hg and a PaO_2 of 240 mm Hg. Hgb and Hct are now 15 and 45 respectively. A repeat chest x-ray is unchanged from admission.

Which ONE one of the following is an acceptable form of therapy for this condition?

a. Hyperbaric oxygen
b. Corticosteroids and "broad spectrum" antibiotics
c. 10% urea
d. Methylene blue
e. Heparin

256. A young man is found on the street in deep coma, breathing slowly, and is admitted to your service. You are unable to evaluate his left pupil because of an old eye injury. The right pupil is 6 mm in diameter and unreactive.

Which ONE of the following is LEAST likely to be the SOLE cause of this finding?

a. Glutethimide (Doriden) poisoning
b. Scopolamine poisoning
c. Right-sided subdural hematoma
d. Left-sided subdural hematoma
e. Damage to the right sixth cranial nerve

257. Which ONE of the following is LEAST helpful in the management of propranolol overdose?

a. Isoproterenol
b. Atropine
c. Glucagon
d. Phentolamine

258. Which ONE of the following is LEAST likely in an 8-year-old child who ingested 12 adult aspirin tablets four hours ago and who now has a plasma salicylate concentration of 80 mg/dl?

a. Decreased whole body potassium content
b. Decreased arterial PCO_2
c. Decreased CO_2 production
d. Decreased bicarbonate concentration
e. Decreased CSF glucose concentration

259. Which ONE of the following statements regarding salicylate poisoning in children is FALSE?

a. Safety closures on containers have significantly decreased the incidence of salicylate poisoning in children.
b. Salicylate elimination is facilitated by alkalinization of the urine.
c. Respiratory acidosis commonly develops early in the course of salicylate intoxication because of a depressive effect on the central nervous system respiratory centers.
d. Glucose administration is an important component of therapy.

260. A 65-year-old male patient with chronic obstructive pulmonary disease (COPD) is admitted to the ICU from the ER where he presented with complaints of anorexia, nausea, headache and tremulousness. His home medications include theophylline, allopurinol and ranitidine. He states that he had been taking more of his "breathing medicine" for a recent worsening of his COPD. He is alert and anxious with a pulse rate of 125. He has a PaO_2 of 65 mm Hg on room air. His theophylline blood level is 80 micrograms per ml. The theophylline is discontinued. Ten minutes after his ICU admission, he has a grand mal seizure.

Which of the following statements describes appropriate therapy in this setting?

a. Charcoal or resin hemoperfusion
b. Activated charcoal 30 grams PO q 2 hours up to 120 grams
c. Discontinue allopurinol and ranitidine and observe.
d. Hemodialysis
e. Both a and b

POISONING/DRUG OVERDOSE

ANSWERS

239-b	240-d	241-b	242-e	243-d	244-b	245-e	246-a
247-e	248-c	249-c	250-e	251-b	252-b	253-c	254-e
255-d	256-e	257-d	258-c	259-c	260-e		

CYANIDE

RATIONALE 239-b

Hydrocyanic acid (prussic acid) and its alkali salts are found in fumigants, insecticides, rodenticides, polishes, and as laboratory reagents. Naturally-occuring nitriles are found in many fruits. Amygdalin, an ingredient in laetrile, is a combination of glucose, benzaldehyde, and hydrogen cyanide found in the seeds of cherry, plum, peach, apricot, apple and pear. Cyanide also is a metabolite of nitroprusside.

Few poisons are as potent or rapid as cyanide. Inhalation of hydrogen cyanide leads to coma in seconds and death in minutes. By ingestion cyanides kill in minutes, and rectal laetrile may be lethal.

Cyanide inhibits cytochrome oxidase, blocking utilization of oxygen. The most sensitive organs are those that are most oxygen dependent, especially the brain and heart. Coma and hypoxic convulsions occur rapidly as do cardiac dysrhythmias, especially bradyarrhythmias. Lactic acidosis and pulmonary edema are common. Arterial oxygen tensions are not reduced.

Cyanide poisoning should be considered in any patient with cellular hypoxia. Few signs are specific. Laboratory tests for cyanide are available, but would hardly be of value in acute poisoning.

Treatment of cyanide poisoning has three aspects. First, oxygen is of value. Oxygen supply to the tissues may be enhanced slightly with inhaled oxygen. More importantly, oxygen may reverse binding of cyanide to cytochrome oxidase and increase conversion of cyanide to the relatively harmless thiocyanate in the presence of thiosulfate.

Second, cyanide detoxification by natural mechanisms may be enhanced. Nitrites (often given as amyl nitrite by inhalation then sodium nitrite by injection) oxidize hemoglobin to methemoglobin and methemeglobin has a high affinity for cyanide. Unfortunately, amyl nitrite will not oxidize much hemoglobin unless given in very large doses. Sodium nitrite is effective, but excessive methemoglobinemia may kill the patient as well. Sodium thiosulfate is injected as a sulfate donor to enhance conversion of cyanide to thiocyanate.

Hydroxocobalamin (vitamin $B_{12}a$) combines with cyanide to form vitamin B_{12}. This drug is highly effective in animals and man with acute (and possible chronic) cyanide poisoining. Toxicity of the chelating hydroxocobalamin is minimal.

REFERENCES

Aitken D, West D, Smith F, et al: Cyanide toxicity following nitroprusside induced hypotension. Can Anaesth Soc J 1977; 24:651

Backer HC, Herbert V: Cyanide poisoning from laetrile in the presence of megadoses of ascorbic acid. JAMA 1979; 241:1891

Buchanan IS, Dhamee MS, Griffiths FE, et al: Abnormal fundal appearances in a case of poisoning by a cyanide capsule. Med Sci Law 1976; 16:29

Cottrell JE, Casthely P, Brodie JD, et al: Prevention of nitroprusside-induced cyanide toxcity with hydroxocobalamin. N Engl J Med 1978; 298:809

Graham DL, Laman D, Theodore J, et al: Acute cyanide poisoning complicated by lactic acidosis and pulmonary edema. Arch Intern Med 1977; 137:1051

Isom GE, Way JL: Effect of oxygen on cyanide intoxication. VI: Reactivation of cyanide-inhibited glucose metabolism. J Pharmacol Exp Ther 1974; 189:235

Ortega JA, Creek JE, et al: Acute cyanide poisoning following administration of Laetrile enemas. J Pediatr 1978; 93:1059

Posner MA, Rodman GH, Klick JM, et al: Cyanide production during nitroprusside therapy in an oliguric patient. Anesth Analg (Cleve) 1977; 56:729

Vesey CJ, Simpson PJ, Adams L, et al: Metabolism of sodium nitroprusside and cyanide in the dog. Br J Anaesth 1979; 51:89

DIGITALIS

RATIONALE 240-d

Toxicity of cardiac glycosides is enhanced by hypercalcemia, hypokalemia, hypomagnesemia, and metabolic alkalosis. Acidosis itself does not increase the frequency of digoxin-induced tachyarrthythmias, but it may lead to loss of intracelluar potassium and increased sympathetic nervous system activity that may increase tachyarrhythmias.

Many patients receive digitalis glycosides before they become critically ill, and the effects of such drugs persist for days even if they are discontinued. Metabolic changes may precipitate digitalis arrhythmias even though the patient has received no digitalis for several days and has "therapeutic" concentrations of digitalis glycosides in serum.

REFERENCES

Arieff AI: Principles of parenteral therapy. In: Clinical Disorders of Fluid and Electrolyte Metabolism. Second Edition. Maxwell MH, Kleeman CK (Eds). New York, McGraw-Hill Book Company, 1972, pp 582-583

Moe GK, Farah AE: Digitalis and allied cardiac glycosides. In: The Pharmacological Basis of Therapeutics. Fifth Edition. Goodman LS, Gilman A (Eds). New York, Macmillan Publishing Co. Inc., 1975, pp 670-671

Nies AS: Heart failure. In: Clinical Pharmacology, Basic Principles in Therapeutics. Melmon KL, Morrelli HF (Eds). New York, Macmillan Publishing Co. Inc., 1978, pp 259-269

RATIONALE 241-b

Digitalis intoxication can be avoided in most patients by careful dosage regulation considering renal function, age, endocrine status, and electrolyte balance. Monitoring of blood concentrations of digitalis glycosides may be of some value. Digitalis causes both impairment of conduction and initiation of abnormal beats. Care must be exercised in suppressing abnormal beats to be certain that there will be normal beats, or any beats, remaining. Phenytoin or bretylium tosylate are the preferred antidysrhythmic agents because they do not directly decrease conduction of normal impulses. Drugs such as quinidine, procainamide, or even lidocaine and propranolol should be avoided for this reason. Atropine might be an appropriate treatment of heart block, in which abnormal beats are seen as an "escape" mechanism. Digitalis impedes conduction and enhances vagal tone; thus, atropine may reverse part or all of digitalis-induced first or second-degree heart block.

Most of the effects of digitalis are caused by inhibition of Na-K-ATPase. This alters the balance of potassium between the inside and outside of myocardial cells, decreasing membrane potential. Lowered membrane potentials cause both impairment of conduction velocity (that is dependent in part on resting membrane potential) and enhancement of ectopic beats (as resting potential approaches threshold potential). In excessive amounts, digitalis also increases the "phase 4" spontaneous diastolic depolarization that may cause ectopic beats. Potassium antagonizes many of these electrical effects, without altering the positive inotropic effects of digitalis. Potassium is an important treatment of digitalis intoxication, even in the presence of impaired conduction, although potassium may worsen heart block in the absence of digitalis intoxication.

Calcium is one of the worst drugs to consider in digitalis intoxication. While calcium enhances the contractility effects of digitalis, it also may dramatically worsen dysrhythmias associated with digitalis toxicity.

REFERENCES

Moe GK, Farah AE: Digitalis and allied cardiac glycosides. In: The Pharmacological Basis of Therapeutics. Fifth Edition. Goodman LS, Gilman A (Eds). New York, Macmillan Publishing Co. Inc., 1975, pp 653-682

Spann JF, Hurst JW: Treatment of heart failure. In: The Heart. Fourth Edition. Hurst JW, Logue RB, Schlant RC, et al (Eds). New York, McGraw-Hill Book Company, 1978, pp 580-606

GLUTETHIMIDE

RATIONALE 242-e

For drugs to be excreted in urine, they must either have an active secretory pathway into the tubule (such as that for penicillin) or they must be filtered at the glomerulus and not extensively reabsorbed. Protein binding diminishes filtration. Lipid solubility favors reabsorption. For drugs that are partially reabsorbed, there are two important determinants of excretion. Increased urine flow generally increases drug excretion in a linear fashion. Urine pH, however, may have a greater effect. Phenobarbital and salicylate clearances are much greater if urine pH is greater than 7.0; alkaline urine promotes ionization of these weak acids. Phencyclidine (PCP) excretion is much greater at urine pH less than 5.5; acid urine promotes ionization, and minimizes reabsorption, of this weak base. For glutethimide, however, diuresis at any urine pH does not lead to appreciable drug elimination because this drug is highly lipid-soluble and extensively reabsorbed in the renal tubules.

Peritoneal dialysis has been employed for removal of drugs, but clearance rates are quite low. If the drug reaches the same concentration in peritoneal dialysis fluid as in blood, and 2 L of fluid are exchanged each hour, clearance may be as great as 33 ml/min. With hemodialysis or hemoperfusion, however, blood may be pumped at rates of 200 ml/min or more through a medium removing all of the drug. Comparisons of peritoneal dialysis with hemodialysis have shown the latter to be much more effective in poisoning.

Hemodialysis with oil was popular in poisoning with lipid-soluble drugs. The rationale of its use was that drug removal might be greater when dialysis is against a fluid in which these drugs are more soluble. However, glutethimide clearances are equal in hemodialysis against water or oil and the limiting factor is not solubility in the dialysis medium, but diffusion across the medium and blood flow through the system.

Hemoperfusion is direct percolation of blood over charcoal or resin. Charcoal hemoperfusion has been used in more patients, but suffers from several disadvantages. It causes greater loss of platelets than resin hemoperfusion, and does not extract some drugs as effectively as resins such as Amberlite XAD-4. In one case, Rosebaum succeeded in removing 37.5 g of glutethimide from one young patient in three episodes of hemoperfusion; hemodialysis generally removes less than 1 g of glutethimide.

When should techniques to hasten drug elimination be used? Even in patients with the deepest coma due to sedative drug overdose, survival is common if the patient has careful supportive critical care. The drugs that cause the longest coma are those that are the most lipid-soluble (such as phenobarbital, glutethimide, and ethchlorvynol). These drugs have large "distribution volumes," meaning that only a small fraction of the total drug is present in blood. Even if diuresis, dialysis, or hemoperfusion were able to rid the blood entirely of drug, only a small fraction of the total body burden would be removed in a few hours. Usually, patients poisoned with such drugs will awaken during hemodialysis or hemoperfusion, only to have coma return quickly when the procedure is stopped. Such awakening occurs because the brain, a repository of lipid-soluble sedative, has high blood flows, and when drug is removed from blood it usually diffuses rapidly from brain. This is not so for the fat and lean body depots of drug. When drugs diffuse slowly from peripheral sites of accumulation, efficacy of removal techniques are limited by slow diffusion. In such cases, removal procedures should be repeated frequently, at intervals of 4-12 hours, so that the drug may diffuse back into the blood before the next procedure.

REFERENCES

Asbach HW, Holz F, Mohring K, et al: Lipid hemodialysis versus charcoal hemoperfusion in imipramine poisoning. Clin Toxicol 1977; 11:211

Brown EA, Kliger AS, Finkelstein FO: Peritoneal dialysis clearances: A practical approach to the measurement of small- and middle-molecule clearances. Nephron 1978; 21:310

Curry SH, Riddall D, Gordon JS, et al: Disposition of glutethimide in man. Clin Pharmacol Ther 1972; 12:849

Gibson TP, Atkinson AJ Jr: Effect of changes in intercompartment rate constants on drug removal during hemoperfusion. J Pharmacol Sci 1978; 67:1178

Goulding R: Experience with hemoperfusion in drug abuse. Kidney Int 1976; 10:S338

Gwilt PR, Perrier D: Plasma protein binding and distribution characteristics of drugs as indices of their hemodialyzability. Clin Pharmacol Ther 1978; 24:154

HYDROCARBONS

RATIONALE 243-d

Poisoning by ingestion of hydrocarbons or inhalation of hydrocarbon fumes is a significant cause of morbidity and mortality in small children. Even when the hydrocarbons are swallowed, pneumonitis can be a significant problem. Pneumonitis commonly results from pulmonary aspiration of hydrocarbon fumes as well as liquid. In the lung, the hydrocarbons markedly decrease surfactant activity, causing severe atelectasis. Hydrocarbon aspiration often causes structural pulmonary damage, making barotrauma with IPPV and CPAP more likely.

Inducing emesis or using gastric lavage after hydrocarbon ingestion is highly controversial. If the patient is fully awake and alert and the ingested agent is noncaustic and is primarily a vehicle for other substances such as insecticides, emetics or gastric lavage may be therapeutic. The presence of an endotracheal tube, even with a tightly inflated cuff, does not ensure against aspiration of low viscosity substances such as petroleum distillates. Therefore, should emesis be induced, it must be done with a great deal of caution. Cathartics have no proven benefit.

REFERENCES

Ashkenazi AE, Berman SE: Experimental kerosene poisoning in rats: Use of C14-labeled bendecane as an indicator of absorption. Pediatrics 1961; 28:642

Beamon RF, Siegal CJ, et al: Hydrocarbon ingestion in children: A six-year retrospective study. JACEP 1976; 5:771

Berman LS: Aspiration of hydrocarbons. Current Reviews in Clinical Anesthesia, Lesson 19, Vol 1, 1981

Gerarde HW: Toxicological studies on hydrocarbons. Toxicol Appl Pharmacol 1959; 1:462,474

Thompson WL: Poisoning: The twentieth-century black death. In: Critical Care: State of the Art. Shoemaker WC, Thompson WL (Eds). Vol 1. Fullerton, CA, Society of Critical Care Medicine, 1980, pp I(N):1-94

EDITORIAL COMMENT

There is no data to support systemic toxicity of absorbed petroleum distillates. The pulmonary toxic effect is secondary to aspiration at the time of ingestion. Therefore, the treatment of choice for hydrocarbon injection is to allow it to pass through the system without reexposing the upper airway to the distillate. The exception to this is when the distillate ingestion is combined with a toxic additional poison. In these cases the options are (1) utilize emesis followed by charcoal, (2) lavage followed by charcoal, or (3) charcoal alone. Choice of treatment modality among these three depends upon the patient's mental status, presence of gag reflex, and propensity of the toxic substance for charcoal. If lavage is performed, an endotracheal tube with adequate cuff seal should be utilized. Recent data indicates that charcoal alone is as effective as emesis induction followed by charcoal, or lavage followed by charcoal in patients who (1) are not obtunded, or (2) who are obtunded and consumed their toxic substances greater than one hour prior to institution of treatment. Consequently, the most appropriate alternative in this patient group is the use of charcoal alone.

ADDITIONAL REFERENCE

Banner W, Walson PD: Systemic toxicity following gasoline aspiration. Am J Emerg Med 1983; 3:292

ISONIAZID

RATIONALE 244-b

The primary manifestations of INH toxicity are recurrent seizures, coma, and metabolic acidosis. INH inhibits activity of brain pyridoxal-5-phosphate which results in decreased levels of gamma-aminobutyric acid (GABA). The reduced level of GABA may lead to seizures. Pyridoxine prevents and ameliorates this decrease in brain GABA. Acidosis associated with INH toxicity is thought to be due to increased lactate from seizure activity. INH may also interfere with the conversion of lactate to pyruvate. Pyridoxine is given intravenously as a single dose, in a gram amount equivalent to the INH ingested. Most patients have cessation of seizures, lightening of coma, and correction of acidosis within two hours. Synergy between phenytoin, diazepam and pyridoxine may occur, and these anticonvulsants may play a secondary role in the management of an INH overdose. Large doses of pyridoxine appear to have few adverse effects although experience in humans is limited.

REFERENCES

Brown CV: Acute isoniazid poisoning. Am Rev Respir Dis 1972; 105:206

Wason S, Laconture PG, Lovejoy FH: Single high-dose treatment of isoniazid overdose. JAMA 1981; 246:1102

OPIOIDS

RATIONALE 245-e

In a patient with decreased respirations who has small pupils and stupor or coma, one must suspect opioid drug intoxication. The pupils may not always be constricted in opioid overdose. They may be dilated by anoxia, brain herniation, or anticholinergic drugs taken together with opioids. Also, the patient may have pupil constriction due to therapeutic use of opioids with coma caused by ingestion of other drugs.

Naloxone, which has almost no agonist actions, is an antagonist of all opioids used clinically, including propoxyphene, pentazocine, diphenoxylate, meperidine, codeine and nalorphine. When given for acute opioid intoxication, the patient often awakens and has improved ventilation. A highly-reliable sign is pupil dilation. Constriction of the pupils is a very unlikely response to naloxone.

If the patient has been a chronic user or abuser of opioids, a withdrawal syndrome may be precipitated with piloerection (especially over the chest), abdominal cramps, diarrhea, and discomfort. Vomiting commonly follows naloxone injections in patients with acute opioid poisoning or in chronic opioid users. Vomiting is a serious side effect of naloxone therapy. Patients with opioid poisoning will survive with ventilation and oxygenation, but aspiration of acidic stomach contents may kill them. Everyone giving naloxone must take responsibility for control of the airway. Some physicians prefer first to insert a nasotracheal or orotracheal tube. An alternative is to put the patient's head down and to one side, continuously cleansing the airway with a large capacity suction device.

It is appropriate to give naloxone intravenously every 5 minutes to adults in doses of 0.4, then 0.8, then 1.6, then 3.2 mg if there has been no response. Some patients who have taken massive overdoses of opioids will respond to the 3.2-mg dose, even though no response has been observed to the 1.6-mg dose. If the patient's pupils dilate, it is certain that the patient has taken an opioid--but it is not proven that opioids are the only poisons present or that the patient's condition is caused by drugs or poisons.

REFERENCES

Arena JM: Poisoning. Third Edition. Springfield, Charles C Thomas, 1974, pp 406-411

Blachly PH: Naloxone for diagnosis in methadone programs. JAMA 1973; 224:334

Jasinski DR, Martin WR, Haertzen CA: The human pharmacology and abuse potential of N-allylnoroxymorphone (naloxone). J Pharmacol Exp Ther 1967; 157:420

Ream NW, Robinson MG, Richter RW, et al: Opiate dependence and acute abstinence. In: Medical Aspects of Drug Abuse. Richter RW (Ed). Hagerstown, MD, Harper and Row, 1975, pp 81-123

EDITORIAL COMMENT

The recommendation for initial management of a comatose child who may have consumed narcotics is an immediate trial dose of .01 mg/kg of naloxone followed in two minutes by .1 mg/kg if no clinical improvement is seen. High doses of naloxone in normal subjects produce only mild subjective side effects and studies have shown the drug is proven safe and effective in narcotic ingestion in children.

Naloxone should not be withheld from the comatose narcotic addict suspected of an opioid overdose. The physician should, however, be aware that withdrawal symptoms may occur.

Propoxyphene may require considerably larger doses of naloxone to reverse its opioid effects.

ADDITIONAL REFERENCES

Handal KA, Schauben JL: Naloxone. Ann Emerg Med 1983; 12:438

Moore RA, Rumack BH, Conner CS, et al: Naloxone. Am J Dis Child 1980; 134:156

PHENOBARBITOL

RATIONALE 246-a

Phenobarbital is a long-acting barbiturate commonly used to treat seizure disorders. It is 40%-60% bound to plasma proteins. The pH of this drug is 7.2 and raising the urine pH greater than 8.0 with bicarbonate administration favors the poorly reabsorbed ionized form, thereby enhancing drug excretion. Charcoal hemoperfusion and hemodialysis are both effective in lowering serum levels. The former is more effective.

REFERENCE

Rall TW, Schleifer LS: Drugs effective in the therapy of the epilepsies. In: The Pharmacologic Basis of Therapeutics. Sixth Edition. Goodman LS, Gilman A (Eds). New York, Macmillan Publishing Co. Inc., 1980

POISONING/GENERAL

RATIONALE 247-e

Acetaminophen, often promoted as a safe substitute for aspirin, may be a treacherous poison, causing few symptoms in the first ten hours after ingestion while it produces irreversible liver damage. Doses as small as 6.5 gm (12 extra strength Tylenol) in the adult have caused liver damage. Acetaminophen (or paracetamol) is metabolized by the P_{450} mixed function oxidase drug-metabolizing enzymes in liver to a toxic metabolite that binds avidly to liver cell proteins causing delayed cell necrosis. Therapeutic doses do not cause toxicity because there is sufficient glutathione in these cells to bind the metabolite; but toxicity occurs when glutathione is depleted, when this mechanism is overwhelmed with large doses, or when acetaminophen metabolism has been accelerated by chronic use of ethanol, sedatives, and other enzyme-inducing drugs. Several antidotes are effective, if given within ten hours of ingestion, in repleting glutathione, binding the toxic metabolite, or inhibiting acetaminophen metabolism. Cysteamine and L-methionine are not readily available, but acetylcysteine (mucomyst) is available and is highly effective when given promptly in oral doses of 140 mg/kg stat and 70 mg/kg every four hours for a total of three days. This patient has ingested a dose of 65 gm of acetaminophen and, without the proper antidote, would be expected to have severe or fatal liver damage (with plasma acetaminophen concentrations > 300 mg/L four hours after ingestion). Naloxone antagonizes the opiate effects of propoxyphene and may be used to enhance spontaneous ventilation or as a diagnostic test, but it is not essential in this patient who is being ventilated adequately. Nalorphine has opiate agonist properties and should be avoided when naloxone is available. Ipecac syrup may cause emesis in 85% of patients to whom it is given, but gavage is more appropriate in a ventilated adult. Recovery of Darvocet four hours after ingestion may be minimal. Methylphenidate is an analeptic, arousing the intoxicated patient, but also causing seizures, enhanced sympathetic nervous system activity, and increased oxygen consumption. In addition, it inhibits metabolism of many drugs, thereby increasing and prolonging their toxic effects. (It is not known if methylphenidate inhibits metabolism of acetaminophen to its toxic metabolite, but there are safer antidotes that are readily available.) Methylphenidate should be avoided in poisoning and intoxication.

REFERENCES

Alsop J: Use of acetylcysteine in acetaminophen poisoning. Hospital Pharmacy 1977; 12:493

Ameer B, Greenblatt DJ: Acetaminophen. Ann Intern Med 1977; 87:202

RATIONALE 248-c

Endotracheal intubation is important in a comatose patient who is known or suspected to have taken a drug overdose. It ensures adequate airway protection, oxygenation, and ventilation. Induction of vomiting in a comatose patient is contraindicated. Even if an endotracheal tube is in place, aspiration is likely to occur in this setting. Placement of an Ewald tube for gastric lavage is important to facilitate the evacuation of larger pills or pill fragments. Administration of an absorbent such as charcoal via a gastric tube decreases the absorption of most drugs except solvents and inorganic salts.

REFERENCES

Thompson WL: Poisoning: The twentieth century black death. In: Critical Care: State of the Art. Vol 1. Shoemaker WC, Thompson WL (Eds). Fullerton, CA, Society of Critical Care Medicine, 1980, pp I(N):1-94

Thompson WL: Recognition, treatment and prevention of poisoning. In: SCCM Textbook of Critical Care. Shoemaker WC, Thompson WL, Holbrook PR (Eds). Philadelphia, WB Saunders Co., 1984, pp 801-832

RATIONALE 249-c

The treatments for acetaminophen, cyanide and propranolol overdose are correctly listed. The therapy for lead poisoning is incorrect. Chelating agents are used for lead poisoning. Although naloxone has now been proven effective for many conditions, lead poisoning is not one of them.

REFERENCES

June CH: Poisoning. In: The Pharmacologic Approach to the Critically Ill Patient. Chernow B (Ed). Baltimore, Williams & Wilkins Co., 1983, pp 661-687

Thompson WL: Poisoning: The twentieth century black death. In: Critical Care: State of the Art. Vol 1. Shoemaker WC, Thompson WL (Eds). Fullerton, CA, Society of Critical Care Medicine, 1980, pp I(N):1-94

RATIONALE 250-e 251-b 252-b

Incomplete combustion of carbon containing compounds, particularly in a relatively closed space, can lead to the production of dangerous levels of carbon monoxide. Symptoms of carbon monoxide poisoning are nonspecific, and patients may escape early diagnosis unless the physician considers this diagnostic possibility in any patient who complains of headache, nausea, vomiting, confusion, or coma. In 1895, Haldane demonstrated that carbon monoxide bound reversibly to hemoglobin, blocking the binding of oxygen to hemoglobin and resulting is tissue hypoxia. He also demonstrated that rats poisoned with potentially lethal concentrations of carbon monoxide survived if treated with hyperbaric oxygenation.

Sources of carbon monoxide exposure in the general environment include automobiles and cigarette smoke. Carbon monoxide is a colorless, odorless gas. The initial toxic effects are often insidious. Carboxyhemoglobin levels of 5%-9% lower exercise threshold for induction of angina in patients with underlying coronary artery disease. At higher levels patients with underlying cardiovascular disease may suffer lethal complications from carbon monoxide exposure. Twenty percent carboxyhemoglobin may cause previously healthy subjects to complain of headache, nausea, vomiting, and loss of manual dexterity. At levels of ≥ 50% most patients are comatose. Seventy percent carboxyhemoglobin is a potentially lethal level. Chronic exposure to carbon monoxide over two to three weeks can lead to a compensatory increase in red cell mass.

The pathogenesis of carbon monoxide toxicity is mainly by decreasing the delivery of oxygen to peripheral tissue. Carbon monoxide has an affinity for the oxygen binding site of hemoglobin 200-240 times greater than that of oxygen. It is important to remember, however, that this binding is dissociable. Carbon monoxide can be competitively removed from hemoglobin by high concentrations of oxygen. The level of carboxyhemoglobin is a function of the level of carbon monoxide exposure and its duration. Once carboxyhemoglobin is formed, hemoglobin becomes unavailable for oxygen transport. However, the evidence of tissue hypoxia for a given carboxyhemoglobin level is more severe than one would expect from reduction of the effective hemoglobin content alone. The interaction of carbon monoxide and hemoglobin interferes with the unloading of oxygen from the normal oxyhemoglobin present, especially at high carboxyhemoglobin concentrations. If carboxyhemoglobin levels are greater than 45%, the oxyhemoglobin dissocation curve is shifted left, interfering with oxygen unloading at peripheral tissues. A tissue oxygen tension lower than normal is required to unload oxygen from normal oxyhemoglobin in the presence of more than 45% carboxyhemoglobin. It appears that the potential for carbon monoxide to interfere with intracellular heme-containing enzyme systems (cytochrome oxidase and cytochrome P_{450} systems) is of theoretical interest, but is not of clinical importance.

The arterial blood gases of the patient with serious carbon monoxide poisoning are characterized by a normal PaO_2, metabolic acidosis (a reflection of tissue hypoxia), hypocarbia (reflecting compensatory hyperventilation secondary to the hypoxia and acidosis), and markedly decreased oxygen content and saturation. Direct analysis of carboxyhemoglobin levels, for example by oximetry, rapidly confirms this diagnosis.

The treatment of choice remains the highest possible concentration of inspired oxygen with adequate minute ventilation. The half-life of carbon monoxide elimination with the patient breathing room air is 240 minutes. If the patient is ventilated with 100% oxygen, this half-life may be decreased to 40 minutes. If one treats a patient in a hyperbaric chamber breathing pure oxygen at two atmospheres, this half-life can be reduced to 25-30 minutes. Under hyperbaric conditions, physically dissolved oxygen may provide most tissue oxygenation needs.

Because breathing 100% oxygen decreases the half-life of carboxyhemoglobin markedly, oxygen therapy is a more rapid and effective treatment than attempting exchange transfusion. (In the future, infusion of fluorocarbon emulsions that transport oxygen may be a useful treatment as rats whose blood is replaced with such emulsions thrive when breathing carbon monoxide at concentrations more than 25%.) Intravenous sodium bicarbonate may correct the metabolic acidosis temporarily. Controlled ventilation, tracheal intubation, and PEEP are probably not indicated in the patient described, as he is already hyperventilating and has a PaO_2 of 110 mm Hg on room air.

CNS damage after acute carbon monoxide poisoning is similar to that after other severe hypoxic ischemic insults. Patients may be comatose with myoclonic jerks and decerebrate rigidity. As they improve, they may have evidence of residual dystonic movements, related to damage to the basal ganglia, as well as cerebellar ataxia and alterations, in both cognitive function and personality. In a three-year follow-up study of patients poisoned with carbon monoxide, Smith and Brandon reported a 13% incidence of neuropsychiatric disorders; 40% of these patients had measurable memory impairment. Patients who have been seriously poisoned with carbon monoxide may develop the rare entity of postanoxic encephalopathy, described in 1962 by Plum, et al. This syndrome has been described only to follow episodes of severe hypoxia which have resulted in an initial period of coma. The syndrome usually begins 7-21 days after the initial insult. Patients initially recover consciousness and may appear to be normal. However, this transient improvement is followed by an abrupt onset of irritability, confusion, decerebrate rigidity--often progressing to coma and death. The prognosis of these patients is grim and no therapy has been efficacious.

REFERENCES

Agostini JC, Ramirez RG, Albert SN, et al: Successful reversal of lethal carbon monoxide intoxication by total body asanguineous hypothermic perfusion. Surgery 1974; 75:213

Ames A III, Wright RL, Kowada M, et al: Cerebral ischemia. II: The no-reflow phenomenon. Am J Pathol 1968; 52:437

Ayres SM, Evans R, Licht D, et al: Health effects of exposure to high concentrations of automotive emissions. Studies in bridge and tunnel workers in New York City. Arch Environ Health 1973;27:168

Geyer RP: Review of perfluorochemical-type blood substitutes. Tenth International Congress of Nutrition: Symposium on Perfluorochemical Artificial Blood, Kyoto, 1975, pp 3-19

Haldane J: The relation of the action of carbonic oxide to oxygen tension. J Physiol (Lond) 1895; 18:201

Nemoto EM, Kofke WA, Kessler P, et al: Studies on the pathogenesis of ischemic brain damage and the mechanism of its amelioration by thiopental. Acta Neurol Scand [Suppl] 1977; 64:142

Plum F, Posner JB, Hain RF: Delayed neurological deterioration after anoxia. Arch Intern Med 1962; 110:18

Safar P, Stezoski W, Nemoto EM: Amelioration of brain damage after 12 minute cardiac arrest in dogs. Arch Neurol 1976; 33:91

Smith JS, Brandon S: Morbidity from acute carbon monoxide poisoning at three-year follow-up. Br Med J 1973; 1:318

RATIONALE 253-c 254-e

The syndrome described for this patient is classic for poisoning by tricyclic antidepressant drugs such as amitriptyline. Acetaminophen causes hepatotoxicity that is delayed. Aspirin may cause coma, but temperature is increased, ventilation is increased, and cardiac conduction problems are not common. Diazepam may cause profound coma with ventilatory depression preceding hypotension, but it does not increase muscle tone, cause extensor plantar responses, or the cardiac conduction abnormalities. Heroin and other opiates depress respiration, and heroin overdose usually causes slow breathing. Pupils are constricted by opiates, though they may be dilated by brain anoxia or other drugs. EKG abnormalities are infrequent in heroin overdose though myocardial infarction can result from the hypoxia.

The tricyclic antidepressants (TCA) have four important classes of actions that may explain some of their therapeutic and toxic effects. First they inhibit reuptake and inactivation of serotonin (5-hydroxytryptamine, 5-HT) in the brain. This may be related to their effects on temperature regulation (hypothermia and hyperthermia), sleep (sedation and REM suppression), and extrapyramidal function (choreoathetosis and myoclonus). This effect is greater with the methylated tricyclic drugs such as imipramine, amitriptyline, and doxepin. Second, they inhibit reuptake and inactiviation of norepinephrine. This may, in part, explain the tachycardia, orthostatic hypotension, and tachyarrhythmias caused by tricyclics. This effect on norepinephrine reuptake is more prominent with the demethylated analogs such as desipramine, nortriptyline, and protriptyline. Third, they have potent anitcholinergic (atropine-like) effects causing dry mouth, urinary retention, blurred vision, constipation, and sinus tachycardia. Fourth, they have "quinidine-like" effects on cardiac electrophysiology causing increased sinus rate, prolonged PR interval, and increased duration of repolarization in the atria and ventricles. The QRS and QT intervals are increased at therapeutic and especially at toxic doses. These latter effects are now being studied for potential therapeutic use in decreasing ventricular tachyarrhythmias.

The patient with severe poisoning with tricyclic antidepressants often has coma, ventilatory insufficiency, abnormal deep tendon reflexes, sinus tachycardia, mild systolic hypotension, and a prolongation of PR, QRS, and QT intervals. These effects correlate with plasma concentrations of tricyclic antidepressants, and the more severely poisoned patient usually has plasma concentrations greater than 1 mg/L. Less common manifestations of tricyclic antidepressant poisoning include grand mal seizures, bundle-branch block, ventricular tachyarrhythmias, and mild hypothermia. All patients ingesting more than 1 g of tricyclic antidepressant acutely will have some toxic manifestations, though seizures and cardiac arrest usually occur after adults ingest doses of about 2.5 g. All patients with plasma concentrations greater than 1 mg/L have QRS durations greater than 100 msec. Although these toxic manifestations are serious, with good critical care the mortality from tricyclic antidepressant poisoning has been reduced.

Atropine, an antagonist of the muscarinic cholinergic receptors, is an effective antidote for poisoning with cholinesterase inhibitors as found in insecticides, but would worsen TCA's atropine-like effects. Epinephrine effects may be potentiated by TCAs and it should be used cautiously. Usually, hypotension is not severe and catecholamines are not required. Naloxone is a nearly pure antagonist of opiate receptors and would reverse coma and ventilatory insufficiency of opiate overdose, but would have no effect in tricyclic antidepressant poisoning.

Physostigmine is an inhibitor of cholinesterase, thereby causing effects similar to those associated with poisoning with insecticides and "nerve gases" that cause miosis, lacrimation, salivation, bronchorrhea, bradycardia, heart block, bladder spasms, defecation, and abdominal cramps. It often reverses the coma, myoclonus, increased deep tendon reflexes, extensor plantar responses, and increased muscle tone, but it does not reliably prevent or reverse grand mal seizures and, in fact, rapid injection of physostigmine may evoke grand mal seizures. Grand mal seizures are best treated with intravenous diazepam.

Ventricular tachyarrhythmias should not be treated with quinidine, procainamide, or lidocaine, that may worsen the basic defect in conduction. Injection of sodium bicarbonate, together with potassium in some cases, has been reported to correct the acute loss of intracellular potassium, improve conduction, and minimize ventricular tachyarrhythmias. The preferred specific antiarrhythmics at present are propranolol, that is useful acutely especially when ventricular tachyarrhythmias are caused by the enhanced norepinephrine actions, and phenytoin that does not usually further depress cardiac electrical conduction. Additional comparative studies are required to define optimal therapy.

Physostigmine has been suggested as a limited diagnostic test for confirmation of TCA poisoning. Arousal, however, does not occur in all patients with tricyclic antidepressant poisoning and may also occur in patients poisoned with methprylon, ethchlorvynol, and perhaps other drugs. The duration of physostigmine effect is short, averaging 30 minutes. Although a constant intravenous infusion of physostigmine may be given, its own toxicity is considerable and this is not recommended. Clearly, physostigmine should be used conservatively, only when the patient is well-protected in a critical care environment.

REFERENCES

Aquilonius SM, Hedstrand U: The use of physostigmine as an antidote in tricyclic antidepressant intoxication. Acta Anaesthesiol Scand 1978; 22:40

Bigger JT Jr, Kantor SJ, Glassman AH, et al: Is physostigmine effective for cardiac toxicity of tricyclic antidepressant drugs? JAMA 1977; 237:1311

Biggs JT, Spiker DG, Petit JM, et al: Tricyclic antidepressant overdose: Incidence of symptoms. JAMA 1977; 238:135

Brorson L, Wennerblom B: Electrophysiological methods in assessing cardiac effects of the tricyclic antidepressant imipramine. Acta Med Scand 1978; 203:429

Burckhardt D, Raeder E. Muller V, et al: Cardiovascular effects of tricyclic and tetracyclic antidepressants. JAMA 1978; 239:213

Burks JS, Walker JE, Rumack BH, et al: Tricyclic antidepressant poisoning: Reversal of coma, choreoathetosis, and myoclonus by physostigmine. JAMA 1974; 230:1405

Nattel S, Bayne L, Ruedy J: Physostigmine in coma due to drug overdose. Clin Pharmacol Ther 1979; 25:96

Newton RW: Physostigmine salicylate in the treatment of tricyclic antidepressant overdose. JAMA 1975; 231:941

Petit JM, Spiker DG, Ruwitch JF, et al: Tricyclic antidepressant plasma levels and adverse effects after overdose. Clin Pharmacol Ther 1977; 21:47

Thorstrand C: Clinical features in poisonings by tricyclic antidepressants with special reference to the ECG. Acta Med Scand 1976: 199:337

Vohra J, Hunt D, Burrows G, et al: Intracardiac conduction defects following overdose of tricyclic antidepressant drugs. Eur J Cardiol 1975; 2:453

RATIONALE 255-d

Normally hemoglobin exists in the reduced (Fe^{+2}) state. When subjected to oxidant stress the heme iron becomes Fe^{+3} (methemoglobin). The Fe^{+3} heme iron is incapable of binding oxygen. As red blood cells circulate a small amount of hemoglobin undergoes oxidation. The methemoglobin formed is reduced enzymatically by methemoglobin reductase.

$$Hb^{+3} + NADH \xrightarrow{\text{Methemoglobin reductase}} Hb^{+2} + NAD$$

Acquired methemoglobinemia is generally due to exposure to significant oxidant stress by drugs or toxins. Individuals heterozygous for methemoglobin reductase deficiency are much more likely to develop methemoglobinemia than normals after oxidant stress. Likewise infants and children may have decreased activity of methemoglobin reductase and, therefore, may be less able than adults to protect hemoglobin against oxidation.

Drugs commonly implicated in acquired methemoglobinemia include:

Nitrites and nitrates
Aniline dyes
Phenacetin and acetanilid
Sulfonamides
Lidocaine, chlorate

Normally less than 1% of total hemoglobin exists as methemoglobin. Clinically obvious cyanosis occurs when methemoglobin levels reach 10%-15% of total hemoglobin. Dyspnea, weakness and tachycardia occur at levels greater than 35%. Arterial blood is chocolate brown in color while the oxygen tension may be normal.

Treatment of methemoglobinemia includes supportive measures and identification and discontinuation of the oxidant stress. Intravenous methylene blue (2 mg/kg initially) reduces methemoglobin to hemoglobin and is used in severe cases.

In this case the 0.5% silver nitrate used for topical burn care provided the oxidant stress. Methemoglobinemia should be considered in any cyanotic patient without obvious cardiopulmonary disease. Another clue in this case is the "very dark" arterial blood gases with oxygen tensions in excess of 100 mm Hg.

REFERENCES

Gibson GR, Hunter JB, et al: Methemoglobinemia produced by high-dose intravenous nitroglycerin. Ann Intern Med 1982; 96:615

Kiese M: Methemoglobinemia: A Comprehensive Treatise. West Palm Beach, CRC Press, 1977

Turnberg JL, Luce E: Methemoglobinemia: A complication of silver nitrate treatment of burns. Surgery 1968; 63:328

RATIONALE 256-e

The comatose patient described has a fixed dilated right pupil and a left pupil that cannot be evaluated. Damage to the right sixth cranial nerve by itself does not explain the coma and is incorrect because the third cranial nerve controls pupil dilatation. However, as trauma or infection is frequently the cause for a sixth nerve paresis, the level of consciousness may be consistent with that possibility. The parasympathetic pupiloconstrictor fibers travel in the third cranial nerve. The pupil dilates after injury to this nerve, either directly or indirectly, as when uncal herniation compresses the nerve against the posterior cerebral artery of tentorium. Involvement of the sixth cranial nerve affects the ability to abduct the right eye (paralysis of right lateral gaze) but does not affect the pupil.

Several drugs such as atropine and scopolamine are known to cause dilated and glutethimide (Doriden) characteristically produces midposition or moderately dilated (4-8 mm) pupils. These may be unequal and can be fixed to light for several hours after ingestion of enough drug to cause coma. Fixed and dilated pupils do not necessarily signify a poor prognosis.

Subdural hematomas have been classified as acute, subacute and chronic. The acute and subacute varieties most often present with alterations in the level of consciousness, whereas headache is the more common presentation in the chronic group. In one large review, pupillary inequality was more common in acute bleeds, and, although in 79% of the cases the dilated pupil was on the side of the lesion (therefore a right-sided subdural would be consistent with this patient's course and findings), in 8% the dilated pupil was on the contralateral side. Therefore, this patient could conceivably have a left-sided subdural. In addition, increased intracranial pressure could cause bilateral pupillary dilation.

REFERENCES

McKissock W, Richardson A, Bloom WH: Subdural hematoma: A review of 389 cases. Lancet 1960; 1:1365

Plum F, Posner JB: The Diagnosis of Stupor and Coma. Second Edition. Philadelphia, FA Davis Co., 1972

EDITORIAL COMMENT

A prospective study comparing (1) charcoal alone vs. (2) ipecac followed by charcoal or gastric lavage followed by charcoal revealed that charcoal alone was equal to standard gastrointestinal elimination methods (ipecac or lavage) followed by charcoal with the exception of obtunded patients who had overdosed within one hour of intervention. Charcoal administration is currently delayed in many patients given ipecac because of nausea and continued emesis.

Renzi et al. presented data from small numbers of patients indicating that, if needed, activated charcoal can be combined with n-acetylcysteine and given orally in patients with acetaminophen overdose. Both of these agents may offer significant benefit in acetaminophen overdose and previous in-vitro data had supported charcoal binding of acetylcysteine. Further corroborative data indicating that these agents can indeed be combined would greatly facilitate the management of the acetaminophen overdose patient. Initial data also support the combination of activated charcoal with ipecac for maximum early absorption of toxic projects without decreasing emesis induction.

Isobutyl nitrite has been known for some time to be associated with methemoglobinemia when abused orally. Methemoglobinemia can also be induced by the more popular inhalation route of substance abuse.

Hyperbaric oxygen therapy has long been recognized for acute carbon monoxide poisoning. This mode of therapy is also effective if neurologic sequelae recur. Recurrent symptomatology may develop between 1 and 21 days after initial exposure and resolves with reinstitution of hyperbaric therapy. Hyperbaric oxygen therapy facilitates rapid removal of carbon monoxide from the hemoglobin and cytochrome systems while reoxygenating compromised tissues. Carboxyhemoglobin levels correlate with presence of carbon monoxide poisoning. There is, however, poor correlation between degree of elevation and severity of clinical findings.

ADDITIONAL REFERENCES

Black M: Acetaminophen hepatotoxicity. Annu Rev Med 1984; 35:577

Guss DA, Normann SA, Manoguerra AS: Clinically significant methemoglobinemia from inhalation of isobutyl nitrite. Am J Emerg Med 1984; 2:518

Kulig K, Bar-Or D, Cantrill SV, et al: Management of acutely poisoned patients without gastric emptying. Ann Emerg Med 1985; 14:562

Meyers RAM, Snyder SK, Emhoff TA: Subacute sequelae of carbon monoxide poisoning. Ann Emerg Med 1985; 14:1163

Norkool DM, Kirkpatrick JN: Treatment of acute carbon monoxide poisoning with hyperbaric oxygen: A review of 115 cases. Ann Emerg Med 1985; 14:1168

Renzi RP, Donovan JW, Martin TG: Concomitant use of activated charcoal and n-acetylcysteine. Ann Emerg Med 1985; 14:568

PROPRANOLOL

RATIONALE 257-d

Propranolol is a nonselective beta-blocker which, when taken in overdose, may cause bradydysrhythmias, hypotension, and cardiovascular collapse. Isoproterenol, a nonselective beta-agonist may, therefore, be useful in counteracting many of the pharmacological effects of propranolol. Atropine increases the heart rate by parasympathetic inhibition. Glucagon is both an inotrope and a chronotrope. Its inotropic properties are distinctly separate from those mediated by beta-receptors, although its chronotropic actions may at least be partially mediated by beta-receptors. However, glucagon has been shown to be effective in cases of propranolol overdose refractory to isoproterenol. Phentolamine is a nonselective alpha-blocker and, therefore, has no place in treatment of propranolol overdose.

REFERENCES

Chernow B, Lake CR: Pharmacologic Approach to the Critically Ill Patient. Baltimore, Williams & Wilkins Co., 1983

Dreisbach RH: Handbook of Poisoning. Eleventh Edition. Los Altos, CA, Lange Medical Publications, 1983, pp 390-392

Halloran TJ, Philips CE: Propranolol intoxication. Arch Intern Med 1981; 141:810

EDITORIAL COMMENT

Glucagon remains the most effective drug in beta-adrenergic blocker overdose. It has a salutary effect on both heart rate and blood pressure. Epinephrine is the second most effective form of treatment. Isoproterenol is minimally effective improving blood pressure in less than 25% and heart rate in only approximately 10% of cases in one study. Atropine has been reported to be the least effective of all treatments. If used, atropine should be given in larger doses than usual. Incremental doses to at least 3 mg may be necessary. Glucagon's effect is mediated through specific receptors in the myocardium which are not blocked by beta-blocking agents. Beta-receptor blockade effect lasts longer than beta-agonist effect and, therefore, repeated dosing is usually required. Intravenous calcium chloride has been successful in reversing the hypotension and bradycardia associated with combined beta-blocker and calcium-channel blocker overdose. Insertion of a transvenous pacemaker may be effective if drug therapy fails.

ADDITIONAL REFERENCES

Hall-Boyer K, Zaloga GP, Chernow B: Glucagon: Hormone or therapeutic agent? Crit Care Med 1984; 12:584

Heath A: Beta-adrenoceptor blocker toxicity: Clinical feature and therapy. Am J Emerg Med 1984; 2:518

Henry M, Kay MM, Viccellio P: Cardiogenic shock associated with calcium-channel and beta-blockers. Am J Emerg Med 1985; 3:334:336

Weinstein RS: Recognition and management of poisoning with beta-adrenergic blocking agents. Ann Emerg Med 1984; 13:1123

SALICYLATES

RATIONALE 258-c 259-c

Salicylates stimulate directly the respiratory center causing hyperventilation and thereby decrease arterial carbon dioxide tension and bicarbonate concentration. Overall metabolic rate is increased, however, with increased oxygen consumption, increased carbon dioxide production, and often hyperpyrexia. Of importance is the effect of salicylates on glucose concentrations in blood and brain. Aspirin was used as an early therapy of diabetes mellitus because it lowers blood sugar, but even when blood sugar is maintained there may be critical reduction of the glucose concentration in brain and cerebrospinal fluid.

Salicylate is still the single most common poison ingested by young children in the United States, although the incidence has fallen four-fold since the introduction of safety containers. Early symptoms of salicylate poisoning include rapid deep breathing which is due to the direct effect of the drug on the medullary respiratory center, causing a respiratory alkalosis. Severe salicylate intoxication uncouples oxidative phosphorylation and profoundly alters carbohydrate, lipid and amino acid metabolism. This causes a significant increase in lactic, pyruvic, and keto acids, resulting in metabolic acidosis. Fluid and electrolyte losses are common. Special attention should be given to intravascular volume and potassium replacement. Treatment with bicarbonate corrects the acidosis and facilitates renal excretion of the drug. Inhibition of Krebs cycle enzymes leads to decreased glucose availability.

REFERENCES

Arena JM: The treatment of poisoning. Clin Symp 1978; 30:20

Finberg L: Salicylate intoxication. In: Pediatrics. Rudolph AM (Ed). New York, Appleton-Century-Crofts, 1977, pp 788-790

Hill JB: Salicylate intoxication. N Engl J Med 1973; 288:1110

Temple AR: Pathophysiology of aspirin overdose toxicity, with implications for management. Pediatrics 1978; 62(Suppl):873

Thompson WL: Recognition, treatment, and prevention of poisoning. In: SCCM Textbook of Critical Care. Shoemaker WC, Thompson WL, Holbrook PR (Eds). Philadelphia, WB Saunders Co., 1984, pp 822-823

Thurston JH, Pollock PG, Warren SK, et al: Reduced brain glucose with normal plasma glucose in salicylate poisoning. J Clin Invest 1970; 49:2139

EDITORIAL COMMENT

Utilizing osmotic diuresis and increasing urine pH to more than 6, the half-life of salicylate can be reduced from 22 hours to 7 hours. Volume deficit must be corrected prior to osmotic diuresis. Bicarbonate is used to alkalinize the urine. Acetazolamide alone is contraindicated because it may enhance the metabolic acidosis seen with salicylates. Vitamin K, 10-20 mg intramuscularly, should be administered prophylactically with significant salicylate overdose. Hemodialysis or peritoneal dialysis can be used for life-threatening salicylate overdoses. Salicylate noncardiac pulmonary edema is more commonly seen in younger patient groups and associated with high morbidity and mortality. Early aggressive detoxification, supportive therapy, and hemodynamic monitoring would appear to be indicated in this group.

ADDITIONAL REFERENCES

Brenner BE, Simon RR: Management of salicylate intoxication. Drugs 1982; 24:335

Fisher CJ, Albertson TE, Foulke GE: Salicylate-induced pulmonary edema: Clinical characteristics in children. Am J Emerg Med 1986; 3:33

Hormaechea E, Carlson RW, Rogove H, et al: Hypovolemia, pulmonary edema and protein changes in severe salicylate poisoning. Am J Med 1979; 66:1046

Proudfoot AT: Salicylates and salicylamides. In: Clinical Management of Poisoning and Drug Overdose. Winchester HH (Ed). Philadelphia, WB Saunders Co., 1983, p 575

THEOPHYLLINE

RATIONALE 260-e

Zwillich described eight patients who sustained seizures secondary to theophylline toxicity. In only one patient were adverse effects secondary to theophylline noted prior to the seizure. Four of these patients died. It is clear, therefore, that nausea and vomiting do not always precede more serious toxicity.

The mortality rate in patients with theophylline-induced seizures is reported to be 50%. Seizures and dysrhythmias secondary to theophylline toxicity are often refractory to therapy.

Parks recommends charcoal or resin hemoperfusion, even in the asymptomatic patient for a level greater than 60 micrograms per ml. Although the subject is controversial, the literature does support the seriousness of theophylline intoxication.

Enteral administration of activated charcoal may also be effective in this setting. Charcoal significantly increases drug clearance in both enteral and parenteral administration of theophylline due to enterohepatic circulation. Activated charcoal may be used in conjunction with hemoperfusion in treatment of the severely intoxicated patient but should not be relied upon as the sole therapy. Peritoneal and hemodialysis do not clear theophylline efficiently and are not adequate for the management of poisoning.

Erythromycin and cimetidine increase theophylline's half-life and may precipitate toxicity. Ranitidine, a new H-2 receptor blocker, when compared to cimetidine, has less effect on theophylline pharmacokinetics.

Allopurinol also increases theophylline's half-life at doses greater than 300 mg per day. The clinical significance of this phenomenon, however, has not been established.

REFERENCES

Levy G: Gastrointestinal clearance of drugs with activiated charcoal. N Engl J Med 1982; 307:676

Mountain RD, Neff TA: Oral theophylline intoxication. Arch Intern Med 1984; 144:724

Park GD, et al: Use of hemoperfusion for treatment of theophylline intoxication. Am J Med 1983; 74:961

True RJ, Berman JM, Mahotte CK: Treatment of theophylline toxicity with oral activated charcoal. Crit Care Med 1984; 12:113

Zwillich MD, et al: Theophylline induced seizures in adults. Ann Intern Med 1975; 82:784

EDITORIAL COMMENT

Two different populations of theophylline overdose patients have been identified, the acute single ingestion patient and the chronic over-medicated patient. One study demonstrated that patients suffering chronic repeated overmedication developed predominantly seizures and serious arrhythmias with serum levels of 28-70 mg/liter. In contrast, single overdose patients were less likely to have seizures and arrhythmias but were easily recognized by the presence of hypotension, hypokalemia, and low serum bicarbonate, features not present in the chronic type patients. Seizures and arrhythmias were seen in the acute single ingestion group when levels exceeded 100 mg/liter.

Although patients with very high theophylline concentrations may not tolerate oral activated charcoal secondary to emesis, those who do benefit from 30 gram doses every 2 hours times 4 due to the entero-hepatic circulation of theophylline.

In patients with preexisting neurologic disease, seizure activity may be seen at theophylline levels much lower than expected. Reports of seizures with theophylline levels of 26 have been reported in this group. Length of therapy in theophylline overdose will be somewhat dependent on the sustained release property of the preparation.

ADDITIONAL REFERENCES

Gal P, Miller A, McCue JD: Oral activated charcoal to enhance theophylline elimination in an acute overdose. JAMA 1984; 251:3130

Olson KR, Benowitz NL, Woo OF, et al: Theophylline overdose: Acute single ingestion versus chronic repeated overmedication. Am J Emerg Med 1985; 3:386

Park GD, Radomski L, Goldberg MJ, et al: Effects of size and frequency of oral doses of charcoal on theophylline clearance. Clin Pharmacol Ther 1983; 34:663

Sawyer WT, Caravati EM, Ellison MJ, et al: Hypokalemia, hyperglycemia, and acidosis after intentional theophylline overdose. Am J Emerg Med 1985; 3:408

Singer EP, Kolischenko A: Seizures due to theophylline overdose. Chest 1985; 87:755

Section 15

PULMONARY

261. All of the following statements about the Adult Respiratory Distress Syndrome (ARDS) are true EXCEPT:

  a. Complement mediated neutrophil aggregation may be a major contributor to the initial pulmonary capillary injury.
  b. Neutrophils release superoxide radicals as well as neutral and acid proteases.
  c. The "capillary leak" is responsible for increased interstitial fibronectin which in turn causes interstitial fibrosis via fibroblast activation.
  d. Factor VIII:antigen may be a sensitive circulating indicator of pulmonary endothelial injury and repair.
  e. Thrombocytopenia is commonly found in this disorder.

262. All of the following are risk factors for the development of the adult respiratory distress syndrome EXCEPT:

  a. Pulmonary contusion
  b. Near drowning
  c. Hypercalcemia
  d. Sepsis
  e. Aspiration of gastric contents

263. Which of the following most closely approximates the expected PaO_2 in a normal individual at sea level breathing 40% oxygen? (Assume $PaCO_2$ = 40 mm Hg).

  a. 120 mm Hg
  b. 150 mm Hg
  c. 180 mm Hg
  d. 230 mm Hg
  e. 300 mm Hg

264. Which ONE of the following statements concerning pulmonary aspiration of gastric contents is TRUE?

  a. Early pulmonary lavage with alkaline or neutral solutions decreases morbidity.
  b. Steroids are the cornerstone of treatment and should be instituted within the first 12 hours after aspiration.
  c. Bronchoscopy should be performed if large aspirated particles are thought to obstruct airways.
  d. Prophylactic antibiotics are indicated to decrease the incidence of bacterial pneumonia.

265. Atelectasis during the first week of life in a premature infant is common because of:

  a. Lower than normal concentrations of surfactant
  b. Alveoli numbering about one-half those found in the adult
  c. Transpulmonary pressures of zero at the end of normal exhalation
  d. All of the above
  e. None of the above

Questions 266-269: Match each of the following patient descriptions with ONE of the options listed in a-d below. Use each letter once.

a. Respiratory therapy monitored-volume quantitated incentive spirometry
b. Fiberoptic bronchoscopy
c. Observation only
d. Intermittent positive pressure breathing

266. Cervical spine injured patient, not intubated, with reduced diaphragm function. Forced vital capacity is 12 cc/kg. Although patient's ventilatory muscle strength is improving, chest radiograph is noted to have a new finding of bibasilar plate-like atelectasis. A-a gradient has widened slightly.

267. Postoperative patient with new onset left lower lobe atelectasis. Arterial blood gases reveal a PaO_2 of 70 mm Hg and a $PaCO_2$ of 38 mm Hg on 4 liters O_2 per nasal cannula. Patient is presently receiving no respiratory therapy.

268. Recently intubated adult patient with viral pneumonia has developed acute onset of total right-lung atelectasis. PaO_2 is 40 mm Hg after FIO_2 has been increased from .5 to .8.

269. Patient improving from status asthmaticus is noted to have right lower lobe collapse.

270. During mechanical ventilation your patient has sudden cyanosis, dyspnea, and hypotension. You find her to have a pneumothorax and insert a chest tube applying 5 mm Hg of suction. It bubbles for 1 hour, but then bubbling ceases. The tube is not obstructed and chest roentgenography reveals it to be in good position with no residual pleural air space.

Which ONE of the following actions is now MOST appropriate?

a. Clamp the chest tube.
b. Remove the chest tube.
c. Reposition or replace the chest tube.
d. Open the chest tube to air without seal.
e. Continue chest tube suction as before.

271. Which ONE of the following statements about the infant or child with acute bronchiolitis is TRUE?

a. Nebulized epinephrine is a very effective bronchodilator.
b. Corticosteroids are of significant benefit and should be routinely used.
c. Coxsackie virus is the most common etiological agent.
d. Children under the age of one are most often affected.
e. The chest radiograph usually reveals diffuse infiltrates.

272. Which ONE of these physiological variables is LEAST likely to be INCREASED in the usual patient with chronic obstructive lung disease?

a. Alveolar ventilation
b. Dead space-to-tidal volume ratio
c. Pulmonary arterial mean pressure
d. Respiratory rate 2 min after moderate exercise

273. Which ONE of the following produces an increase in lung compliance?

a. Emphysema
b. Supine position
c. General anesthesia
d. Decreased functional residual capacity (FRC)
e. Left ventricular failure

Questions 274-277 refer to the following patient: A 50-year-old male patient has been mechanically ventilated for 14 days. He was a victim of a motor vehicle accident and sustained lung contusions and a flail chest injury. He has a tracheal tube and is paralyzed. Pressures measured proximally in the ventilator circuit are shown below.

Peak inspiratory pressure (PIP) = 50 cm H_2O
Plateau pressure (PP) = 40 cm H_2O

The patient's PaO_2 subsequently deteriorates. Each of the items listed below may cause such a deterioration. Match each of the following items with the appropriate pair of remeasured airway pressures (a-d). Each pair of pressures may be used once, more than once, or not at all.

274. Bronchospasm

275. Pneumothorax

276. Left ventricular failure

277. Bronchial mucus plugging

a.	b.	c.	d.
PIP 50 cm H_2O	PIP 80 cm H_2O	PIP 80 cm H_2O	PIP 30 cm H_2O
PP 40 cm H_2O	PP 40 cm H_2O	PP 70 cm H_2O	PP 20 cm H_2O

278. All of the following statements regarding the control of ventilation are true EXCEPT:

a. Peripheral chemoreceptors are responsible for all of the increase in ventilation that occurs in man in response to arterial hypoxemia.
b. Central chemoreceptors are located near the ventral surface of the medulla, close to the exit of the 9th and 10th cranial nerves.
c. Peripheral chemoreceptor response to arterial PCO_2 is significantly more important than that of the central chemoreceptor.
d. Molecular CO_2 diffuses across the blood-brain barrier much more rapidly than H+ or HCO_3^- ions.
e. Central chemoreceptors respond to changes in brain extracellular fluid H+ concentration.

279. Arterial oxygen tension is LEAST directly influenced by:

a. Inspired oxygen tension
b. Alveolar oxygen tension
c. Mixed venous oxygen tension
d. Venoarterial admixture proportion of cardiac output
e. Venous hematocrit

280. A patient is paralyzed with pancuronium and mechanically ventilated with a constant tidal volume (500 ml). Increasing the ventilatory rate from 12 to 16 per minute will MOST likely increase which ONE of the following?

a. Cerebral blood flow
b. Plasma bicarbonate concentration
c. Venoarterial admixture
d. Dynamic lung compliance
e. Total dead-space ventilation

281. A previously-healthy patient weighing 170 pounds is lying quietly in bed receiving controlled mechanical ventilation via an endotracheal tube at a rate of 16/min with tidal volume 700 ml.

Which ONE of the following events is MOST likely to increase arterial $PaCO_2$ from 25 mm Hg to 50 mm Hg?

a. Addition of 150 ml of dead space
b. Decreasing ventilatory rate to 12/min
c. Decreasing tidal volume to 500 ml
d. Shivering
e. None of the above

282. Which ONE of the following is NOT characteristically seen in the Adult Respiratory Distress Syndrome (ARDS)?

a. Early loss of both type I and type II alveolar cells (leaving a denuded basement membrane), followed by proliferation and repopulation of the alveoli by the type I alveolar cells.
b. Alveolar and interstitial edema with alveolar septal thickening and capillary congestion during the initial stages of ARDS.
c. Disruption of the alveolar-capillary membrane with increased capillary permeability leading to exudation of fluid and protein into the alveoli and interstitial spaces at relatively low hydrostatic pressures.
d. Complement-mediated neutrophil aggregation in the pulmonary capillaries with the release of superoxide radicals and proteases.
e. All of the above statements are correct.

283. All the following statements about pulmonary oxygen toxicity are true EXCEPT:

a. Oxygen in high concentration is toxic to the lung through the generation of superoxide radicals and other reactive oxidant molecules.
b. High concentration oxygen impairs adherence of Gram-negative organisms to lower respiratory tract epithelium and enhances migration of alveolar macrophages.
c. Mucociliary clearance is impaired.
d. Pulmonary antiprotease defense mechanisms are deactivated.
e. Chemotaxins are released from alveolar macrophages.

284. A 32-year-old female has a bacterial pneumonia requiring ventilator support. A left-sided pleural effusion develops and a thoracentesis is performed.

All of the following necessitate chest tube drainage of the pleural space EXCEPT:

a. A pleural fluid WBC count of 18,000
b. A positive gram stain
c. A positive culture
d. A pH of 6.8 with a normal blood pH
e. A pleural fluid glucose of 30 mg/dl with a normal blood glucose

285. Which ONE of the following antibiotics is MOST effective in treating Legionnaires' disease?

a. Cephalothin
b. Clindamycin
c. Erythromycin
d. Tobramycin
e. Vancomycin

286. Which ONE of the following statements is MOST correct about Legionnaires' disease?

a. Caused by an anaerobic Gram-positive bacillus
b. Organism first caused disease in the summer of 1976
c. Disease only occurs in epidemics
d. More than one strain of causative organism has been identified
e. Usual presentation is with bloody sputum and physical signs of lung consolidation

287. Which ONE of the following statements concerning bacterial pneumonia in the intensive care unit is INCORRECT?

a. Individuals with upper airway colonization by Gram-negative bacilli are at increased risk of developing Gram-negative pneumonia.
b. Elastic fibers in pulmonary secretions may be indicative of a necrotizing pneumonia.
c. Prophylactic antibiotics are associated with development of drug resistant strains of bacteria.
d. Bacteremia is a more common cause of bacterial pneumonia than is aspirated material.
e. Removal of excessive oropharyngeal and tracheobronchial secretions is an essential component of preventative therapy.

288. Which ONE of the following is MOST likely to yield a specific etiological diagnosis in a patient with hospital-acquired bacterial pneumonia?

a. Percutaneous fine needle lung aspiration (FNLA)
b. Flexible fiberoptic bronchoscopy with transbronchial biopsy
c. Plugged telescoping catheter (PTC) brush
d. Endotracheal tube suction specimen

289. In a mechanically ventilated patient receiving positive end-expiratory pressure (PEEP) with normal coagulation, which ONE of the following is MOST likely to produce significant morbidity?

a. Percutaneous fine needle lung aspiration (FNLA)
b. Flexible fiberoptic bronchoscopy with transbronchial biopsy
c. Plugged telescoping catheter (PTC) brush
d. Endotracheal tube suction specimen

290. Theoretical goals of PEEP therapy include all of the following EXCEPT:

a. Increased oxygen transport
b. Reduced work of breathing
c. Increased functional residual capacity
d. Reduced dead space
e. Improved lung compliance

291. In a patient with ARDS requiring an FIO_2 of 0.45 and a PEEP of 15 cm H_2O, a drop in PaO_2 from 70 mm Hg to 50 mm Hg may result from which of the following?

a. An increase in $\dot{Q}s/\dot{Q}t$
b. A decrease in cardiac output
c. A rise in pulmonary artery occlusion pressure
d. A fall in pulmonary artery occlusion pressure
e. All of the above

292. Which ONE of the following is LEAST likely to result from institution of positive pressure ventilation and PEEP?

a. Increase in venous return resulting in a rise in right atrial pressure
b. Impairment of the normal chronotropic response of the heart
c. Decrease in left ventricular stroke volume for a given filling pressure
d. Decrease in left ventricular afterload

293. Positive end-expiratory pressure (PEEP) may result in all of the following physiologic effects in patients with adult respiratory distress syndrome EXCEPT:

a. Increased functional residual capacity (FRC)
b. Reduction of lung water
c. Reduced intrapulmonary shunting ($\dot{Q}s/\dot{Q}t$)
d. Decreased oxygen delivery to peripheral tissues
e. Correction of low ventilation/perfusion ($\dot{V}/\dot{Q}$) areas

294. The protein content of lymph from the lung is increased MOST when:

a. Plasma colloidal osmotic pressure is < 10 mm Hg.
b. Pulmonary artery occlusion pressure is > 10 mm Hg.
c. Pseudomonas aeruginosa organisms are injected.
d. Lung minute volume of ventilation is increased.

295. The LEAST likely result of measurement of arterial blood gases in a patient with acute pulmonary edema breathing room air is:

a. $PaCO_2$ = 20 mm Hg
b. $PaCO_2$ = 40 mm Hg
c. $PaCO_2$ = 60 mm Hg
d. pH = 7.40
e. PaO_2 = 95 mm Hg

296. All of the following statements regarding the forces governing fluid exchange in the lung are true EXCEPT:

a. Normally there is a net filtration of fluid from the intravascular to extravascular space.
b. The sum of pressures in the Starling equation is greater than zero under normal conditions.
c. Lung lymph flow increases approximately linearly as left atrial pressure increases.
d. The protein osmotic pressure of lung lymph increases approximately linearly as left atrial pressure increases.
e. Hydrostatic and osmotic pressures are active determinants of lung fluid exchange.

297. Which ONE of the following statements regarding neurogenic pulmonary edema (NPE) is FALSE?

a. NPE usually occurs in the absence of underlying cardiac or pulmonary disease.
b. NPE can develop within seconds after CNS injury.
c. Experimental studies suggest that NPE is largely mediated by the sympathetic nervous system, specifically the alpha-adrenergic system.
d. A typical radiographic appearance helps distinguish NPE from other causes of pulmonary edema.

298. Low arterial oxygen tensions in a fireman who collapsed while working in a burning plastics (vinyl chloride) factory are LEAST likely to be caused by:

a. Inhaled carbon monoxide
b. Bronchospasm
c. Upper airway obstruction due to edema and laryngospasm
d. Ventilation-perfusion inequality
e. Pulmonary irritation from toxic products of plastics combustion

299. Which of the following is most likely to be indicated in the initial management of inhalation injury?

a. Corticosteroids
b. Prophylactic antibiotics
c. Tracheostomy
d. Fiberoptic bronchoscopy

300. A 28-year-old male inmate is admitted to the ICU after being overcome by smoke in a jail cell fire. He has no evidence of external burns. He is confused but his vital signs are stable. A persistent productive cough is noted.

Which ONE of the following is most likely to be TRUE?

a. Upper airway injury is unlikely.
b. A normal PaO_2 negates the need for supplemental oxygen therapy at this time.
c. Lower airway injury is unlikely.
d. Bronchoscopy may yield valuable information in this patient.
e. Antibiotics should be initiated.

301. Which ONE of the following findings is LEAST likely in a patient with massive pulmonary embolization breathing room air?

a. Arterial PaO_2 = 85 mm Hg
b. Arterial $PaCO_2$ = 20 mm Hg
c. Arterial pH = 7.5
d. Right atrial pressure = 5 mm Hg
e. Pulmonary artery pressure = 35/15 mm Hg

302. Which of the following findings is least compatible with the diagnosis of pulmonary embolism?

a. A chest radiograph demonstrating an elevated hemidiaphragm only
b. A room air PaO_2 of greater than 90 mm Hg
c. A normal physical examination of the chest
d. An electrocardiogram showing sinus tachycardia only

303. Following a life-threatening pulmonary embolism, thrombolytic therapy (streptokinase/urokinase) may be used MOST safely in which ONE of the following settings?

a. Two months following an intracerebral hemorrhage
b. Two months following a craniotomy for removal of a brain tumor
c. Twenty days following an uncomplicated vaginal delivery
d. Active hemorrhage from a gastric ulcer

ANSWERS

261-c	262-c	263-d	264-c	265-d	266-d	267-a	268-b
269-c	270-e	271-d	272-a	273-a	274-b	275-c	276-c
277-b	278-c	279-e	280-e	281-d	282-a	283-b	284-a
285-c	286-d	287-d	288-a	289-a	290-d	291-e	292-a
293-b	294-c	295-e	296-d	297-d	298-a	299-d	300-d
301-a	302-b	303-c					

ADULT RESPIRATORY DISTRESS SYNDROME

RATIONALE 261-c

Complement mediated neutrophil aggregation is thought to be a major contributor to the initial pulmonary capillary injury in ARDS. Complement activation with C5a generation may be responsible for the neutrophil aggregation. Neutrophils are capable of producing both endothelial and interstitial pulmonary injury through the release of superoxide radicals as well as neutral and acid proteases.

Thrombocytopenia is often present in patients with ARDS even in the absence of disseminated intravascular coagulation. A reduced platelet life span and platelet deposition in the lungs and reticulo-endothelial system have been demonstrated.

Several markers of pulmonary microvascular injury have recently been reported including Factor VIII:antigen and the fibrin/fibrinogen degradation product "D antigen."

No connection between the capillary leak phenomenon and the fibrotic response has been demonstrated. Fibronectin is an adhesive glycoprotein that is responsible in part for the architecture of connective tissue. It is in fact destroyed by neutral acid proteases in this condition.

REFERENCES

Carvalho CA, Bellman BS: Altered Factor VIII in acute respiratory failure. N Engl J Med 1982; 307:1113

Haynes JB, Hyers TM: Elevated fibrin(ogen) degradation products in adult respiratory distress syndrome. Am Rev Respir Dis 1980; 122:841

Hosea S, Brown E: Role of complement activation in a model of adult respiratory distress syndrome. J Clin Invest 1980; 66:375

Hyers TM: Pathogenesis of adult respiratory distress syndrome. Current concepts. Semin Respir Med 1981; 2:104

McDonald JA, Baum BJ: Destruction of a major extracellular adhesive glycoprotein (fibronectin) of human fibroblasts by neutral proteases from polymorphonucler leukocyte granules. Lab Invest 1979; 40:350

Rinaldo JE, Rogers RM: Adult respiratory distress syndrome: Changing concepts of lung injury and repair. N Engl J Med 1982; 306:900

Schneider RC, Zapol WM, Carvalho CA: Platelet consumption and sequestration in severe acute respiratory failure. Am Rev Respir Dis 1980; 122:445

RATIONALE 262-c

Direct pulmonary injury as a result of pulmonary contusion, near drowning, and aspiration has been correlated with increased risk for development of ARDS. Diffuse bilateral pneumonias may also increase risk. Sepsis is by far the most commonly associated risk factor for development of this syndrome. Hypercalcemia is not a singular risk factor for ARDS.

REFERENCES

Fein AM, Lippmann M, Holtzman H, et al: The risk factors, incidence, and prognosis of ARDS following septicemia. Chest 1983; 83:40

Hudson LD: Causes of the adult respiratory distress syndrome - Clinical recognition. Clin Chest Med 1982; 3:195

Loyd JE, Newman JH, Brigham KL: Permeability pulmonary edema - Diagnosis and management. Arch Intern Med 1984; 144:143

Pepe PE, Potkin RT, Reus DH, et al: Clinical predictors of the adult respiratory distress syndrome. Am J Surg 1982; 144:124

Shoemaker WC: Circulatory pathophysiology of ARDS and its fluid management. In: Textbook of Critical Care. Shoemaker WC, Thompson WL, Holbrook PR (Eds). Philadelphia, WB Saunders Co., 1984, p 310

EDITORIAL COMMENT

Great energy is being devoted to exploring the etiology of acute lung injury. Adult respiratory distress syndrome (ARDS) remains the clinical model for acute lung injury. The importance of oxygen-free radical injury and the possibility of preventing this by increasing levels of native antioxidants such as superoxide dismutase is an exciting area of research. Oxygen-free radicals include superoxide (O_2^-), hydrogen peroxide (H_2O_2), and hydroxyl radical (OH^-).

Antioxidants may block oxygenation of arachidonic acid preventing generation of peroxy radicals.

The role of platelet activating factor and serotonin in acute lung injury continue to be investigated.

A variety of injurious agents can stimulate an uncontrolled and generalized injurious lung parenchymal reaction. Mediators carried in leukocytes and platelets can lead to generalized pulmonary injury and modification of this inflammatory response can occur at numerous stages and offers hope in the treatment of adult respiratory distress syndrome.

In postoperative and septic patients early correction of hypovolemia, pulmonary vasoconstriction, suboptimal myocardial performance, and reduced oxygen delivery and consumption relative to the increased needs of the hypercatabolic state may prevent the development of ARDS and decrease its mortality.

Clinical and experimental studies indicate that complement activation may play a significant role in the development of pulmonary vascular injury. There is now preliminary evidence that oxygen radicals have the ability to generate chemotactic activity that is related to the 5th component of complement. Xanthine dehydrogenase is converted during ischemia to xanthine oxygenase, which then has the potential to generate superoxide in tissues. The possibility of allopurinol interrupting this cycle is being investigated.

In polytrauma patients and postoperative patients with ARDS, a significant correlation exists between immunoreactive trypsin and ARDS. Many of these patients also have abnormal amylase levels raising the possibility of a pancreatic etiology of the immunoreactive trypsin.

Although increased pulmonary vascular resistance in ARDS may be due to sequestration of leukocytes and platelets or extrinsic compression due to interstial edema, the possibility that it may be secondary to vasoconstriction which could be ameliorated by prostaglandin is being studied.

ADDITIONAL REFERENCES

Andreadis N, Petty TL: Adult respiratory distress syndrome: Problems and progress. Am Rev Respir Dis 1985; 132:1344

Bertrand Y: Oxygen-free radicals and lipid peroxidation in adult respiratory distress syndrome. Intensive Care Med 1985; 11:56

Dupont GD, Hass M, Pincemail J, et al: Immunoreactive trypsin in the adult respiratory distress syndrome. Intensive Care Med 1984; 10:7

Glauser FL, Fairman RP: The uncertain role of the neutrophil in increased permeability pulmonary edema. Chest 1985; 88:601

Hechtman HB, Valeri R, Shepro D: Role of humoral mediators in adult respiratory distress syndrome. Chest 1984; 86:623

Mosher DF: Physiology of fibronectin. Annu Rev Med 1984; 35:561

Shoemaker WC, Appel PL: Pathophysiology of adult respiratory distress syndrome after sepsis and surgical operations. Crit Care Med 1985; 13:166

Woodcock TE: Prostacyclin and ARDS (Letter). Intensive Care Med 1985; 11:273

ALVEOLAR AIR EQUATION

RATIONALE 263-d

The alveolar air equation is written: $P_AO_2 = (P_B - P_{H_2O})\ FIO_2 - \frac{PaCO_2}{0.8}$

In this case $P_AO_2 = (760 - 47) \times 0.4 - \frac{40}{0.8}$

$P_AO_2 = 235$ mm Hg

The normal (A-a) gradient is 5 to 10 mm Hg

235 - 5 = 230 mm Hg

REFERENCE

Shapiro BA, Harrison RA, Trout CA: Clinical Applications of Respiratory Care. Second Edition. Chicago, Year Book Medical Publishers, 1980

ASPIRATION

RATIONALE 264-c

If a patient is suspected of having aspirated large particulate matter, and evidence of volume loss exists on chest radiograph, bronchoscopy should be performed. Bronchoscopy in the setting of severe respiratory distress is, however, a formidable and hazardous procedure. Since damage to the lung by acid is almost instantaneous and is buffered by tissue protein, lavage is not useful and may be harmful in this setting. There are no conclusive clinical or experimental data which document that steroids are beneficial for aspiration pneumonitis unless given prophylactically. In fact, steroids administered after aspiration of food stuff may interfere with normal healing. Infection in the aspirated patient is difficult to document. Leukocytosis, fever, and pulmonary infiltrates are nonspecific responses and may be seen in uncomplicated chemical pneumonitis. Prophylactic antibiotic effectiveness is doubtful, and antibiotics should be withheld pending clinical evidence of infection.

REFERENCES

Modell JH, Boysen PG: Pulmonary aspiration of stomach contents. In: SCCM Textbook of Critical Care. Shoemaker WC, Thompson WL, Holbrook PR (Eds). Philadelphia, WB Saunders Co., 1984, pp 273-274

Murray HW: Antimicrobial therapy in pulmonary aspiration. Am J Med 1979; 66:188

Wolfe JE, Bone RC, Ruth WE: Effects of corticosteroids in the treatment of patients with gastric aspiration. Am J Med 1977; 63:719

Wynne JW, Modell JH: Respiratory aspiration of stomach contents. Ann Intern Med 1977; 87:466

ATELECTASIS

RATIONALE 265-d

Atelectasis is a common problem in the premature infant and is caused by all three factors named. Surfactant production is often reduced, making the alveolar surfaces "sticky." The smaller number of alveoli and their small size predispose to alveolar closure. At the end of normal exhalation the premature infant has a zero transpulmonary pressure, thereby allowing alveolar closure to occur.

REFERENCES

Avery ME, Fletcher BD: The Lung and its Disorders in the Newborn Infant. Third Edition. Philadelphia, WB Saunders Co., 1974

Sykes MK, McNicol MW, Campbell EJM: Respiratory Failure. Second Edition. Philadelphia, JB Lippincott Co., 1976, p 305

RATIONALE 266-d 267-a 268-b 269-c

Management of atelectasis in the ICU is a difficult and controversial problem. Marini et al. prospectively demonstrated that for routine lobar atelectasis in the postoperative patient, vigorous respiratory therapy alone was as good as bronchoscopy plus respiratory therapy. However, the numbers of patients were small and the atelectasis was treated soon after diagnosis. It seems reasonable, however, to treat recently developed lobar atelectasis in patients who are not receiving vigorous respiratory therapy with an adequate regimen consisting of a minimum of q 2h volume-monitored incentive spirometry with the possible addition of chest percussion and postural drainage (CPPD) in those patient groups who can be shown to generate 30 cc of sputum or greater per day.

O'Donohue presents good reasoning for using IPPB in those patients with atelectasis who are unable to obtain adequate vital capacity readings with incentive spirometry, particularly if improvement in respiratory strength is expected. It is important that volumes be measured with IPPB and only continued if there is a 25% or greater increase in a patient's vital capacity when compared to incentive spirometry inflation volume.

Patients receiving mechanical ventilation who develop atelectasis can be treated with periodic bag inflation and suction with the possible addition of CPPD. Patients who develop sudden massive atelectasis, particularly whole-lung, especially when associated with marked oxygenation defects, are candidates for fiberoptic bronchoscopy. The scenario in case 3 fits this description.

Atelectasis associated with severe asthma attacks is not unusual. Bronchoscopy in asthmatics has been associated with increased complications and should be avoided unless strong indications exist. In a patient who is improving after status asthmaticus with acceptable ABGs and is noted to have lobar or segmental atelectasis, most would recommend expectantly observing this atelectatic area for several weeks or longer before considering intervention. Since the asthmatic patient already has hyperinflated lungs, incentive spirometry would not be indicated.

REFERENCES

Mahajan VK, Catron PW, Huber GL: The value of fiberoptic bronchoscopy in the management of pulmonary collapse. Chest 1978; 73:817

Marini JJ, Pierson DJ, Hudson LD: Acute lobar atelectasis: A prospective comparison of fiberoptic bronchoscopy and respiratory therapy. Am Rev Respir Dis 1979; 119:971

O'Donohue WJ Jr: Maximum volume IPPB for the management of pulmonary atelectasis. Chest 1979; 76:683

O'Donohue WJ Jr: National survey of the usage of lung expansion modalities for the prevention and treatment of postoperative atelectasis following abdominal and thoracic surgery. Chest 1985; 87:76

O'Donohue WJ Jr: Perioperative measures for lung expansion. In: Current Advances in Respiratory Care. Park Ridge, IL, American College of Chest Physicians, 1984, pp 10-20

Schmidt-Nowara WW, Altman AR: Atelectasis and neuromuscular respiratory failure. Chest 1984; 85:792

EDITORIAL COMMENT

The treatment of atelectasis remains somewhat controversial, but generally accepted guidelines are that chest physiotherapy is the recommended initial approach and flexible bronchoscopy is reserved for refractory atelectasis. The potential usefulness and safety of the pediatric flexible bronchoscope for refractory atelectasis in small children has recently been demonstrated.

ADDITIONAL REFERENCES

Hedenstierna G, et al: New aspects on atelectasis during anesthesia. Clin Physiol 1985; 5(Suppl 3):127

Kirilloff L: Does chest physical therapy work? Chest 1985; 88:436

Nussbaum E: Pediatric flexible bronchoscopy and its application in infantile atelectasis. Clin Pediatr 1985; 24:379

Tisi GM: Atelectasis after abdominal surgery - Mechanism and prevention. Pulmonary Perspectives 1985; 2:3

BAROTRAUMA

RATIONALE 270-e

Suction should be continued for 18-36 hours. Within this period of time, pneumothorax often recurs. Clamping or removing the chest tube would permit pneumothorax to recur and not protect against the development of a tension pneumothorax. There is no evidence that the chest tube needs repositioning or replacement. If bubbling has ceased, and there is not residual pleural air, the pleural leak has closed. Opening the chest tube to air without a seal would only be safe if a constant positive pressure was maintained in the alveoli.

One of the important complications of mechanical ventilation is pneumothorax. It occurs more frequently in patients with diseased lungs, the use of high ventilatory pressures, and PEEP. Any unexplained sudden hypotension, dyspnea or cyanosis in a patient who is being ventilated mechanically should be regarded as a sign of pneumothorax until proven otherwise. The diagnosis frequently can be made by listening for unilateral hyperresonance or decrease in breath sounds. If time permits, a chest x-ray may be taken for confirmation. A pneumothorax in a patient mechanically ventilated should be treated with a chest tube. In a supine patient, this tube should be inserted in the second interspace at the anterior axillary line.

REFERENCES

Green RA, Johnston RF: Pneumothorax. In: Textbook of Pulmonary Diseases. Second Edition. Baum GL (Ed). Boston, Little, Brown and Co., 1974, p 992

Takaro T: The pleura and empyema. In: Davis-Christopher Textbook of Surgery. Eleventh Edition. Sabiston DC Jr (Ed). Philadelphia, WB Saunders Co., 1977, p 2091

EDITORIAL COMMENT

Patients who have a pneumothorax or large pleural effusion (with pulmonary collapse) present for periods longer than three days are at risk for developing reexpansion hypotension and pulmonary edema following rapid evacuation of fluid or air from the fluid cavity. Risk factors additionally include arterial hypoxemia during the pneumothorax, an elevated and rising hemoglobin level and the development of respiratory distress following insertion of a pleural drain. Slow evacuation of pneumothoracies by underwater drainage alone or by repeated aspiration of less than 1,000 ml of fluid or air are less likely to precipitate pulmonary edema. Both reexpansion edema and reexpansion hypotension may be seen alone or in combination.

ADDITIONAL REFERENCES

Christman BW, Marini JJ: Pneumothorax and barotrauma: Diagnosis and management. Pulmonary Clinical Update 1985; 1:1

Pavlin DJ, Raghu G, Rogers TR, et al: Reexpansion hypotension - A complication of rapid evacuation of prolonged pneumothorax. Chest 1986; 89:70

BRONCHIOLITIS

RATIONALE 271-d

Bronchiolitis most often affects infants under the age of one year. The disease is usually caused by the respiratory syncytial virus and has an overall mortality of about 1%. Cyanosis is an infrequent finding although variable degrees of arterial hypoxemia are often present during the acute phase of the illness. The disease primarily affects the small bronchioles and causes plugging from inspissated secretions, fibrin, and cellular debris. This leads to regional atelectasis and decreased compliance in some areas while other areas become hyperinflated. Physical findings include tachypnea, chest retractions, and wheezing which do not respond to bronchodilators. The chest radiograph usually reveals hyperinflation with minimal infiltrates. These infants should be closely monitored with arterial or transcutaneous oxygen measurements and treated with intravenous hydration and oxygen enriched humidified gas. Corticosteroids are of no proven benefit and antibiotics should be used only when bacterial infections are present. Endotracheal intubation and mechanical ventilation may become necessary if hypercapnia develops. Nondepolarizing muscle relaxants which improve chest wall compliance and decrease peak airway pressures may also be required for adequate ventilation. Neither alpha-adrenergic nor beta-adrenergic agonists administered by nebulization will reduce pulmonary resistance.

REFERENCES

Heiser MS, Downs JJ: Acute respiratory failure in infants and children due to lower respiratory tract obstructive disease. In: Textbook of Critical Care. Shoemaker WC, Thompson WL, Holbrook PR (Eds). Philadelphia, WB Saunders Co., 1984, pp 247-248

Wohl MEB, Chernick V: Bronchiolitis. Am Rev Respir Dis 1978; 118:759

CHRONIC OBSTRUCTIVE PULMONARY DISEASE

RATIONALE 272-a

Severe chronic obstructive lung disease is frequently complicated by clinically significant alveolar hypoventilation (increased $PaCO_2$). Large areas of the lung become underventilated because of alveolar destruction and small airway dysfunction. The residual volume of the lung increases and further interferes with the ability of inspired air to take up oxygen and clear carbon dioxide. When the arterial carbon dioxide is used to calculate dead space from the Bohr equation, a large percentage of the total lung volume is found to be dead space, the so-called physiological dead space.

The emphysematous lung is characterized by areas of poor alveolar ventilation and also by regions that have poor ventilation relative to capillary perfusion. When both alveolar ventilation and capillary perfusion decrease in parallel, little change in arterial blood gases occur until a major amount of tissue is lost; one lung can be lost surgically without changing resting arterial oxygen and carbon dioxide tensions. When perfusion persists through underventilated areas, however, the resultant decrease in ventilation/perfusion leads to lower oxygen and higher carbon dioxide tensions.

While occasional "pink-puffers" hyperventilate relative to their metabolic needs and may exhibit carbon dioxide tensions between 30-40 mm Hg, most patients with lung disease have normal or decreased alveolar ventilation. The use of tranquilizers, excessive oxygen, or the presence of respiratory infection may lead to additional hypoventilation. An increase in carbon dioxide tends to buffer the respiratory center so that the respiratory response to carbon dioxide is blunted and an additional component of respiratory center malfunction is superimposed. The final stages of alveolar hypoventilation in chronic pulmonary disease are characterized by substantial carbon dioxide retention, hypoxia, pulmonary hypertension, right ventricular failure, polycythemia, and somnolence.

Both destruction of the pulmonary vascular bed and chronic hypoxemia produce increases in pulmonary artery pressures. Inadequate respiratory reserve is unmasked with exercise and associated with inappropriate early rise in respiratory rate.

REFERENCES

Briscoe WA, Cree EM, Filler J, et al: Lung volume, alveolar ventilation and perfusion interrelationships in chronic pulmonary emphysema. J Appl Physiol 1960; 15:785

Macklem PT: The pathophysiology of chronic bronchitis and emphysema. Med Clin North Am 1973; 57:669

COMPLIANCE

RATIONALE 273-a 274-b 275-c 276-c 277-b

Lung compliance is defined as a change in volume with respect to a change in pressure.

$$C = \Delta V/\Delta P$$

More compliant lungs require less pressure to produce a set volume change. Less compliant lungs, conversely, require more pressure to produce a set volume change. The term total compliance refers to total system compliance (chest wall compliance + lung compliance). Chest wall compliance in a given patient is usually constant. Lung compliance is derived by measuring the change in lung volume with respect to the change in transpulmonary pressure. Transpulmonary pressure is defined as the pressure difference between the mouth and the intrapleural space. It is measured directly with an intrapleural catheter or indirectly with an esophageal balloon.

Emphysema breaks down lung tissue, decreases elasticity and lung recoil and, therefore, increases compliance. This loss of elastic tissue also causes early airway collapse and obstruction on exhalation. Lung compliance is decreased as one moves from the upright to the supine position, probably secondary to a decrease in functional residual capacity (FRC). General anesthesia decreases compliance, even beyond that produced by the decrease in FRC, for reasons that are not totally defined. Decreasing FRC decreases compliance and makes the lungs stiffer, classic examples being ARDS and interstitial fibrosis. The increased lung water seen with left ventricular failure also decreases lung compliance.

Normal FRC is associated with ideal lung compliance curve characteristics. At this point, work-of-breathing is minimized. As FRC decreases, however, compliance decreases, the lungs become stiffer, and the work-of-breathing increases.

Strictly speaking, compliance ($C = \Delta V \Delta P$) is a static measurement made in the absence of flow. In the dynamic state (during gas flow), the airway pressure generated depends not only upon total system compliance but also upon airway resistance to gas flow. Assuming a constant chest wall compliance, airway pressure (which is referenced to atmospheric pressure) is routinely used in mechanically ventilated patients to estimate changes in lung compliance and airway resistance.

Peak inspiratory pressure (PIP) reflects both total system compliance and airway resistance.

At end inspiration, just following the cessation of gas flow, airway pressure declines. If the expiratory limb of the ventilator circuit is momentarily occluded, the airway pressure will drop and reach a plateau. This plateau pressure (PP) represents the pressure required to distend the lungs and chest wall with a given volume of gas. Because no gas is flowing during this measurement and because chest wall compliance is usually constant, this measurement reflects true static lung compliance.

Those pathologic conditions that increase airway resistance such as mucus plugging or bronchospasm generally increase PIP only. Those that effect lung parenchyma, such as increased lung water or pneumothorax, increase both PIP and PP.

REFERENCES

Bates DV, Macklem PT, Christie RV: Respiratory Function in Disease. Philadelphia, WB Saunders Co., 1971, pp 29-31

Bone RC: Diagnosis of causes for acute respiratory distress by pressure volume curves. Chest 1976; 70:740

Connors AF, McCaffree DR, Rogers RM: The adult respiratory distress syndrome. DM 1981; 27:47,61

Downs JB, Douglas ME: Applied physiology and respiratory care. In: Critical Care: State of the Art. Vol 3. Shoemaker WC, Thompson WL (Eds). Fullerton, CA, Society of Critical Care Medicine, 1982, pp III(E):1-35

Shapiro BA, Harrison RA, Trout CA: Clinical Applications of Respiratory Care. Second Edition. Chicago, Year Book Medical Publishers, 1980

EDITORIAL COMMENT

Most new mechanical ventilators have automatic devices incorporated into the ventilator circuit to measure effective compliance. When these measurements are compared with the more traditional super-syringe measurements to construct the static compliance PV curve, the correlation appears to be good and allows reliance on ventilator measured compliance in the ICU setting.

ADDITIONAL REFERENCE

Mancebo J, Calaf N, Benito S: Pulmonary compliance measurement in acute respiratory failure. Crit Care Med 1985; 13:589

CONTROL OF VENTILATION

RATIONALE 278-c

Chemoreceptors respond to changes in the composition of the fluid that surrounds them. The central chemoreceptors are located in the ventral surface of the medulla close to the exit of the 9th and 10th cranial nerves. A decrease in the pH of the fluid surrounding these chemoreceptors increases ventilation while an increase in pH decreases ventilation.

Peripheral chemoreceptors are located at the bifurcation of the common carotid arteries and just above and below the aortic arch. They are responsible for all of the increase in ventilation that occurs in response to arterial hypoxemia. The response of the peripheral chemoreceptors to changes in arterial $PaCO_2$ and pH is much less important than that of the central chemoreceptors.

REFERENCES

Berger AJ, Mitchell RA, Severinghaus JW: Regulation and respiration. N Engl J Med 1977; 297:2,92

Civetta JM: Invasive catheterization. In: Critical Care: State of the Art. Vol 1. Shoemaker WC, Thompson WL (Eds). Fullerton, CA, Society of Critical Care Medicine, 1980, pp I(B):1-47

HYPOXEMIA

RATIONALE 279-e

Arterial oxygen tension (i.e., the partial pressure of oxygen in arterial blood) is directly related to inspired and alveolar oxygen tensions. Arterial hypoxemia is caused by reduced inspired oxygen tensions (e.g., at high altitudes) or reduced alveolar oxygen tensions (e.g., with high carbon dioxide tensions in alveoli). Venoarterial admixture (shunting) reduces arterial oxygen tensions by admixture of relatively less oxygenated venous blood. Low mixed venous oxygen tensions lower arterial oxygen especially when venoarterial admixture is increased. Venous (or arterial) hematocrit values do not directly influence oxygen tensions, though the hemoglobin concentration does determine the oxygen content.

REFERENCES

Martin L: Respiratory failure. Med Clin North Am 1977; 61:1369

Shapiro BA, Harrison RA, Walton JR: Clinical Application of Blood Gases. Second Edition. Chicago, Year Book Medical Publishers, 1977, p 90

Sykes MK, McNicol MW, Campbell EJM: Respiratory Failure. Second Edition. Philadelphia, JB Lippincott Co., 1976

West JB: Ventilation/Blood Flow and Gas Exchanges. Third Edition. Oxford, England, Blackwell Scientific Publications, 1977

MECHANICAL VENTILATION

RATIONALE 280-e

Increasing the rate of mechanical ventilation in a paralyzed patient increases alveolar ventilation, lowers arterial carbon dioxide tensions, and reduces cerebral blood flow. Plasma bicarbonate concentration would be reduced in compensation for the hypocapnia. Venoarterial admixture and "dynamic lung compliance" would change little. However, dead-space ventilation each minute would be increased as this is the product of dead space and ventilatory rate.

RATIONALE 281-d

Arterial carbon dioxide partial pressure (i.e., concentration) is a linear function of the ratio of carbon dioxide production to alveolar ventilation. For the concentration to double the alveolar ventilation must be halved. In a 170 pound patient the usual dead space is about 170 ml and may be halved by an endotracheal tube. Thus the alveolar ventilation is about 16 x (700 - 85) =

9.84 L/min. Adding 150 ml of dead space will reduce alveolar ventilation to 16 x (700 - 85 - 150) = 7.44 L/min and would be predicted to increase $PaCO_2$ from 25 to 33 mm Hg (25 x 9.84/7.44) = 33. Decreasing rate from 16 to 12 will reduce alveolar ventilation by 25% and increase $PaCO_2$ to about 33 mm Hg. Decreasing tidal volume to 500 ml will decrease alveolar ventilation to about 6.6 L/min and increase $PaCO_2$ to about 37 mm Hg. Thus none of the interventions will sufficiently reduce alveolar ventilation to cause a doubling of carbon dioxide concentration. However, shivering or major motor seizures will double or triple oxygen consumption and carbon dioxide production, thereby causing the increment in arterial $PaCO_2$. In the patient with controlled ventilation, the carbon dioxide concentration may be changed greatly by struggling, shivering, seizures, and efforts to breath.

REFERENCES

Martin L: Respiratory failure. Med Clin North Am 1977; 61:1369

Singleton GJ, Olsen R, Smith RL: Corrections for mechanical dead space in the calculation of physiological dead space. J Clin Invest 1972; 51:2768

West JB: Pulmonary Pathophysiology. The Essentials. Baltimore, Williams & Wilkins Co., 1977

Wilson RF: Principles and Techniques of Critical Care. Kalamazoo, MI, The Upjohn Co., 1978

RATIONALE 282-a

ARDS can be characterized pathologically into 3 phases: the exudative phase (24-96 hours), the early proliferative phase (3-10 days), and the late proliferative phase (7-10 days). During the exudative phase, type I alveolar cells die and are later replaced by proliferating cuboidal type II alveolar cells which are more resistant to injury. In addition, the integrity of capillary wall intercellular junctions is impaired, leading to exudation of contents into interstitial and alveolar spaces. Hyaline membranes are formed. In the early proliferative phase, type II alveolar cells rapidly proliferate, altering gas exchange across the alveolar-capillary surfaces. Hyaline membranes organize and inflammatory infiltrates develop in the alveolar septae. The late proliferative phase is characterized by widespread fibrosis. Complement-mediated neutrophil aggregation and release of their destructive contents is seen in all phases, but is felt to be a major contributor to the initial endothelial injury.

REFERENCES

Bachofen M, Weibel ER: Structural alterations of lung parenchyma in the adult respiratory distress syndrome. Clin Chest Med 1982; 3:35

Coalson JJ: Pathophysiologic features of respiratory distress in the infant and adult. In: Critical Care: State of the Art. Vol 3. Shoemaker WC, Thompson WL (Eds). Fullerton, CA, Society of Critical Care Medicine, 1982, pp III(A):1-28

Connors AF, et al: The adult respiratory distress syndrome. DM 1981; 27:4

Rinaldo JE, Rogers RM: Adult respiratory distress syndrome: Changing concepts of lung injury and repair. N Engl J Med 1982; 306:900

EDITORIAL COMMENT

Patients who are not chronic CO_2 retainers and who present with early acute respiratory failure usually demonstrate hypocapnia reflecting an increased minute volume. Overzealous controlled mechanical ventilation may be associated with respiratory alkalosis causing a detrimental shift in the oxyhemoglobin dissociation curve to the left thus inhibiting release of oxygen to the tissues. Hypoxemia may often be treated with supplemental oxygen alone. Mechanical ventilation may not be necessary or desirable.

Carbon dioxide removal is proportional to the fresh tidal volume that contacts the alveolar capillary membrane over time. Assuming no change in CO_2 production or dead-space ventilation, changes in $PaCO_2$ can be roughly predicted by ventilator rate and tidal volume. However, if CO_2 production or dead space change, this relationship will not necessarily apply. The patient's work of breathing and comfort may significantly alter CO_2 production. Progression of lung disease or changes in flows, pressures or volumes may alter dead-space ventilation.

ADDITIONAL REFERENCES

Macintyre NR: Mechanical Ventilation. Pulmonary Clinical Update. American College of Chest Physicians 1985; 1:1

Norwood SH, Civetta JM: Ventilatory support in patients with ARDS. Surg Clin North Am 1985; 64:895

OXYGEN TOXICITY

RATIONALE 283-b

High concentration oxygen deactivates antiprotease defense mechanisms, impairs mucociliary clearance, increases adherence of Gram-negative organisms to lower respiratory tract epithelium and impairs migration of alveolar macrophages. Oxygen in high concentration is toxic to the lung through the generation of superoxide radicals and other reactive oxidant molecules. The combination of acute lung injury and high concentration oxygen may be synergistic in the development of oxygen toxicity. In addition, oxygen poisoning causes release of chemotaxins from alveolar macrophages which in turn enhances the inflammatory response and promotes lung injury.

REFERENCES

Develse SM, Fanburg BL. Normobaric oxygen toxicity of the lung. N Engl J Med 1980; 303:76

Fisher AB. Oxygen therapy: Side effects and toxicity. Am Rev Respir Dis 1980; 5(part 2):122

McCord JM, Fridovich I: The biology and pathology of oxygen radicals. Ann Intern Med 1978; 89:122

Rinaldo IE, Rogers RM. Adult respiratory distress syndrome: Changing concepts of lung injury and repair. N Engl J Med 1982; 306:900

PLEURAL EFFUSION

RATIONALE 284-a

Approximately 40% of documented bacterial pneumonias are associated with parapneumonic effusions. Of these, only a small percentage require chest tube drainage. Criteria for chest tube insertion are those that indicate bacterial invasion of the pleural space. These include a positive gram stain, a positive culture, a pleural fluid glucose less than 40 mg/dl with normal or increased blood glucose, or gross purulence (empyema). High WBC counts with a PMN predominance can be seen in parapneumonic effusions that do not require chest tube drainage and, therefore, should not be used as criteria for chest tube insertion unless gross purulence is present. Pleural fluid pH is also utilized to make decisions on chest tube insertion. The fluid should be collected anaerobically in a heparinized syringe and immediately placed on ice. A parapneumonic effusion with a pH less than 7.0 (given a normal blood pH) requires chest tube drainage. Nonparapneumonic effusions may also have a very low pH. Examples include pleural effusions associated with malignancy, tuberculosis, and rheumatoid arthritis. The same is true for a glucose less than 40 mg/dl which can be seen in nonparapneumonic effusions such as rheumatoid arthritis and malignancy.

REFERENCES

Light RW, Girard WM, Jenkinson SG, et al: Parapneumonic effusions. Am J Med 1980; 69:507

Light RW: Management of parapneumonic effusions. Arch Intern Med 1981; 141:1339

PNEUMONIA

RATIONALE 285-c

By the agar dilution technique, the minimal inhibitory concentrations (MICs) of cephalothin, clindamycin, and vancomycin for Legionella were found by Thornsberry et al. to be greater than the range usually associated with susceptibility. Sensitivity of Legionnaires' agent to aminoglycosides was tested by Fraser et al., using gentamicin in a guinea pig intraperitoneal injection model. Gentamicin was unsuccessful in preventing guinea pig death in this study.

The agent of choice in the management of Legionnaires' disease is erythromycin. This is based on suggestive data from the 1976 outbreak in Philadelphia, and on more definitive bacteriological studies in animals after the agent was identified. The death rate among patients receiving erythromycin or tetracycline in the 1976 epidemic was about one-half of that of untreated patients, and less than that of patients treated with other antibiotics, including cephalothin and gentamicin. The dosage of erythromycin that has been used in the management of Legionnaires' disease is variable, and there is some evidence that an intravenous dose of 2-4 g/day may be necessary. Combining erythromycin with rifampin may be more effective than erythromycin alone.

REFERENCES

Fraser DW, Wachsmuth IK, Bopp C, et al: Antibiotic treatment of guinea pigs infected with agent of Legionnaires' disease. Lancet 1978; 1:175

Sanford JP: Legionnaires' disease: The first thousand days. N Engl J Med 1979; 300:654

Scully RE, Galdabini JJ, McNeely BU: Case records of the Massachusetts General Hospital: Weekly clinicopathological exercises (case 17-1978). N Engl J Med 1978; 298:1014

RATIONALE 286-d

The agent responsible for Legionnaires' disease was isolated in 1977. It was found to be aerobic and Gram-negative, and was given the name: Legionella pneumophila. After the causative agent was identified, a plethora of reports showed serological evidence that it caused previous outbreaks of undiagnosed diseases. The disorder may occur in both sporadic cases and epidemics, and both of these have been reported to occur most often between June and November. The usual presentation is with constitutional symptoms, including malaise, headache, and myalgia, and although the sputum is sometimes bloodtinged, it is rarely grossly bloody. The serological diagnosis of Legionnaires' disease has resulted in the identification of distinct strains or serotypes: the Philadelphia, Togus, Wadsworth VA, and Bloomington strains.

REFERENCES

Edelstein PH, Meyer RD, Finegold SM: Isolation of a new serotype of Legionnaires' disease bacterium. Lancet 1978; 2:1172

McDade JE, Shepard CC, Fraser DW, et al: Legionnaires' disease: Isolation of a bacterium and demonstration of its role in other respiratory disease. N Engl J Med 1977; 297:1197

Sanford JP: Legionnaires' disease: The first thousand days. N Engl J Med 1979; 300:654

Scully RE, Galdabini JJ, McNeely BU: Case records of the Massachusetts General Hospital: Weekly clinicopathological exercises (case 17-1978). N Engl J Med 1978; 298:1014

Terranova W, Cohen ML, Fraser DW: 1974 outbreak of Legionnaires' disease diagnosed in 1977: Clinical and epidemiological features. Lancet 1978; 2:122

RATIONALE 287-d

Patients who have oropharyngeal colonization with Gram-negative rods are at an increased risk for development of Gram-negative pneumonia. Aspiration of infected material is the most common cause of pneumonia. Inability to clear airway secretions predisposes to aspiration and atelectasis. Use of prophylactic antibiotics has been associated with development of drug resistant bacteria. Elastic fibers in the sputum are associated with necrotizing pneumonias. Secretion retention leads to mucus plugging and predisposition to bacterial pneumonia.

REFERENCES

de Jongh CA, Caplan ES, Schimpff SC: Infections in the critical care patient. In: Textbook of Critical Care. Shoemaker WC, Thompson WL, Holbrook PR (Eds). Philadelphia, WB Saunders Co., 1984, pp 505-517

Johanson WG, Pierce AK, Sanford JP: Changing pharyngeal bacterial flora of hospitalized patients. Emergence of Gram-negative bacilli. N Engl J Med 1969; 281:1137

Klastersky J, Huysmans E, Weerts D, et al: Endotracheally administered gentamicin for the prevention of infections of the respiratory tract in patients with tracheostomy. A double blind study. Chest 1974; 65:650

Wolinsky E: Pulmonary infection in critical care medicine. In: Textbook of Critical Care. Shoemaker WC, Thompson WL, Holbrook PR (Eds). Philadelphia, WB Saunders Co., 1984, pp 576-579

RATIONALE 288-a 289-a

Percutaneous fine needle lung aspiration (FNLA) is most likely to yield a specific diagnosis in bacterial pneumonia. FNLA may, however, on occasion fail to demonstrate bacterial pathogens even if they are present within the pulmonary parenchyma.

FNLA is also most likely to produce significant morbidity. Pneumothorax commonly occurs following this procedure in non-mechanically ventilated patients and, therefore, is relatively contraindicated in mechanically ventilated patients and perhaps absolutely with PEEP.

An endotracheal tube suction specimen is least likely to yield a specific diagnosis. The endotracheal tube and upper airway of mechanically ventilated patients become rapidly colonized with oral flora. Correlation of specimen findings with parenchymal organisms is poor.

Transbronchial biopsy is helpful in diagnosis of invasive opportunistic infection. It is of no value, however, in diagnosis of nonopportunistic nosocomial pneumonia because specimens are contaminated with upper airway secretions. Although barotrauma and hemorrhage may occur with this technique, it is usually tolerated quite well and its associated morbidity is expected to be less than FNLA in the mechanically ventilated patient receiving PEEP with normal coagulation.

The plugged telescoping catheter brush is currently being investigated for the diagnosis of bacterial pneumonias. Although showing promise of allowing guidance in antibiotic therapy, its sensitivity and specificity in this setting remain to be determined. The procedure is generally well tolerated.

REFERENCES

Chastre JS, Vian F, Brun P, et al: Concise clinical studies: Prospective evaluations of the protected specimen brush for the diagnosis of pulmonary infections in ventilated patients. Am Rev Respir Dis 1984; 130:924

Fossieck BE Jr, Parker RH, Cohen MH, et al: Fiberoptic bronchoscopy and culture of bacteria from the lower respiratory tract. Chest 1977; 72:5

Moser KM, Mauer J, Jassy L, et al: Sensitivity, specificity, and risk of diagnostic procedures in a canine model of streptococcus pneumoniae pneumonia. Am Rev Respir Dis 1982; 125:436

Repsher LH, Levin DC, Matthay RA, et al: Transbronchial lung biopsy via the fiberoptic bronchoscope in the diagnosis of diffuse pulmonary infiltrates in the immunosuppressed host. Natl Cancer Inst Monogr 1976; 43:127

Rinke CM: Diagnosis of acute, diffuse pulmonary infiltrates. JAMA 1984; 252:2044

Tobin MJ, Grenvik A: Nosocomial lung infection and its diagnosis. Crit Care Med 1984; 12:191

Wimberley N, Faling LJ, Bartlett JG: A fiberoptic bronchoscopy technique to obtain uncontaminated lower airway secretions for bacterial culture. Am Rev Respir Dis 1979; 119:337

Zucker A, Pollack M, Katz R: Blind use of the double-lumen plugged catheter for diagnosis of respiratory tract infections in critically ill children. Crit Care Med 1984; 12:867

EDITORIAL COMMENT

Bacterial culture of expectorated sputum and endotracheal tube suctioned sputum (even if gathered in a sterile manner) is unreliable for predicting the infecting organism in patients with pneumonia. Gram stain may be helpful to direct therapy but is not a diagnostic gold standard. Although additional studies touting the value of the protected telescoping brush catheter in the management of bacterial pulmonary infection in intubated patients have been published, validation of this procedure awaits further prospective well-designed comparative studies with gold standard diagnosis.

The evaluation of pulmonary infection is often complex and associated with many variables in the immunocompromised patient. In general, early aggressive tissue diagnosis is preferred. The choice of a transbronchial or an open lung biopsy procedure depends on the condition of the patient and the location and character of the disease process. Often the patient cannot tolerate transbronchial biopsy because of a bleeding diathesis. In patients in whom there is a high suspicion of virus, fungus, or parasitic pneumonia, immediate definitive tissue diagnosis is preferred. Antibiotic therapy should not be withheld awaiting biopsy. Twenty-four hours of antibiotic therapy will not effect biopsy diagnosis of fungal, viral, or parasitic pneumonia. In the adult acute leukemia patient, diffuse pulmonary infiltrates require an earlier, more aggressive approach when compared to localized infiltrates in which empiric therapy may be fruitful. Papin et al. have demonstrated relative safety of transbronchial biopsy in mechanically ventilated patients (some with up to PEEP of 10).

Typical pneumocystis pneumonia presents with diffuse bilateral alveolar and intersitial shadowing beginning in the perihilar area and later coalescing and spreading into a butterfly pattern. Many atypical radiographic features have been described, however, and absence of this classic presentation cannot be relied upon as an indicator for absence of pneumocystis pneumonia.

It must be remembered that in the immunocompromised host up to 25% of pulmonary complications are not infectious.

Pulmonary infection in the Acquired Immunodeficiency Syndrome (AIDS) is a challenge for the critical care physician. It appears now that the diagnosis of pneumocystis pneumonia, the most common pulmonary infection in this group, can be made by bronchoalveolar lavage in most patients. Increased yield by combining lavage with transbronchial biopsy and brushing has been shown. Diagnosis may also be made on exam of sputum in this group. Since patients with AIDS may have pneumocystis carinii pneumonia even in the absence of chest x-ray abnormalities, if a significant increase in the alveolar-arterial oxygen gradient is present, it is recommended that fiberoptic bronchoscopy with lavage, brush, and biopsy be entertained early. Patients with pneumocystis pneumonia invaribly have positive gallium lung scans even when the chest radiograph is normal if the patient has significant pulmonary symptoms.

ADDITIONAL REFERENCES

Berger R, Arango L: Etiologic diagnosis of bacterial nosocomial pneumonia in seriously ill patients. Crit Care Med 1985; 13:833

Catterall JR, Potasman I, Remington JS: Pneumocystis carinii pneumonia in the patient with AIDS. Chest 1985; 88:758

Hartman B, Koss M, Hui A, et al: Pneumocystis carinii pneumonia in the acquired immunodeficiency syndrome (AIDS). Chest 1985; 87:603

Horsburgh CR: Pulmonary infection in the immunocompromised host. Pulmonary Clinical Update. American College of Chest Physicians 1985; 1:1

MacFarlane JT, Finch RG: Pneumocystis carinii pneumonia. Thorax 1985; 40:561

Papin TA, Brum CA, Weg JG: Transbronchial biopsy during mechanical ventilation. Chest 1986; 89:168

Pitchenik AE, Parvin G, Torres A, et al: Sputum examination for the diagnosis of pneumocystis carinii pneumonia in AIDS. Am Rev Respir Dis 1986; 133:226

Rosen MJ, Tow TW, Steirstein AS, et al: Diagnosis of pulmonary complications of the acquired immune deficiency syndrome. Thorax 1985; 40:571

Rosenow EC, Wilson WR, Cockerill FR: Pulmonary disease in the immunocompromised host (first of two parts). Mayo Clin Proc 1985; 60:473

Suffredini AF, Tobin MJ, Wajszczuk CP, et al: Acute respiratory failure due to pneumocystis carinii pneumonia: Clinical, radiographic, and pathologic course. Crit Care Med 1985; 13:237

Torzillo PJ, McWillian DB, Young IH, et al: Use of protected telescoping brush system in the management of bacterial pulmonary infection in intubated patients. Br J Dis Chest 1985; 79:125

Wardman AG, Milligan DW, Child JA, et al: Pulmonary infiltrates and adult acute leukaemia: Empiric treatment and survival related to the extent of pulmonary radiological disease. Thorax 1984; 39:568

POSITIVE END-EXPIRATORY PRESSURE

RATIONALE 290-d

Positive end-expiratory pressure (PEEP) increases functional residual capacity (FRC). It is most efficacious in those disease states characterized by decreased FRC, increased $\dot{Q}s/\dot{Q}t$ and decreased pulmonary compliance. By raising FRC, atelectatic alveoli are recruited for oxygen exchange decreasing $\dot{Q}s/\dot{Q}t$. This allows for an increased PaO_2 with a decreased FIO_2. Just as PEEP will increase ventilation to areas of low $\dot{V}/\dot{Q}$, it may increase ventilation to areas of normal to high $\dot{V}/\dot{Q}$ and subsequently increase dead-space ventilation. As PEEP increases FRC toward normal, the compliance of the lung increases and, therefore, decreases the work of breathing.

REFERENCES

Downs J, Modell J: Patterns of respiratory support aimed at pathophysiologic conditions. ASA Refresher Courses in Anesthesiology, Vol 5, Chap 6, 1977

Hammon JW, et al: The effect of PEEP on regional ventilation and perfusion in the normal and injured primate lung. J Thorac Cardiovasc Surg 1976; 72:680

Suter PM, Fairley HB, Isenberg M: High level PEEP in acute respiratory insufficiency. N Engl J Med 1975; 292:284

RATIONALE 291-e

In a patient with a significant intrapulmonary shunt, a drop in PaO_2 may result from either an increase in $\dot{Q}s/\dot{Q}t$ or a decrease in cardiac output.

Changes in pulmonary artery occlusion pressure affect the hydrostatic forces governing the movement of fluid into the lung and, as such, may increase or decrease $\dot{Q}s/\dot{Q}t$. However, changes in PAOP may also have dramatic effects on cardiac output, especially in patients on high levels of PEEP. Therefore, a given change in PAOP may increase or decrease PaO_2 depending on which factor (CO or $\dot{Q}s/\dot{Q}t$) is affected most.

REFERENCES

Cheney F, Colley P: The effect of cardiac output on PaO_2. Anesthesiology 1980; 52:496

Dantzker D, Lynch J, et al: Depression of cardiac output is a mechanism of shunt reduction in the therapy of acute respiratory failure. Chest 1980; 77:5,636

Wilson RS, Pontoppidan H: Acute respiratory failure: Diagnostic and therapeutic criteria. Crit Care Med 1974; 2:293

RATIONALE 292-a

Neither positive pressure ventilation (PPV) nor PEEP should increase venous return. Positive pressure ventilation and PEEP raise intrathoracic pressure resulting in: (a) reduction in venous return, and (b) change in the compliance of the right and left atrium altering atrial transmural pressure. Consequently, right atrial pressures may stay the same or rise in spite of a drop in venous return. PPV also impairs the normal chronotropic response of the heart. This dampened response is well documented but poorly understood. It is thought to be induced by lung expansion and mediated through the vagus nerve. Elevated airway pressures increases pulmonary vascular resistance and increases right ventricular afterload. This causes a shift in the interventricular septum compressing the left ventricular cavity altering left ventricular pressure-volume characteristics. Left ventricular afterload has two components: (1) peripheral resistance, and (2) the ventricular transmural pressure. Increases in pleural pressure increase the transmural pressure and "assist" ventricular contraction, thus reducing afterload.

REFERENCES

Buda, et al: Effects of intrathoracic pressure on left ventricular performance. N Engl J Med 1979; 301:453

Goldberg HS, Rabson J: Control of cardiac output by systemic vessels. Am J Cardiol 1981; 47:696

Jardin, et al: Influence of PEEP on left ventricular performance. N Engl J Med 1981; 304:421

Weber RT, Janicke JS, et al: Contractile mechanics and interaction of right and left ventricles. Am J Cardiol 1981; 47:686

RATIONALE 293-b

PEEP improves hypoxemia in the adult respiratory distress syndrome by reversing abnormally decreased FRC. This occurs by opening previously collapsed alveoli and subsequently decreasing intrapulmonary shunting. It also may improve ventilation in areas of low ventilation to perfusion ratios. This results in an improved pulmonary venous admixture ($\dot{Q}s/\dot{Q}t$). Increased levels of PEEP may produce a net reduction in oxygen delivery to the tissues by decreasing the cardiac output. This may occur even if PaO_2 is increased. This effect is primarily caused by a decrease in venous return and can usually be counterbalanced with volume expansion. Occasionally inotropic support may be beneficial. PEEP does not reduce lung water in patients with acute respiratory failure or in experimental models.

REFERENCES

Demling RH, Staub NC, Edmunds HL: Effect of end-expiratory airway pressure on accumulation of extravascular lung water. J Appl Physiol 1975; 38:907

Divertie MB: The adult respiratory distress syndrome. Mayo Clin Proc 1982; 57:371

Jardin F, Farcot JC, Boisante L, et al: Influence of positive end-expiratory pressure on left ventricular performance. N Engl J Med 1981; 304:387

Lind T, McDonald JA, Avioli LV: Adult respiratory distress syndrome. Arch Intern Med 1981; 141:1749

Millard WC, Rice DL, Unger KM, et al: Effect of PEEP on lung water content in experimental noncardiogenic pulmonary edema. Crit Care Med 1981; 9:7

EDITORIAL COMMENT

Using an animal model, the effect of positive end-expiratory pressure (PEEP) vs. mean airway pressure on gas exchange in ARDS was studied. Increasing mean airway pressure was a major determinant in improving oxygenation. Pflex is defined as the pressure at which a major change occurs in the slope of the inspiratory limb of the respiratory volume-pressure curve. It was shown that to optimize oxygenation it was necessary at a given mean airway pressure for the PEEP to be greater than the Pflex. Further increases of PEEP above Pflex had little effect on oxygenation.

Increasing PEEP in the presence of asymmetric lung disease (such as lobar collapse) may decrease arterial oxygen tension due to an increased proportion of cardiac output being diverted to the collapsed lung. One must be very cautious to follow effects of PEEP when it is instituted in patients with asymmetric lung disease. With whole lung asymmetry in ARDS, dual lung ventilation with unilateral PEEP may be beneficial. Both PEEP and continuous positive airway pressure (CPAP) have been utilized in attempts to prophylax against adult respiratory distress syndrome. A recent study failed to show any beneficial effect of 8 centimeters H_2O PEEP when utilized in patients with risk factors for adult respiratory distress syndrome. This study however only looked at one level of PEEP, and the patients were already intubated and mechanically ventilated.

Mask CPAP has been shown to be an effective treatment for postextubation hypoxemia in surgical patients.

It is well documented that levels of PEEP of 15 centimeters or greater may significantly decrease cardiac index. Although left ventricular preload is decreased, right and left ventricular performance are usually unchanged. Myocardial metabolic studies by measurement of lactate in coronary sinus blood suggest that patients may develop cardiac ischemia with PEEP therapy without hemodynamic alterations. It is reasonable, therefore, to employ PEEP with caution in patients at risk for myocardial ischemic injury.

ADDITIONAL REFERENCES

Dehaven CB, Hurst JM, Branson RD: Postextubation hypoxemia treatment with a continuous positive airway pressure mask. Crit Care Med 1985; 13:46

De Leon RS, Orchard C, Sykes K, Brajkovich I: Positive end-expiratory pressure may decrease arterial oxygen tension in the presence of a collapsed lung region. Crit Care Med 1985; 13:392

Kirby RR: Continuous positive airway pressure: To breathe or not to breathe. Anesthesiology 1985; 63:578

Norwood SH, Civetta JM: Ventilatory support in patients with ARDS. Surg Clin North Am 1985; 65:895

Pepe PE, Hudson LD, Carrico J: Early application of positive end-expiratory pressure in patients at risk for the adult respiratory distress syndrome. N Engl J Med 1984; 311:281

Pesenti A, Marcolin R, Prato P, et al: Mean airway pressure vs. positive end-expiratory pressure during mechanical ventilation. Crit Care Med 1985; 13:34

Tittley JG, Fremes SE, Weisel RD, et al: Hemodynamic and myocardial metabolic consequences of PEEP. Chest 1985; 88:496

PULMONARY EDEMA

RATIONALE 294-c

The protein content of lung lymph, that reflects lung capillary permeability, is increased when sheep are injected intravenously with pseudomonas aeruginosa bacteria. Although increased hydrostatic pressures or decreased plasma colloidal osmotic pressure will increase lymph flow, they do not greatly change lymph protein content. Ventilatory pattern does not ordinarily change lymph protein content.

Pulmonary edema is caused by four mechanisms: decreased lymph drainage, increased hydrostatic pressures, decreased plasma colloidal osmotic pressures, and increased pulmonary capillary permeability. Treatment should be individualized and, if possible, directed at the proximate cause.

REFERENCES

Brigham KL, Woolverton WC, Blake LH, et al: Increased sheep-lung vascular permeability caused by pseudomonas bacteremia. J Clin Invest 1975; 54:792

Katz S, Aberman A, Frand VI, et al: Heroin pulmonary edema: Evidence for increased pulmonary capillary permeability. Am Rev Respir Dis 1972; 106:472

RATIONALE 295-e

Acute pulmonary edema is associated with acidosis in more than two-thirds of patients. Metabolic acidosis is common, due to the hypoxemia, hypoperfusion, and increased work of breathing. In the hypoxemic acidotic patient, a $PaCO_2$ of 40 mm Hg is inappropriate, but some patients under-ventilate further with elevation of carbon dioxide tensions and respiratory acidosis. A normal or alkalotic blood pH is seen in less than one-third of patients with pulmonary edema, but a normal arterial oxygen tension during breathing of room air would be distinctly abnormal. In general, the effects of pulmonary edema are manifest most quickly and dramatically on arterial oxygenation, next on roentgenography, and last and least on audible signs of rales and wheezes.

REFERENCES

Aberman A, Fulop M: The metabolic and respiratory acidosis of acute pulmonary edema. Ann Intern Med 1972; 76:173

Laver MB, Hallowell P, Goldblatt A: Pulmonary dysfunction secondary to heart disease: Aspects relevant to anesthesia and surgery. Anesthesiology 1970; 33:161

Robin ED, Cross CE, Zelis R: Pulmonary Edema. N Engl J Med 1973; 288:239,292

RATIONALE 296-d

The general fluid transport equation (Starling's equation) may be used to describe fluid filtration in the lung. The equation is written:

$$\dot{Q}f = Kf\ (Pmv - Ppmv) - \sigma\ Kf\ (\pi mv - \pi pmv),$$

where $\dot{Q}f$ is the net fluid flux; σ is the plasma protein reflection coefficient at the microvascular membrane; P refers to hydrostatic fluid pressure and π refers to protein osmotic pressure in the microvascular (mv) and perimicrovascular (pmv) compartments. It has been demonstrated by Staub and Erdman in sheep with lung lymph fistulas that there is normally a net outward filtration of fluid (intravascular to extravascular). In order for an outward filtration of fluid to occur, the sum of the pressures in the above equation must be greater than zero. Under the same experimental conditions it has been demonstrated that lung lymph flow increases (approximately linearly) while lung lymph protein osmotic pressure decreases (approximately linearly) with elevation of left atrial pressure.

REFERENCES

Erdman AI, Vaughan TR, et al: Effect of increased vascular pressure on lung fluid balance in unanesthetized sheep. Circ Res 1975; 37:271

Staub NC: The forces regulating fluid filtration in the lung. Microvascular Research 1978; 15:45

RATIONALE 297-d

Neurogenic pulmonary edema (NPE) is a variety of pulmonary edema associated with acute, often fatal neurological injury. It generally occurs in the absence of underlying cardiac or pulmonary disease, and within seconds to minutes after CNS injury. Montier in 1918 noted the occurrence of CNS injury and pulmonary edema. Carlson noted the onset of systemic and pulmonary hypertension and rapid accumulation of edema fluid in a patient with an intracranial hemorrhage. Theodore and Rubin have summarized the pathogenesis of pulmonary edema following central nervous system injury. The initial phase results from a centrally mediated sympathetic nervous system discharge. This results in generalized, but transient, vasoconstriction with fluid shifts from high-resistance to low-resistance areas such as the pulmonary circulation. The subsequent increase in pulmonary vascular pressure and volume results in the generation of hydrostatic pressures sufficient to cause pulmonary edema. In addition, pulmonary hypertension and hypovolemia injure blood vessels which results in altered permeability and lung hemorrhage. After the systemic response abates, the patient is left with abnormal pulmonary capillary permeability so that pulmonary edema persists in the face of normal hemodynamics and normal cardiac function.

There are, however, no radiographic features which distinguish NPE from other causes of noncardiac pulmonary edema.

REFERENCES

Carlson RW, Schaeffer RC, Michaels SG, Weil MH: Pulmonary edema following intracranial hemorrhage. Chest 1979; 75:731

Fein IA, Rackow EC: Neurogenic pulmonary edema. Chest 1982; 81:318

Rubin EG, Theodore J: Speculations on neurogenic pulmonary edema. Am Rev Respir Dis 1976; 113:405

EDITORIAL COMMENT

Pulmonary capillary pressure (Pc) is the major pressure determinant in the formation of pulmonary edema. Routinely we measure pulmonary artery occlusion pressure (PAOP) with a pulmonary artery catheter and assume that this reflects pulmonary capillary pressure. However, this is not always true. After pulmonary artery occlusion the pulmonary artery pressure falls rapidly due to the pressure gradient reflected by precapillary resistance. This value is best equated with Pc. The pressure then subsequently falls more slowly to PAOP as pulmonary capillaries which are served by the occluded artery empty until the pressure corresponds to PAOP. The Pc-PAOP pressure gradient reflects post-capillary resistance. A significant Pc-PAOP gradient will lead to pulmonary wedge pressure underestimating the true pulmonary capillary pressure. If a patient's wedge pressure is then used to diagnose noncardiogenic pulmonary edema, it may be an incorrect assumption. A technique now exists using the inflection point of the PAOP tracing to accurately estimate the pulmonary capillary pressure when there is a significant difference between PAOP and pulmonary capillary pressure.

Although lung lymph flow is an accurate estimate of pulmonary edema in the animal model, it is not available in humans. A sensitive indicator of pulmonary edema in the human subject is an increase in extravascular lung water traditionally measured by the thermal-dye double-indicator dilution technique. Recently an indicator dilution technique utilizing thermal indicator alone has shown reproducible and accurate results for measuring extravascular lung water.

Neurogenic pulmonary edema has been associated with various acute processes including subarachnoid hemorrhage, trauma, cerebral ischemia, cerebral herniation secondary to brain tumors, and high-altitude cerebral edema. It is rarely seen in reversible neurologic injury and most often seen in fatal neurologic disease. Animal studies suggest that the etiology is secondary to a massive alpha-adrenergic discharge which either directly effects pulmonary vasculature or indirectly produces left heart failure.

ADDITIONAL REFERENCES

Albertine KH: Ultrastructural abnormalities in increased-permeability pulmonary edema. Clin Chest Med 1985; 6:345

Allison RC, Carlile PV, Gray BA: Thermodilution measurement of lung water. Clin Chest Med 1985; 6:439

Baudendistel LJ, Kaminski DD, Dahms TE: Evaluation of extravascular lung water by single thermal indicator. Crit Care Med 1986; 14:52

Colice GL: Neurogenic pulmonary edema. Clin Chest Med 1985; 6:473

Cope DK, Allison RC, Parmentier JL, et al: Measurement of effective pulmonary capillary pressure using the pressure profile after pulmonary artery occlusion. Crit Care Med 1986; 14:16

Laine GA: Pulmonary capillary pressure? Crit Care Med 1986; 14:76

Matthay MA: Pathophysiology of pulmonary edema. Clinics in Chest Medicine 1985; 6:301

Wohns RN, Tamas L, Pierce KR, et al: Chlorpromazine treatment for neurogenic pulmonary edema. Crit Care Med 1985; 13:210

SMOKE INHALATION

RATIONALE 298-a

Arterial hypoxemia in patients within burning buildings is caused by bronchospasm, mechanical obstruction of the upper airways, inequality of ventilation and perfusion, and pulmonary irritation from toxic products of burning plastics. Carbon monoxide has an affinity for hemoglobin 260 times greater than that of oxygen, and low concentrations of carbon monoxide in inspired air (1 mm Hg) half-saturate hemoglobin (as would oxygen at PaO_2 = 26.6 mm Hg). In addition, carbon monoxide increases the affinity of hemoglobin for oxygen so that in tissues the PaO_2 must be very low for sufficient oxygen to be removed from hemoglobin. Although carbon monoxide also binds to heme-containing tissue enzymes, these effects must be less important because rats, whose blood is replaced by oxygen-carrying perfluorocarbons, function normally while breathing high concentrations of carbon monoxide. However, carbon monoxide does not reduce greatly the tension of oxygen in blood. It reduces the content and capacity.

In evaluating a patient removed from a burning building, consider oxygen content and delivery as well as arterial oxygen tension. Measuring mixed venous oxygen tensions may detect the effects of carbon monoxide poisoning, because of its combined effects on arterial oxygen content and P_{50}, but carbon monoxide should be measured directly and such patients should be hyperventilated with oxygen at high tensions that can eliminate half the carbon monoxide in approximately 45 minutes.

REFERENCES

Jackson DL, Beraducci A: Accidental carbon monoxide poisoning: A growing home hazard. Med Times 1978; 106:28

Roughton FJW: Comparison of the O_2HB and CoHB dissociation curves of the human blood. In: Oxygen Affinity of Hemoglobin and Red Cell Acid Base Status. Third Edition. Rorth M, Astrup P (Eds). New York, Academic Press, 1972, pp 84-92

RATIONALE 299-d

Inhalation injury has become one of the primary determinants of early mortality following burn injury. Fiberoptic bronchoscopy represents a useful and reliable method of diagnosing this disorder. Laryngeal, tracheal or bronchial inflammation or edema (with or without mucosal necrosis or ulceration) and the presence of carbonaceous material in the airway is highly suggestive of inhalation injury. Supraglottic edema may lead to complete upper airway obstruction. This usually occurs within the first 24 hours after injury. In the presence of significant inhalation injury, endotracheal intubation is the initial treatment of choice. The supraglottic edema may resolve within 3-4 days after injury making routine tracheostomy unnecessary. In addition, tracheostomy has been associated with increased morbidity, including tracheopharyngeal fistula and tracheal stenosis. Tracheostomy also permits direct contamination of the airway from the burn surface. Antibiotics are not recommended unless bacterial pneumonia develops. Should an infectious pneumonic process develop, the most common etiologic organisms are coagulase positive Staphylococcus aureus, Aerobacter, Escherichia coli, and Pseudomonas aeruginosa. Prophylactic use of antibiotics in inhalation injury is unnecessary and may select for more resistant strains of organisms. Some studies have shown corticosteroids to increase the mortality rate in inhalation and burn injury.

REFERENCES

Bartlett RH, Niccole M, Tauis MJ, et al. Acute management of the upper airway in facial burns and smoke inhalation. Arch Surg 1976; 112:744

Hunt JL, Agee RN, Pruitt BA: Fiberoptic bronchoscopy in acute inhalation injury. J Trauma 1975; 15:641

Moylan JA, Abib K, Birnbaum M: Fiberoptic bronchoscopy following thermal injury. Surg Gynecol Obstet 1975; 140:541

Moylan JA, Chou CC: Inhalation injury - An increasing problem. Ann Surg 1978; 183:34

Moylan JA, West JT, et al: Tracheostomy in thermally injured patients, a review of five years experience. Ann Surg 1972; 38:119

RATIONALE 300-d

Fire victims may have either thermal injury or chemical injury to upper airways. Lower airway damage is generally due to chemical injury with gases such as nitrous oxides and aldehydes. Occasionally, however, lower airway damage may be produced by steam inhalation. Without external evidence of burns, this patient would not be expected to have thermal upper airway injury; but chemical upper and lower airway injury is certainly possible. Building materials, particularly plastics, release severely caustic gases which react with the moisture in the airways, producing toxic chemicals such as hydrochloric acid.

Carbon monoxide poisoning is the most immediate life-threatening problem in the smoke inhalation victim. It may be associated with a normal PaO_2 as carbon monoxide poisoning has little effect on dissolved oxygen tension. Mild cases of carbon monoxide poisoning may be treated with supplemental oxygen. A carboxyhemoglobin level greater than 25% or cerebral dysfunction are indications for hyperbaric oxygen therapy.

If either thermal or chemical injury to the upper airways is considered, fiberoptic bronchoscopy should be performed early. If significant injury is noted, the patient should be prophylactically intubated over the bronchoscope. This aggressive approach prevents subsequent upper airway obstruction due to increase in swelling of the inflamed tissue. The endotracheal tube facilitates removal of retained secretions and allows application of continuous positive airway pressure. Prophylactic antibiotics are not indicated as they predispose to colonization with resistant organisms.

REFERENCES

Achower BM, Allyn PA, Furnas DW: Pulmonary complications of burns: The major threat to the burn patients. Ann Surg 1973; 177:311

Cahalane M, Demling RH: Early respiratory abnormalities from smoke inhalation. JAMA 1982; 6:771

Hunt JL, et al: Fiberoptic bronchoscopy in acute inhalation injury. J Trauma 1975; 15:641

Venus B, Matsuda T, Copiozo J, et al: Inhalation injury in burn victims. Crit Care Med 1981; 7:520

EDITORIAL COMMENT

Carbon monoxide poisoning is a serious complication of patients involved in smoke inhalation injuries. Any patient who is injured in a closed-space fire or has singed nasal hair or soot in the pharynx is at high risk for carbon monoxide poisoning as well as upper airway obstruction secondary to irritation from toxic gases. If carboxyhemoglobin levels can be obtained, a level higher than 8% in a smoker or a 4% in a non-smoker is reason for admission. Recent data supports that cyanide may play a significant role in mortality secondary to closed fire smoke inhalation.

Using an animal model of smoke inhalation, a recent study showed increased survival in steroid-treated smoke inhalation without any amelioration of lung injury by histopathological scoring. It was postulated that the benefit may be due to better maintenance of lung reflexes matching ventilation and perfusion after lung injury. These animals had no external burns.

ADDITIONAL REFERENCES

Beeley JM, Crow J, Jones JG, et al: Mortality and lung histopathology after inhalation lung injury. Am Rev Respir Dis 1986; 133:191

Myers RA, Messier LD, Jones DW, Cowley RA: New directions in the research and treatment of carbon monoxide exposure. Am J Emerg Med 1983; 2:226

THROMBOEMBOLISM

RATIONALE 301-a

In the two major multiclinic trials of heparin and thrombolytic drugs in pulmonary embolism, 6213 patients were screened and 327 were admitted to the trial with positive pulmonary angiograms for massive or submassive embolization. The symptoms and signs that were more prevalent in the 197 patients with massive embolization than in the 130 with submassive embolization were: pleuritic chest pain (present in 64% of massive and 85% of submassive embolism), apprehension (65%, 50%), increased pulmonary component of the second heart sound (58%, 45%), hemoptysis (23%, 40%), gallop rhythm (39%, 25%), diaphoresis (42%, 27%), heart murmur (27%, 16%), cyanosis (25%, 9%), and syncope (20%, 4%). In addition, 60% of patients with massive emboli had been immobilized, but only 46% of those with submassive emboli had this predisposing condition. Factors that were equally prevalent in these two groups were dyspnea (84%), cough (53%), sweats (27%), tachypnea (more than 16 breaths/min, 92%), rales (58%), tachycardia (pulse more than 100/min, 44%), fever (temperature more than 37.8°C, 43%), phlebitis (32%), edema (24%), current venous disease (49%), and heart failure and chronic lung disease (38%). Hemodynamic data and arterial PaO_2 were measured in most patients with angiographically-proven submassive or massive pulmonary emboli:

	RA	RVS	RVD	PA	PVR	PaO_2
No.	288	269	267	292	194	222
Mean	6.07	45.46	8.55	26.63	377.3	60.80
SD	3.80	16.83	7.31	17.22	268.6	11.73

(RA = mean right atrial pressure [mm Hg]; RVS, RVD = right ventricular systolic and diastolic pressures [mm Hg]; PA = mean pulmonary arterial pressure [mm Hg]; PVR = pulmonary vascular resistance [dyne•sec/cm^5); PaO_2 = systemic arterial oxygen [mm Hg]).

REFERENCES

Bell WR, Simon L, DeMets L: The clinical features of submassive and massive pulmonary emboli. Am J Med 1977; 62:355

Bell WR, Simon TL: A comparative analysis of pulmonary perfusion scans with pulmonary angiograms. Am Heart J 1976; 92:700

Robin ED: Overdiagnosis and overtreatment of pulmonary embolism: The emperor may have no clothes. Ann Intern Med 1977; 87:775

Sasahara, AA: The urokinase pulmonary embolism trial: A national cooperative study. Circulation 1973; 47(Suppl 2):1

USPET Group: Urokinase-streptokinase embolism trial: Phase 2 results: A cooperative study. JAMA 1974; 229:1606

RATIONALE 302-b

The diagnosis of pulmonary embolism may be difficult. With the exception of dyspnea there are no symptoms consistently associated with embolism. Similarly, the only consistent physical findings are tachypnea and tachycardia which may be evanescent. Rales are present in about half the cases of angiographically proven pulmonary embolism while decreased breath sounds and wheezing are uncommon. Although a room air PaO_2 greater than 80 mm Hg does not rule out pulmonary embolism, it makes the diagnosis unlikely. A normal chest radiograph is the most common radiographic finding in this setting. This may be somewhat dependent on whether the radiograph is prospectively or retrospectively evaluated. Tachycardia and nonspecific ST-T changes are the most common electrocardiographic findings in pulmonary embolism.

REFERENCES

Bell WR: The clinical features of submassive and massive pulmonary emboli. Am J Med 1977; 62:355

Moser K: Pulmonary embolism. Am Rev Respir Dis 1977; 115:829

RATIONALE 303-c

The three absolute contraindications for thrombolytic therapy are: (1) an active internal bleeding state, (2) acute cerebrovascular disease within 2 months, or (3) a cerebrovascular procedure within two months. Since it is not known when a "safe" period begins in those with cerebrovascular disease or following a neurosurgical procedure, lytic therapy should not be considered unless approximately two months have elapsed. Even after two months, the patient should be considered to have a strong relative contraindication. Other relative contraindications include the postpartum period (less than 10 days), recent (less than 10 days) surgery, organ biopsy or puncture of a noncompressible vessel, recent serious internal trauma, uncontrolled coagulation defects, pregnancy, cardiopulmonary resuscitation with rib fracture, thoracentesis, paracentesis, lumbar puncture, or other conditions which place the patient at risk for bleeding. The clinician may decide to proceed with lytic therapy in patients with relative contraindications in the setting of life-threatening pulmonary embolism. Because adequate pressure hemostasis cannot be assured, procedures or punctures of femoral, subclavian, or jugular vessels also constitute relative contraindications.

REFERENCES

Bell WR, Meek AG: Current concepts: Guidelines for the use of thrombolytic agents. N Engl J Med 1979; 301:1266

Marder IM: The use of thrombolytic agents: Choice of patient drug administration, laboratory monitoring. Ann Intern Med 1979; 90:802

Sasahara AA, Sharma GVRK, Tow DE, et al: Clinical use of thrombolytic agents in venous thromboembolism. Arch Intern Med 1982; 142:684

Sherry S, Bell WR, Duckert FH, et al: Thrombolytic therapy in thrombosis. National Institutes of Health Consensus Development Conference Summary 1980; 3:1

EDITORIAL COMMENT

Repeat angiographic evaluations of treated pulmonary emboli reveal that resolution occurs over a two to five week interval in most patients. There is usually only minimal angiographic evidence of resolution at 7 days. For periods longer than 7 days, a perfusion scan showing a defect increases the likelihood of angiographic documentation.

A normal perfusion scan eliminates the possibility of clinically significant pulmonary embolism. A high probability ventilation perfusion scan, best defined as multiple segmental or larger perfusion defects with normal ventilation (unmatched defects), allow a diagnosis of pulmonary embolus in the patient with moderate or high risk. Small subsegmental defects defined as 25% or less of a segment are low probability for pulmonary embolus but do not rule out the diagnosis. All other ventilation perfusion scanning combinations including matched defects of any size or number are most helpful in predicting pulmonary embolism. Pulmonary emboli rarely predominate in upper lung zones and are rarely single.

If one obtains a low probability scan in a patient at high risk, a high probability scan in a patient at low risk, or an indeterminant scan in any patient, a pulmonary angiogram should be obtained. Alternatives are radionuclide venography or contrast venography. If the venogram is positive, then the patient should be treated. If the venogram is negative, then it seems reasonable to closely follow the patient with low probability scan, and angiogram the patient with a high probability scan. In the patient with an indeterminant scan and negative venogram, obtaining an angiogram depends upon risk factors and stability of the patient. The lack of cardiopulmonary reserve in the unstable patient makes angiographic documentation of presence or absence of embolus more pressing.

Impedance plethysmography (IPG) is very useful in patients with no history of deep venous disease of the legs. In these patients a positive IPG allows one to assume acute deep vein thrombosis. A positive IPG in patients with chronic deep venous disease may reflect chronic or acute changes. In these patients even a contrast venogram may not allow differentiation between acute and chronic changes.

The finding of a ventilation perfusion match on $\dot{V}/\dot{Q}$ scanning does not rule out pulmonary embolism nor does a ventilation perfusion mismatch rule in a diagnosis of pulmonary embolism without consideration of the size and number of defects.

ADDITIONAL REFERENCES

Benotti JR, Dalen JE: The natural history of pulmonary embolism. Clin Chest Med 1984; 5:403

Duroux P, Simonneau G, Petitpretz P, et al: Therapeutic approach to acute pulmonary embolism. Intensive Care Med 1984; 10:99

Goodman PC: Pulmonary angiography. Clin Chest Med 1984; 5:465

Hall R: Difficulties in the treatment of acute pulmonary embolism. Thorax 1985; 40:729

Huet Y, Lemair F, Brun-Buisson CB, et al: Hypoxemia in acute pulmonary embolism. Chest 1985; 88:829

Hull RD, Hirsh J, Carter CJ, et al: Diagnostic value of ventilation-perfusion lung scanning in patients with suspected pulmonary embolism. Chest 1985; 77:819

Hull RD, Raskob GE, LeClere JR, et al: The diagnosis of clinically suspected venous thrombosis. Clin Chest Med 1984; 5:439

Lemaire F: Pulmonary embolism: What is known, what remains unsolved? Intensive Care Med 1984; 10:79

Ozier U, Dubourg O, Farcot JC, et al: Circulatory failure in acute pulmonary embolism. Intensive Care Med 1984; 10:91

Polak JF, McNeil BJ: Pulmonary scintigraphy and the diagnosis of pulmonary embolism: A perspective. Clin Chest Med 1984; 5:457

Sors J, Safran D, Stern M, et al: An analysis of the diagnostic methods for acute pulmonary embolism. Intensive Care Med 1984; 10:81

Section 16

304. Which ONE of the following conditions is LEAST likely to be demonstrated by ultrasonography (Echo)?

a. Pericardial effusion of 100 ml
b. Aortic and mitral candida endocarditis
c. Left ventricular wall dyskinesia
d. Pancreatic pseudocyst of 200 ml
e. Hemothorax

305. A 56-year-old man with metastatic adenocarcinoma of the colon is admitted to the ICU with dyspnea, tachypnea, tachycardia and hypotension. He has no previous history of heart disease. A narrowed pulse-pressure, jugular venous distension and a normal lung examination are noted. Heart sounds are distant. A chest radiograph obtained 3 days previously is normal. His chest radiograph obtained on the day of ICU admission is shown in Figure 6.

Which ONE of the following M-mode echocardiograms (a-d) is most likely to be obtained in this patient at this time? Each of these echocardiographic projections has been obtained at or close to the mitral valve between positions A and B as shown in the orientation figure.

Orientation Figure:

CW = chest wall
S = sternum
RV = right ventricle
IVS = interventricular septum
AO = aortic outflow
MV = mitral valve
LA = left atrium
PLV = posterior left ventricle

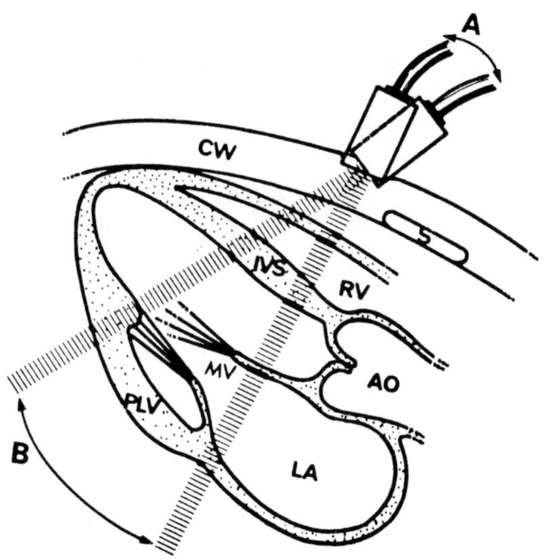

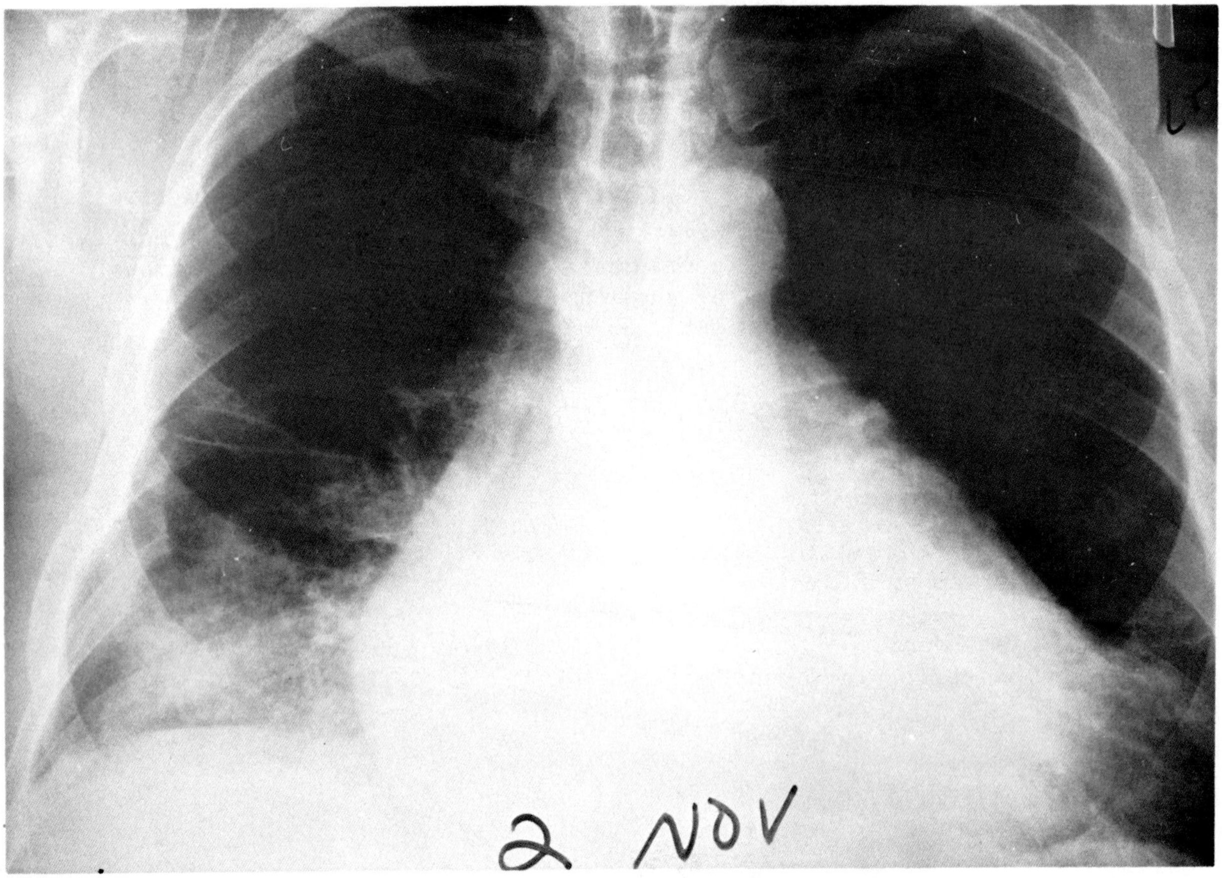

Figure 6

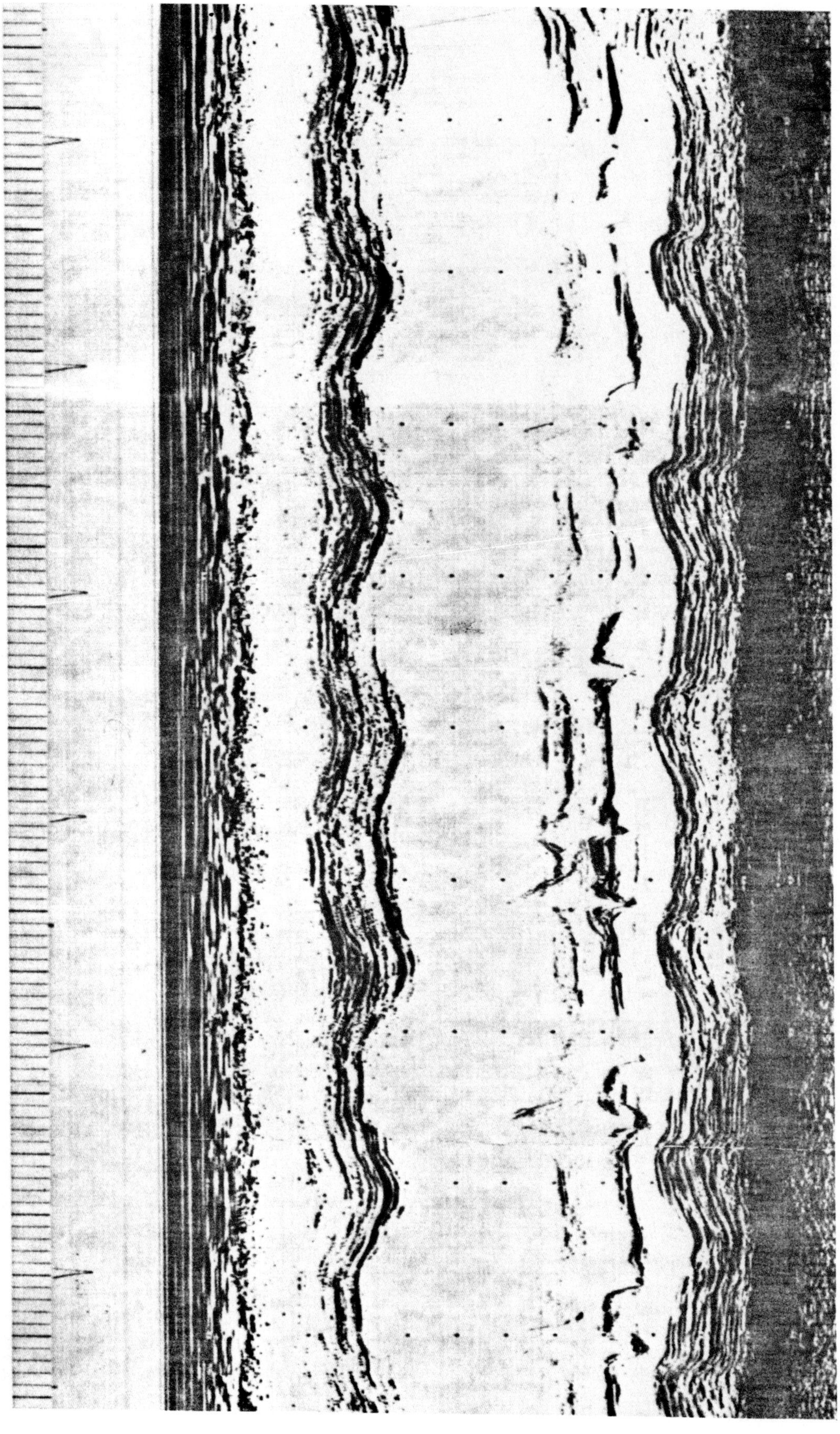

Echocardiogram - a

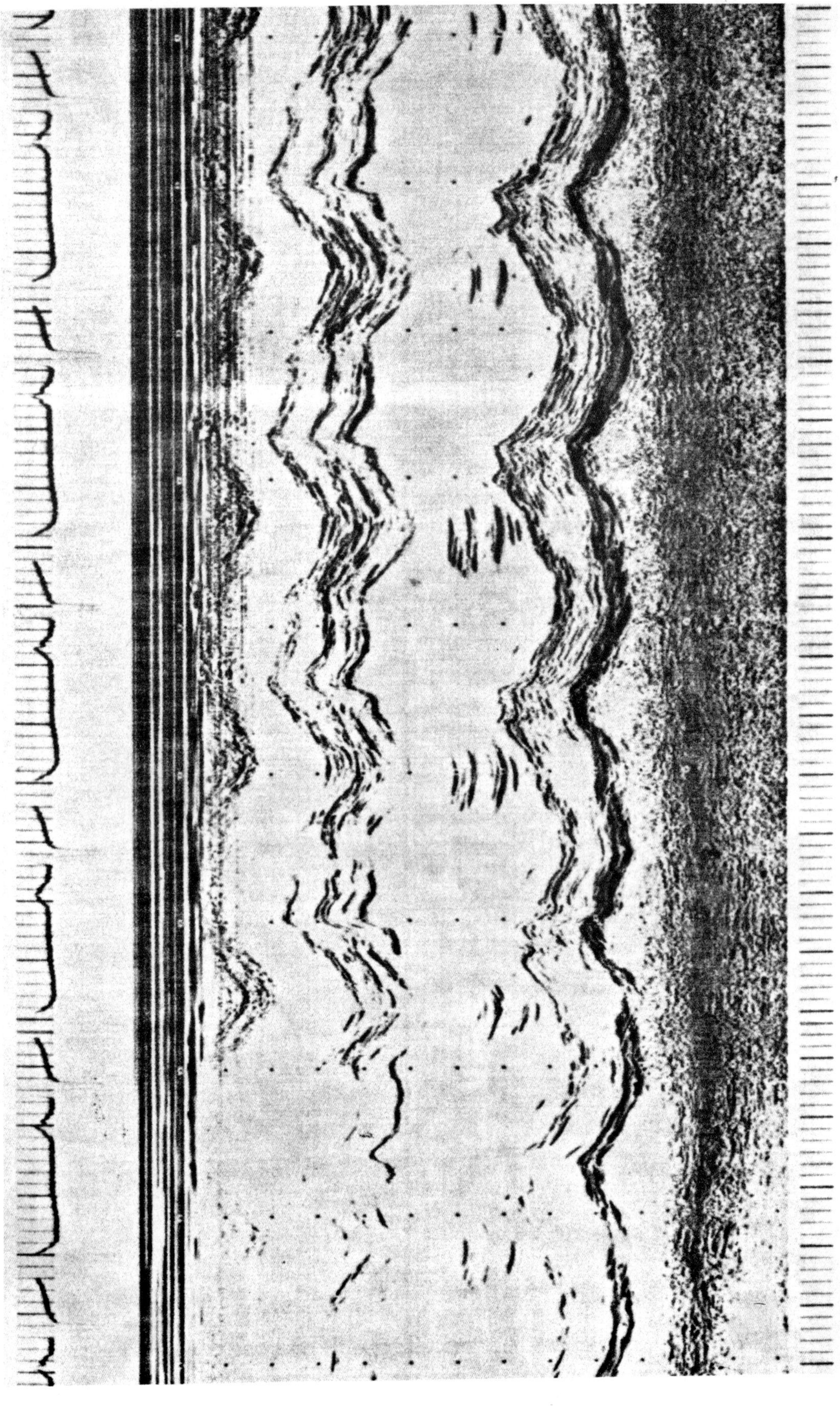

Echocardiogram - b

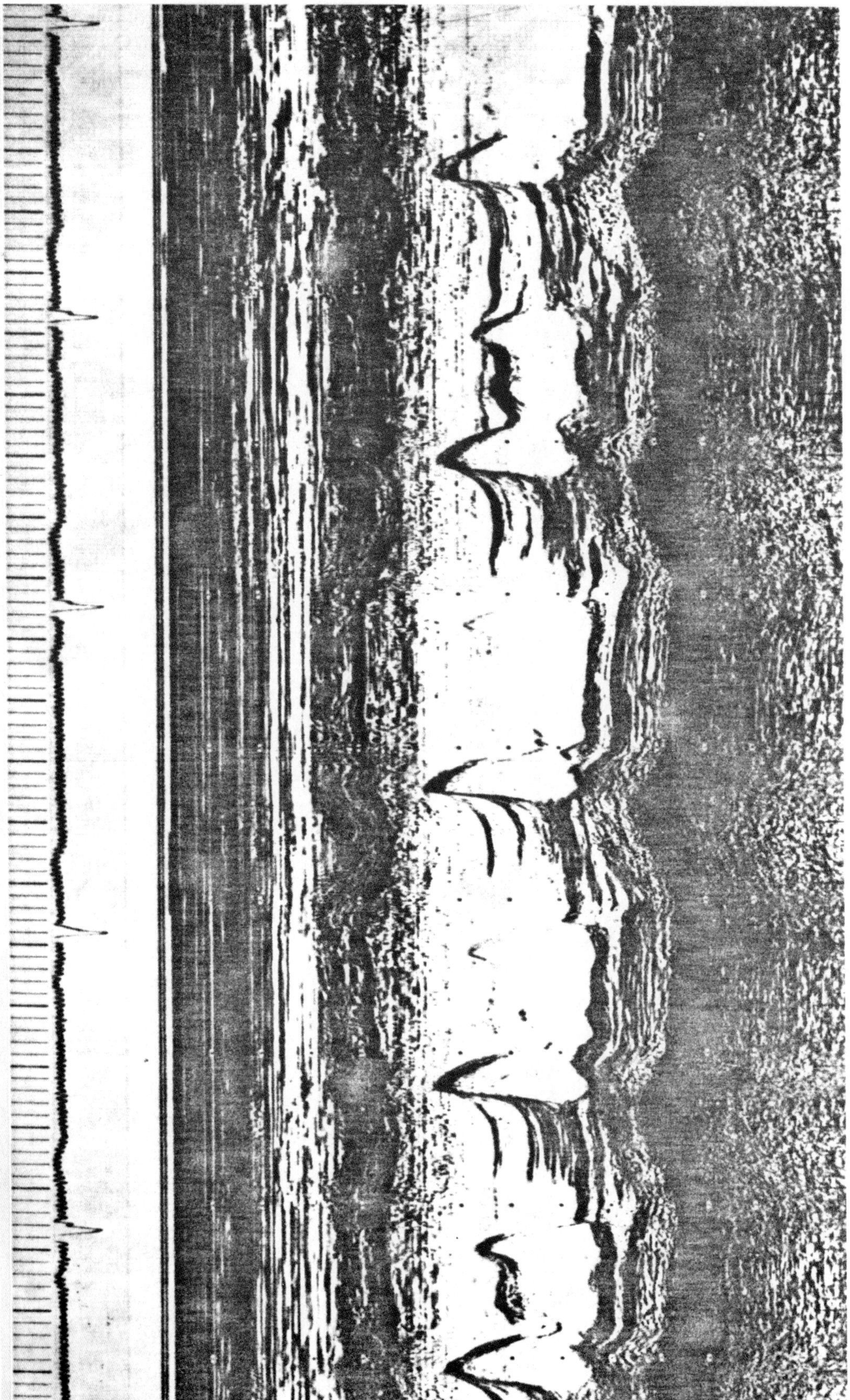

Echocardiogram - c

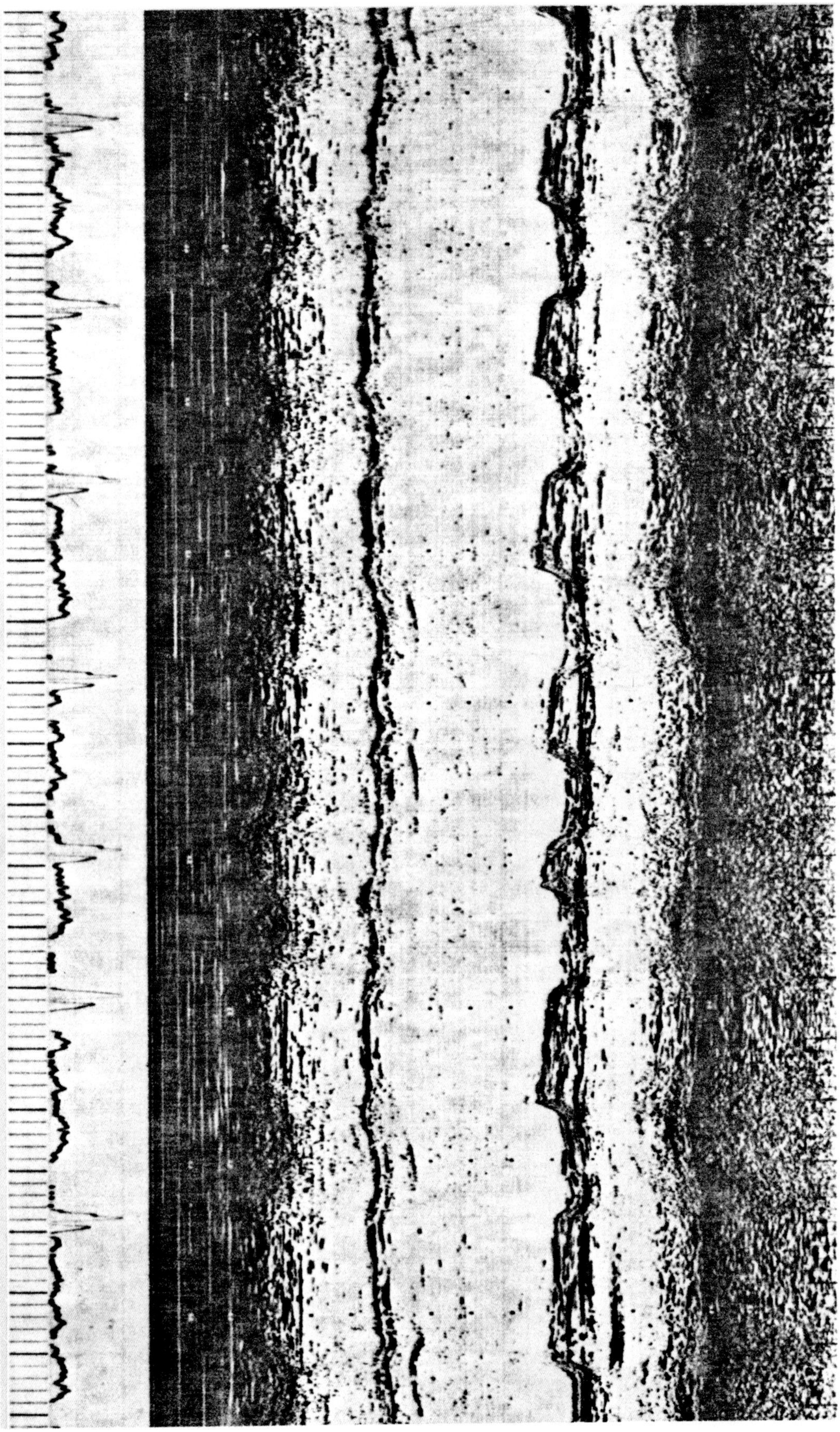

Echocardiogram - d

306. Which ONE of the following statements regarding the portable AP chest radiograph shown in Figure 7 is CORRECT?

a. The endotracheal tube, pulmonary artery catheter and catheter introducer positions are typical.
b. The endotracheal tube position is inadequate; however, the pulmonary artery catheter and catheter introducer positions are typical.
c. The endotracheal tube position is adequate; however, the pulmonary artery catheter and introducer positions are atypical.
d. The endotracheal tube position is inadequate and the pulmonary artery catheter and introducer positions are atypical.

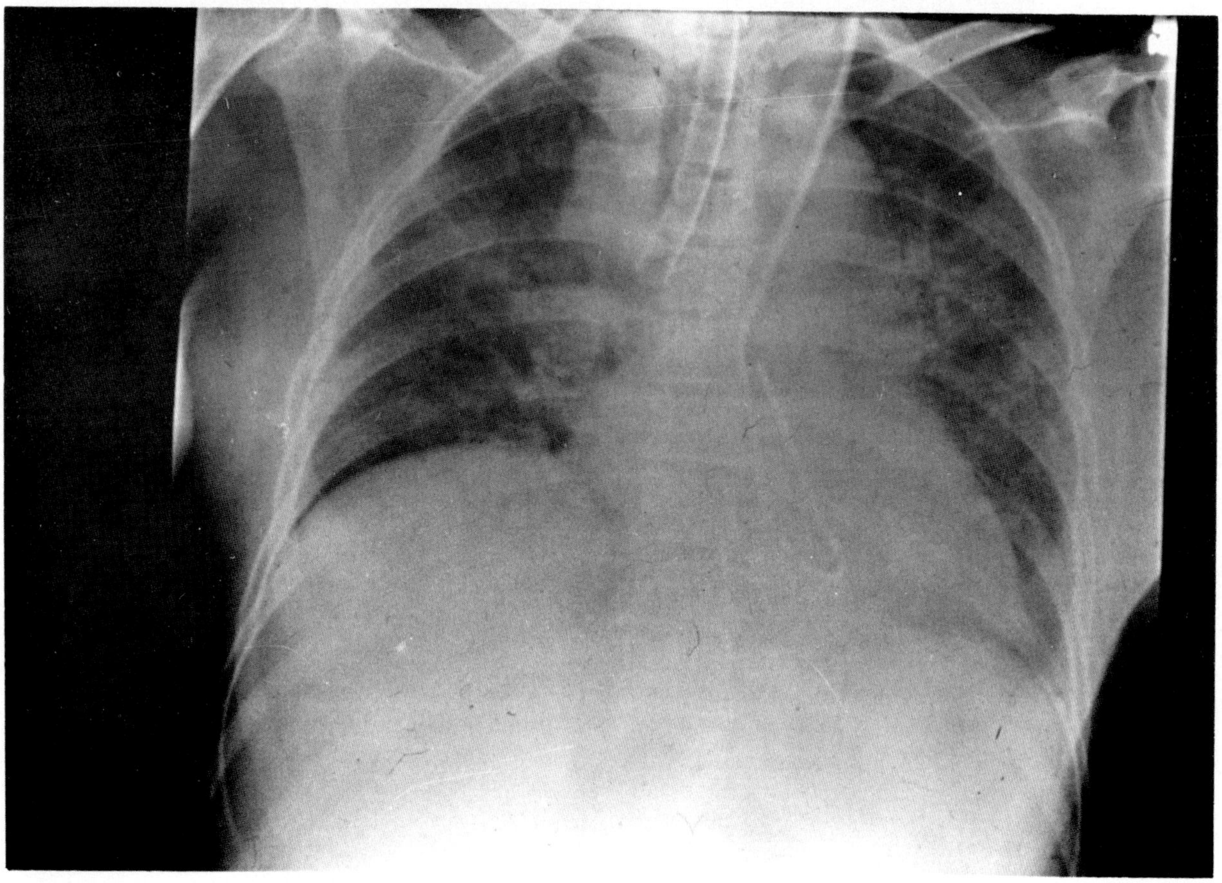

Figure 7

307. A 40-year-old male is admitted to the ICU with sudden onset of respiratory distress. He is hypotensive and hypoxemic. His chest radiograph is shown in Figure 8. Which ONE of the following statements is MOST correct?

a. An emergent pulmonary arteriogram should be performed.
b. After intravascular volume replacement, rigid bronchoscopy should be performed for foreign body removal.
c. A catheter should be placed in the left 2nd intercostal space in the midclavicular line.
d. The patient's trachea should be intubated and positive pressure ventilation with positive end-expiratory pressure should be instituted.

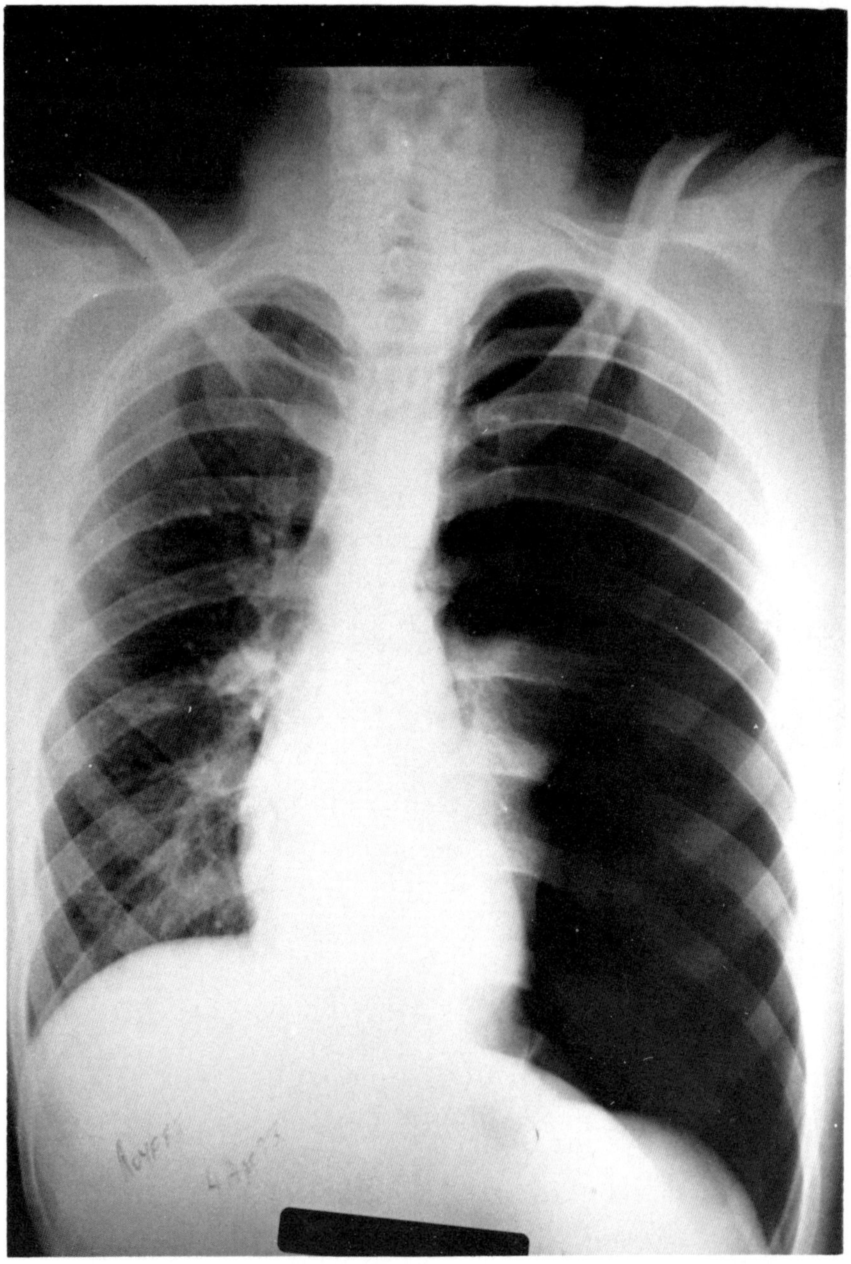

Figure 8

308. Which ONE of the following is MOST likely to have caused the abnormal findings demonstrated in the upright portable chest radiograph shown in Figure 9?

a. Pneumocystoides intestinales
b. Positive pressure ventilation with positive end-expiratory pressure
c. Gas gangrene
d. Loculated subpulmonic pneumothorax
e. Situs inversus

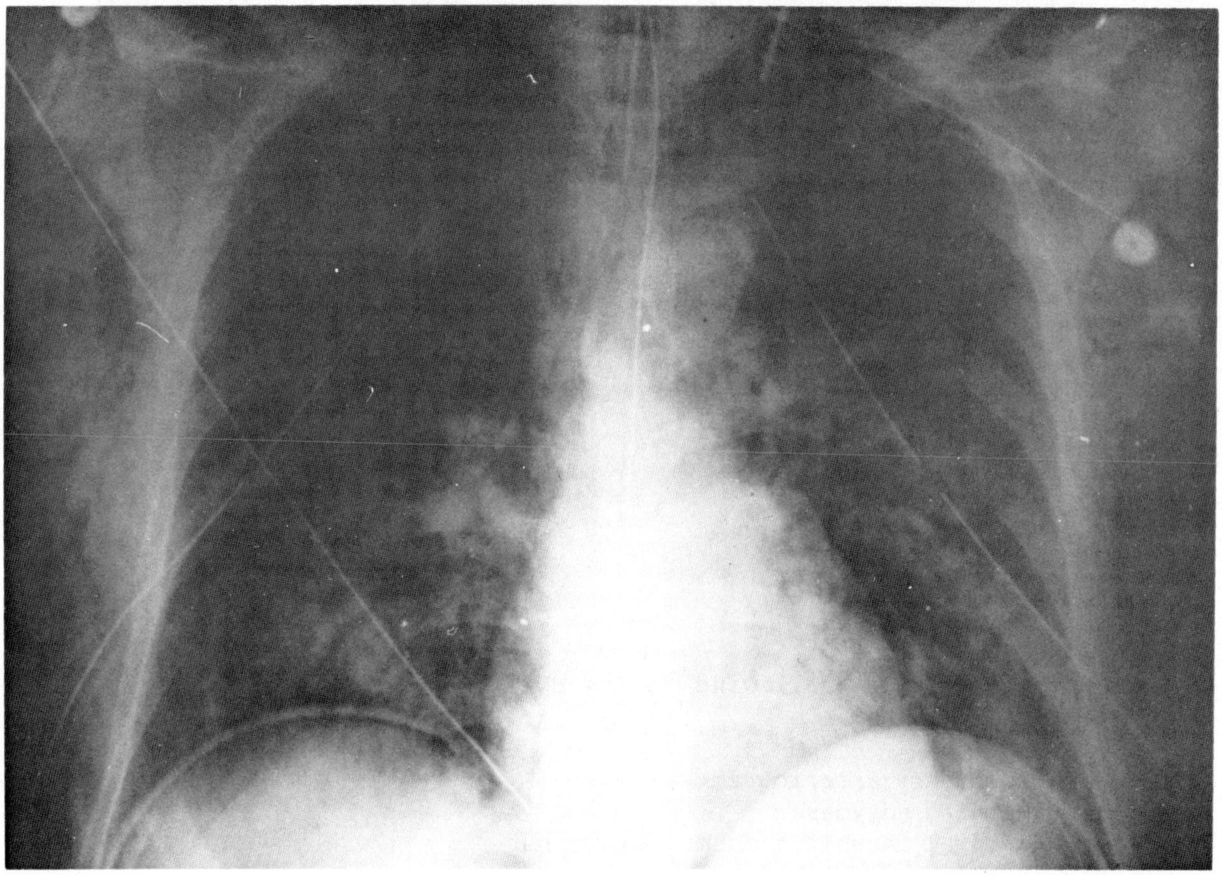

Figure 9

309. A right subclavian catheter was inserted in a patient with Crohn's disease for parenteral alimentation. A chest radiograph was obtained following the procedure and is shown in Figure 10. Four hours later, the patient developed shortness of breath and chest pain. A 12 lead electrocardiogram and a repeat chest radiograph were obtained and are shown below and in Figure 11 respectively.

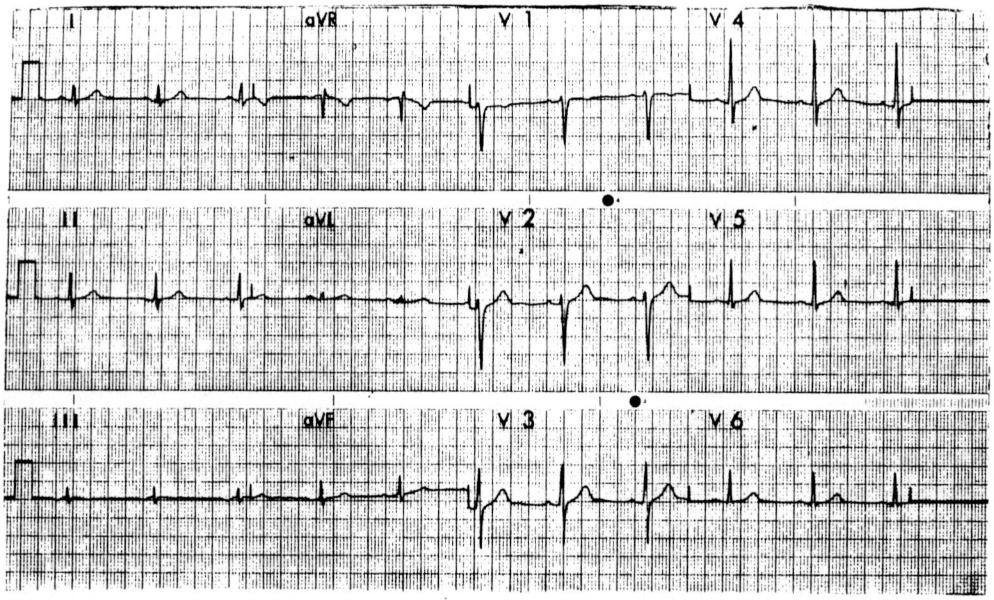

Which ONE of the following is the MOST appropriate diagnostic or therapeutic procedure?

a. Pulmonary arteriogram
b. Cardiac enzymes
c. Lateral decubitus chest radiograph
d. Sublingual nitroglycerin
e. Cross table lateral radiographs of the abdomen

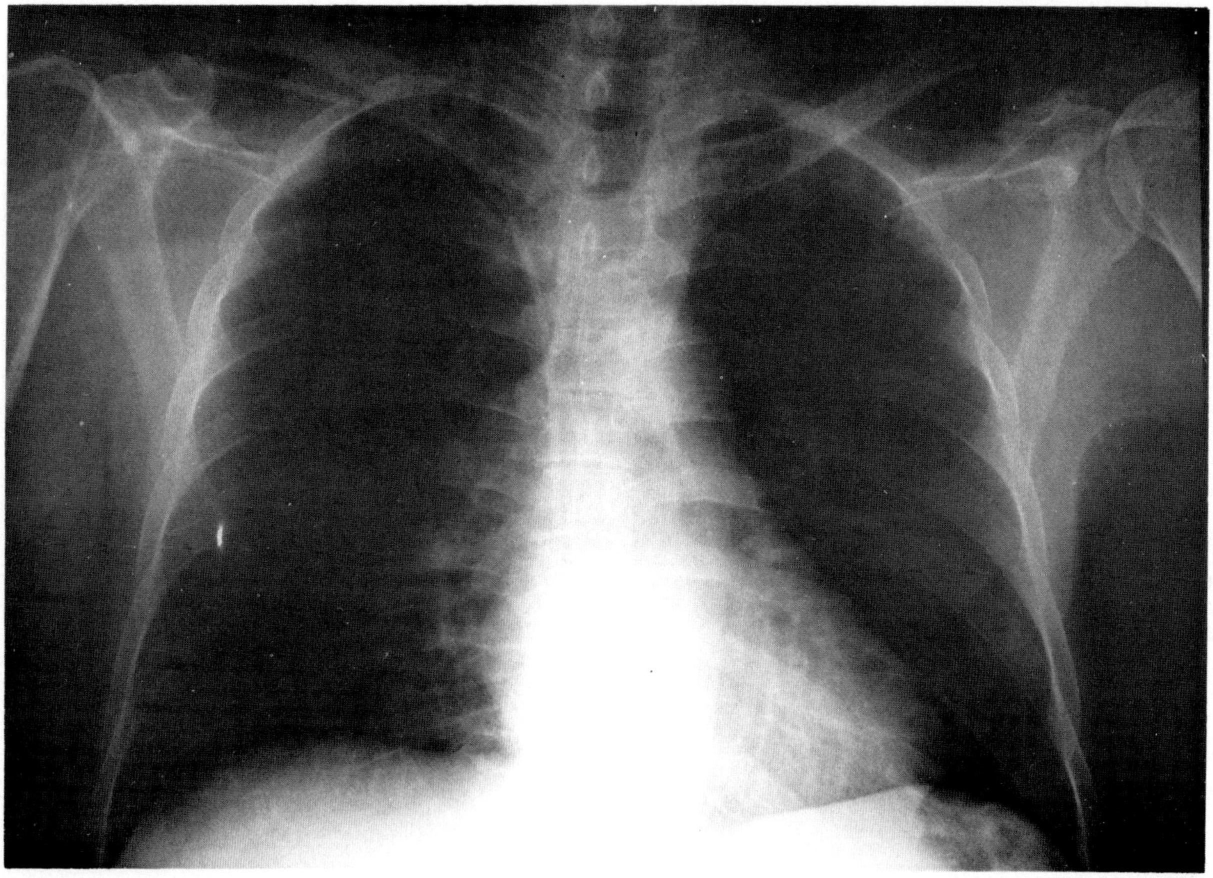

Figure 10

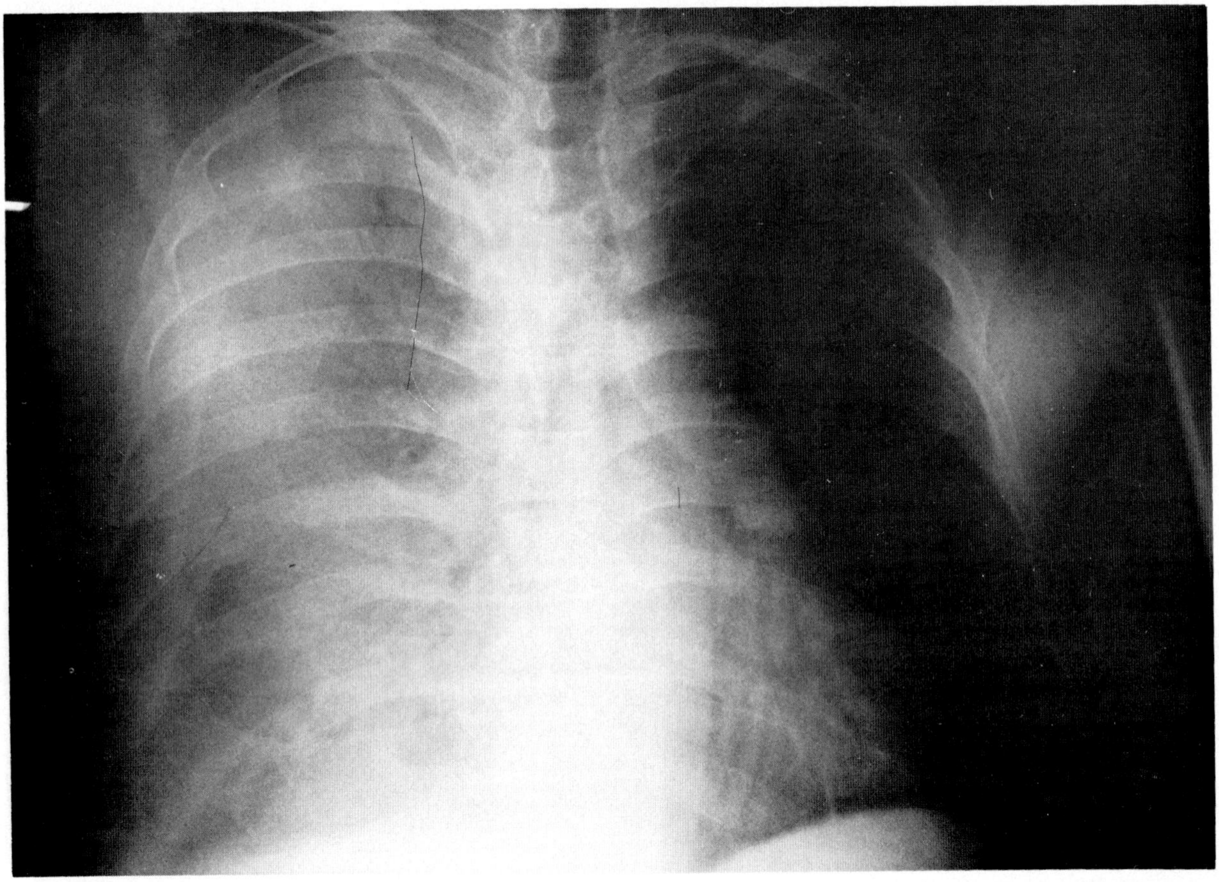

Figure 11

310. Radiographic signs of pericardial effusions include all but which ONE of the following?

a. Cardiomegaly with clear lung fields
b. Straightening of the left heart border shadow
c. Bulging of the right heart border shadow
d. Prominence of the left atrial appendage shadow
e. Alterations in size of the vascular pedicle shadow with changes in patient position

311. A 64-year-old patient with emphysema has acute respiratory failure with an apparent viral pneumonia. On controlled ventilation via an endotracheal tube he appears stable, but after several days, his abdomen becomes distended and on roentgenography he has free air under his diaphragm with a small amount of mediastinal emphysema. He is afebrile and has no abdominal pain. His bowel sounds are slightly hypoactive.

Which ONE of the following is MOST correct?

a. Prompt laparotomy for perforated ulcer
b. Nasogastric suction for perforated ulcer
c. Celiac and mesenteric angiography to confirm mesenteric ischemia
d. Antibiotics for peritonitis that caused his respiratory failure
e. Attempt maneuvers to decrease inspiratory pressure suspecting pneumoperitoneum secondary to mechanical ventilation

312. While reviewing an ICU AP chest radiograph for information on endotracheal tube position, the endotracheal tube tip was noted to be significantly closer to the carina when compared to the previous day's film.

Which ONE of the following is MOST likely to have produced this change?

a. Neck flexion or a larger inspiration
b. Neck extension or a smaller inspiration
c. Neck extension or a larger inspiration
d. Neck flexion or a smaller inspiration

313. A fifteen-month-old previously healthy male has the sudden onset of respiratory distress while playing unobserved at home. Blood gas analysis reveals arterial hypoxemia. Inspiratory (Figure 12) and expiratory (Figure 13) chest radiographs are obtained.

Which ONE of the following is the MOST likely diagnosis?

a. Foreign body aspiration
b. Right lung pneumonia
c. Left unilateral hypolucent lung
d. Tension pneumothorax
e. None of the above

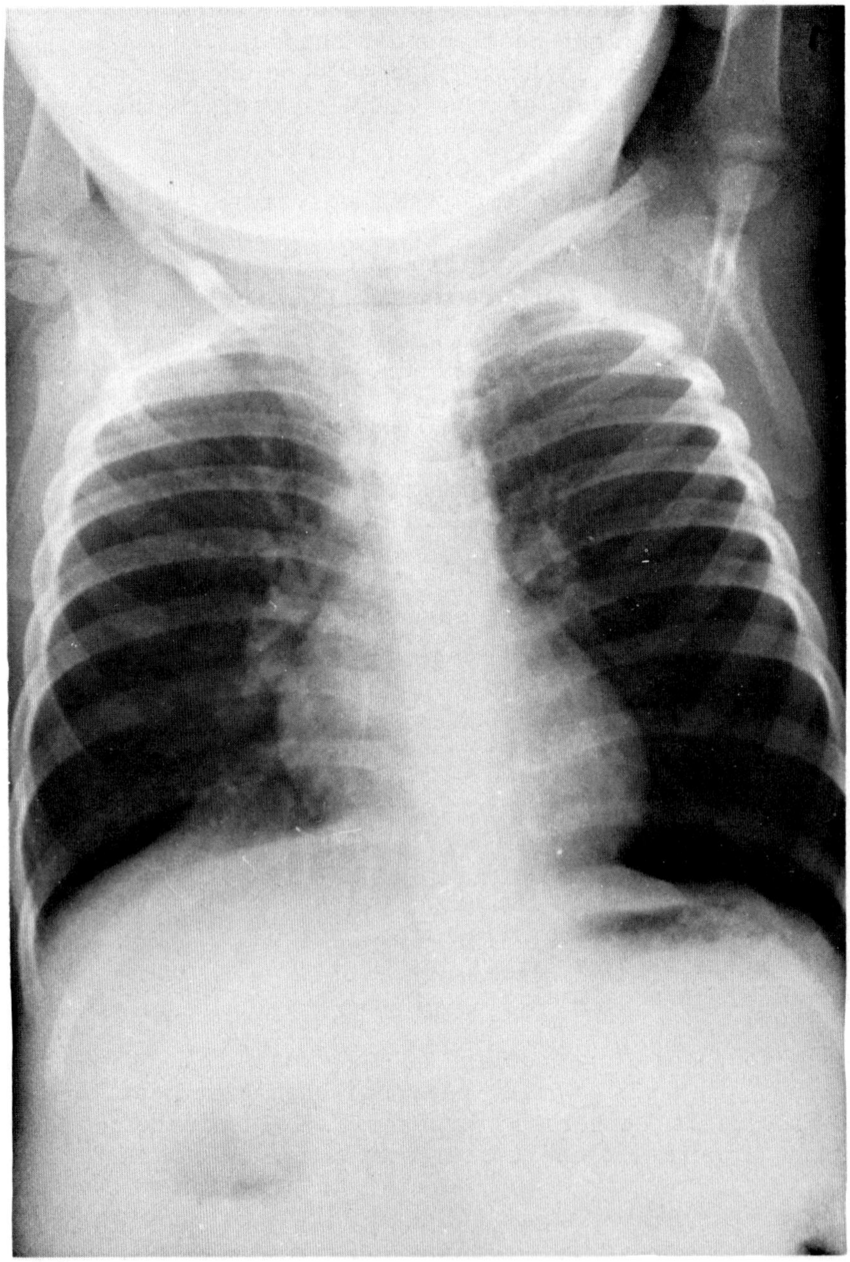

Figure 12

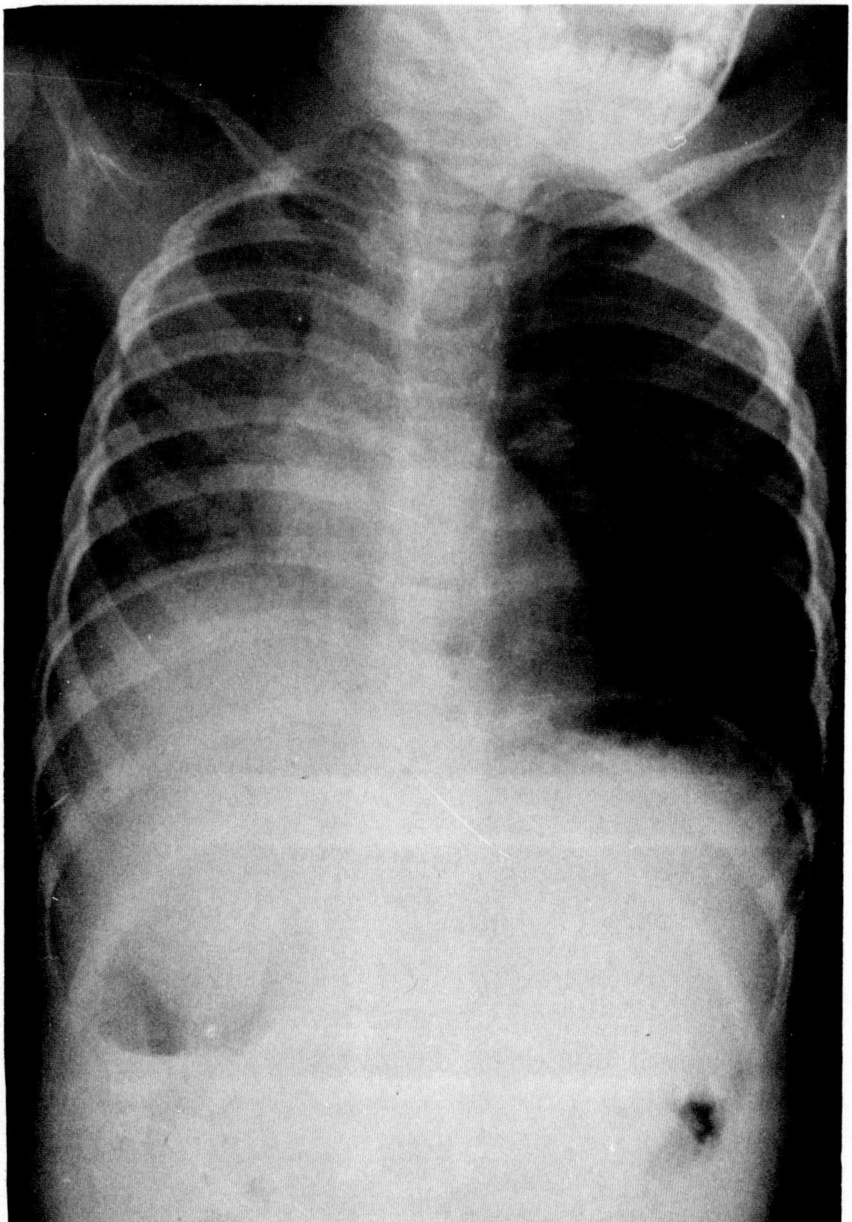

Figure 13

314. The portable upright chest radiograph shown in Figure 14 was obtained two days following an esophageal resection in a 45-year-old male with adenocarcinoma of the esophagus.

Which ONE of the following would be MOST helpful in establishing the ETIOLOGY of the abnormality found in the right hemithorax on this film?

a. Computed tomography of the thorax
b. Diagnostic thoracentesis
c. Ultrasound
d. Indium-labeled white blood cell scan

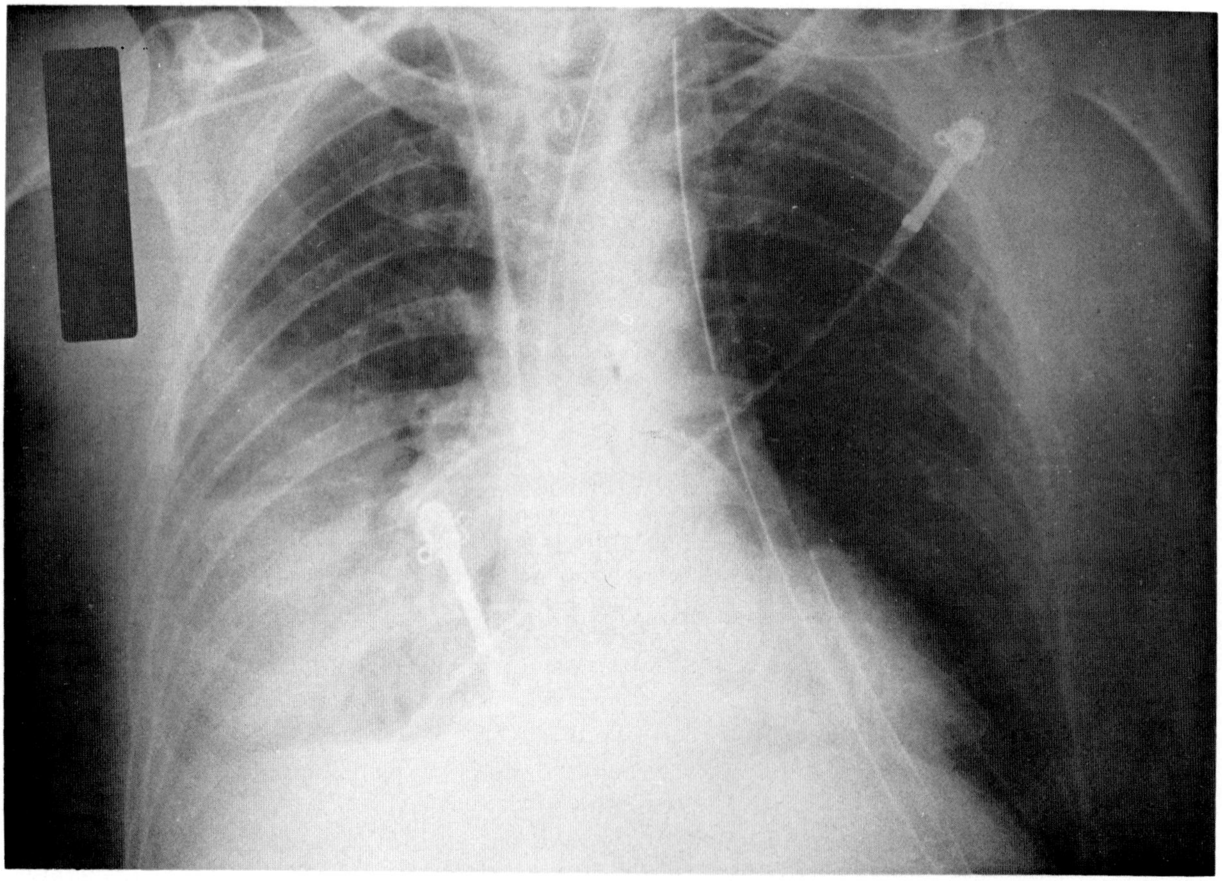

Figure 14

315. Figure 15 demonstrates a radiograph obtained in a patient who sustained abdominal and thoracic trauma in an automobile accident. An exploratory laparotomy is planned.

Based on this radiograph, which ONE of the following actions is MOST accepted?

a. Preoperative aortogram
b. Preoperative pericardiocentesis
c. Postoperative electrocardiographic monitoring for at least 48 hours
d. Preoperative computed tomography of the thoracic spine

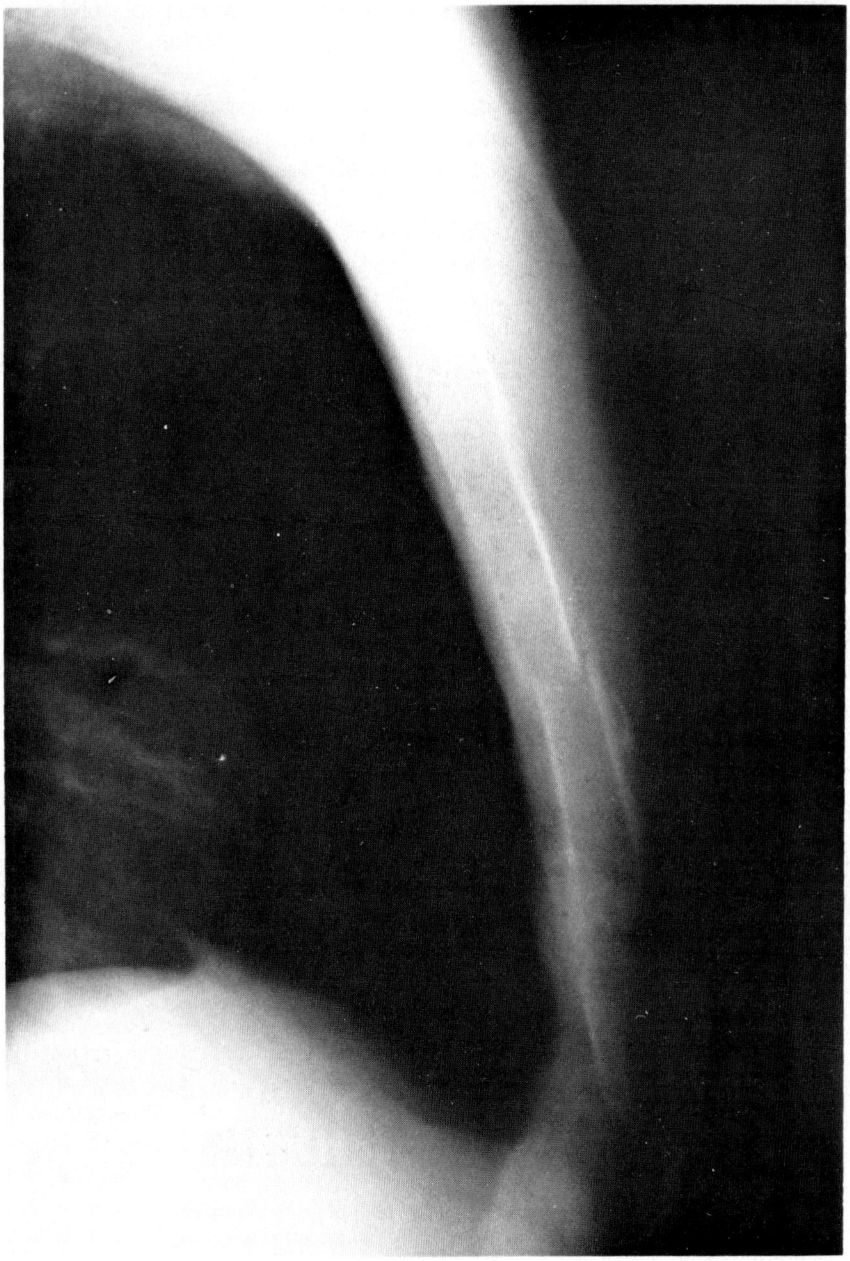

Figure 15

316. A 37-year-old female was admitted to the ICU following a cardiorespiratory arrest. She had been hospitalized 4 days previously because of a right femur fracture sustained during an automobile accident. Two hours prior to her ICU admission, she complained of chest tightness and was noted to be tachypneic and tachycardic. Arterial blood gases were obtained while the patient was breathing room air (pH 7.52, PaO_2 45 torr, $PaCO_2$ 25 torr). Ventilation-perfusion lung scintigraphy was performed (Figures 16 and 17). The patient suffered a cardiorespiratory arrest several minutes after the scan. She was successfully resuscitated and her vital signs are now stable. An AP portable chest radiograph (Figure 18) was obtained following her ICU admission.

Which ONE of the following statements regarding this case is MOST correct?

a. Broad spectrum antibiotics should be promptly instituted.
b. Corticosteroids will improve survival.
c. Fiberoptic bronchoscopy and transbronchial biopsy will likely yield a diagnosis.
d. Anticoagulation therapy is indicated.
e. Emergent thoracotomy is the treatment of choice.

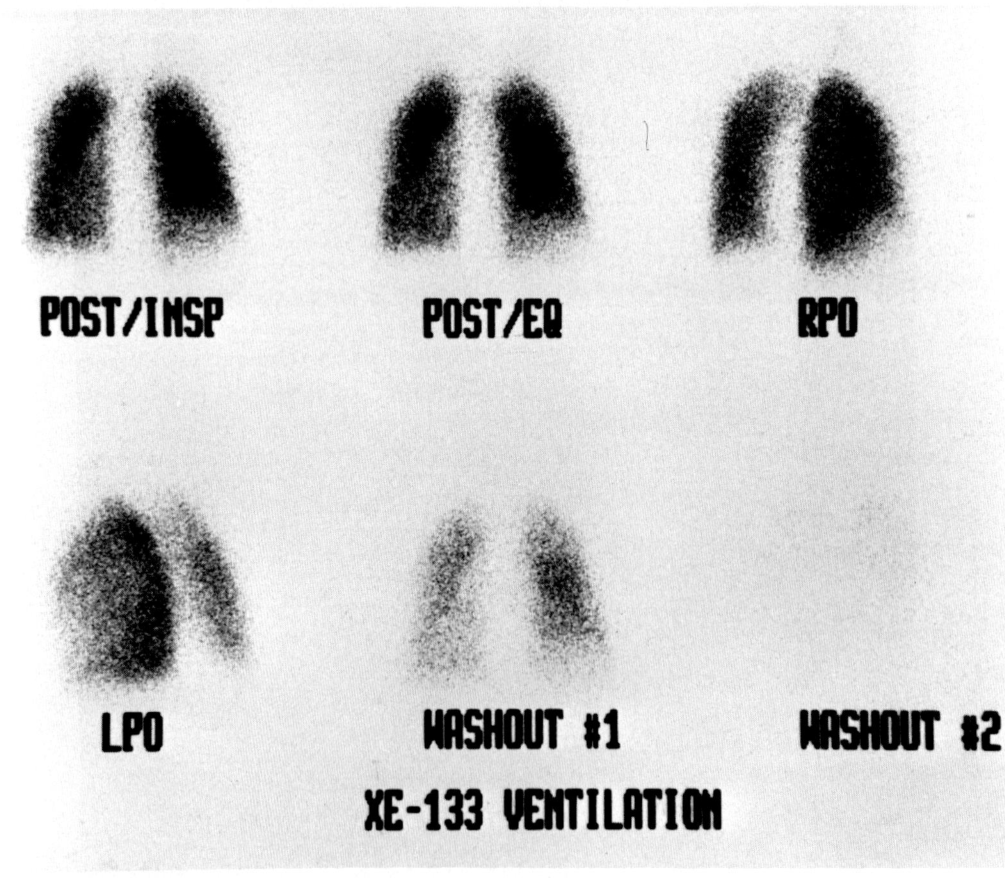

Figure 16

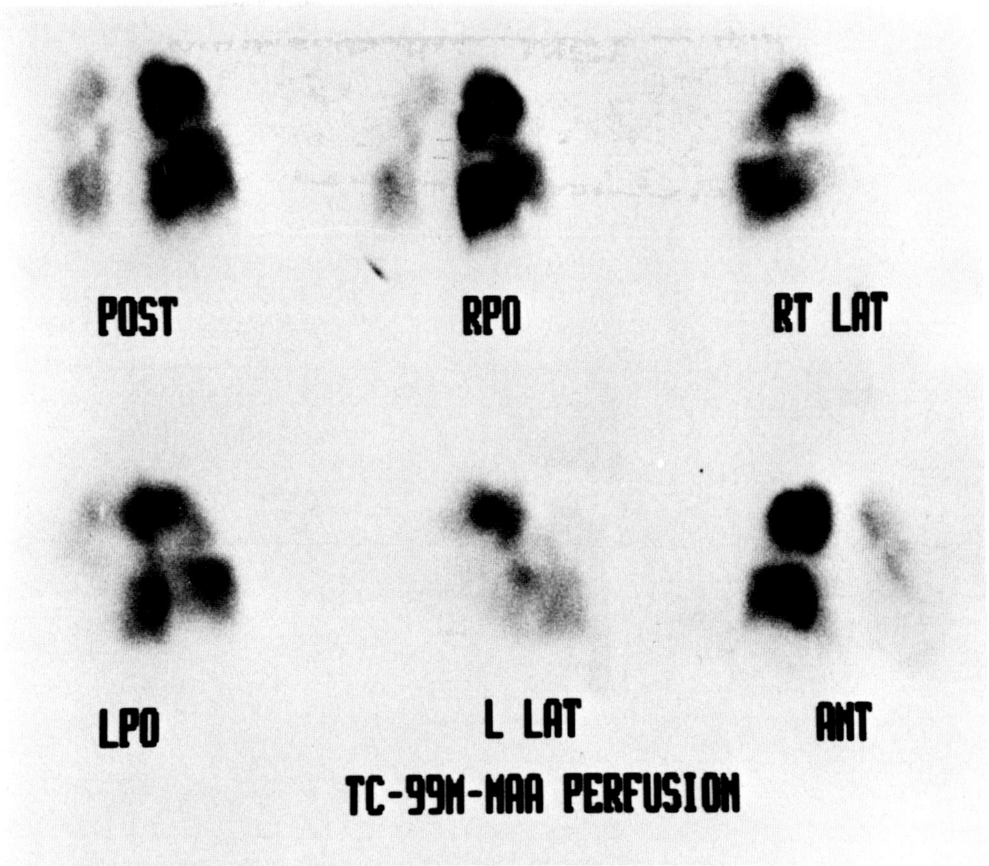

Figure 17

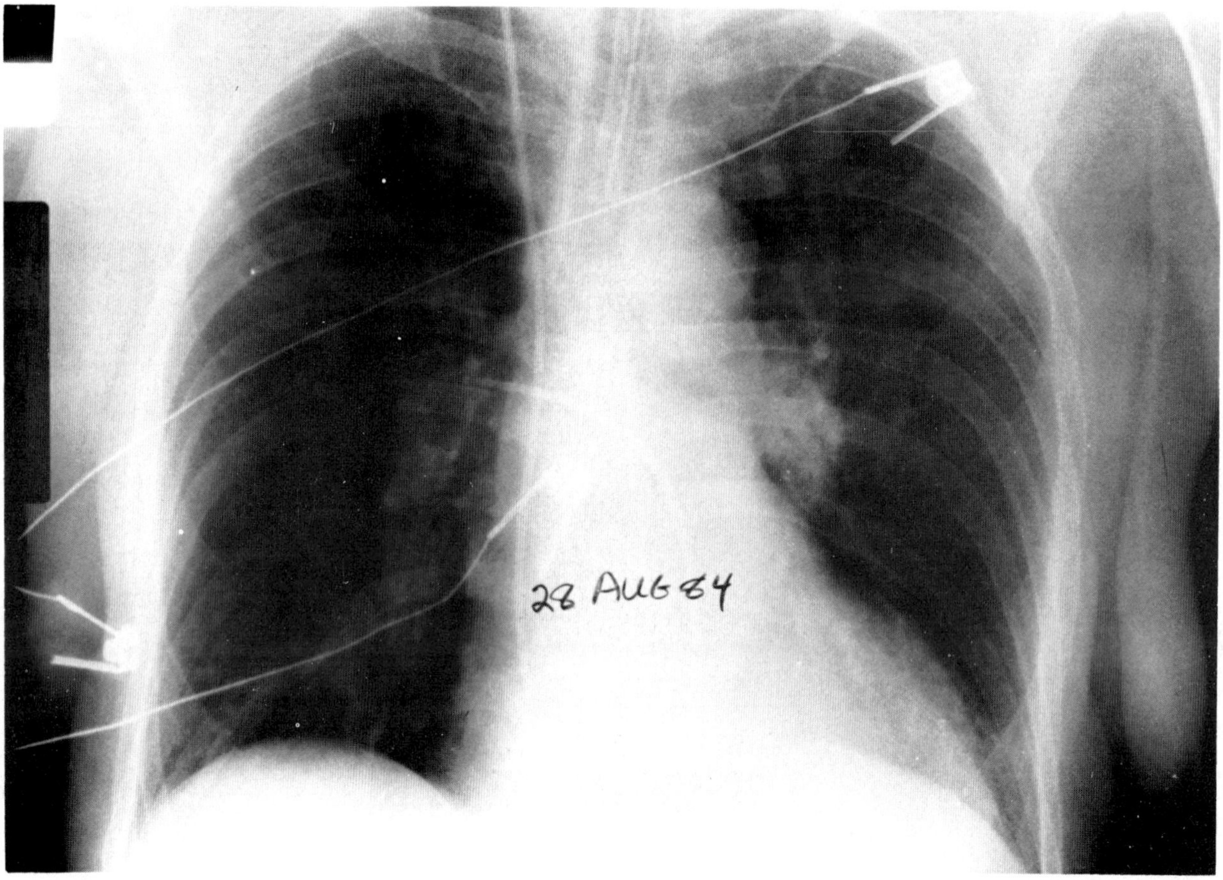

Figure 18

317. A 34-year-old female was admitted to the ICU following ingestion of large quantities of alcohol and diazepam in a suicide attempt. She has been a heavy smoker since age 14. Her only prescribed medication is an oral contraceptive. After 36 hours of supportive therapy, arterial blood gases obtained without supplemental oxygen revealed:

pH 7.49 PaO_2 75 torr $PaCO_2$ 30 torr

A chest radiograph is normal and unchanged from admission. Ventilation-perfusion lung scintigraphy was obtained and is shown in Figures 19 and 20.

Which ONE of the following options is MOST correct in this case?

a. Administer streptokinase.
b. Administer heparin.
c. Administer clindamycin.
d. Observe patient and treat symptomatically.
e. Insert an inferior vena cava filter.

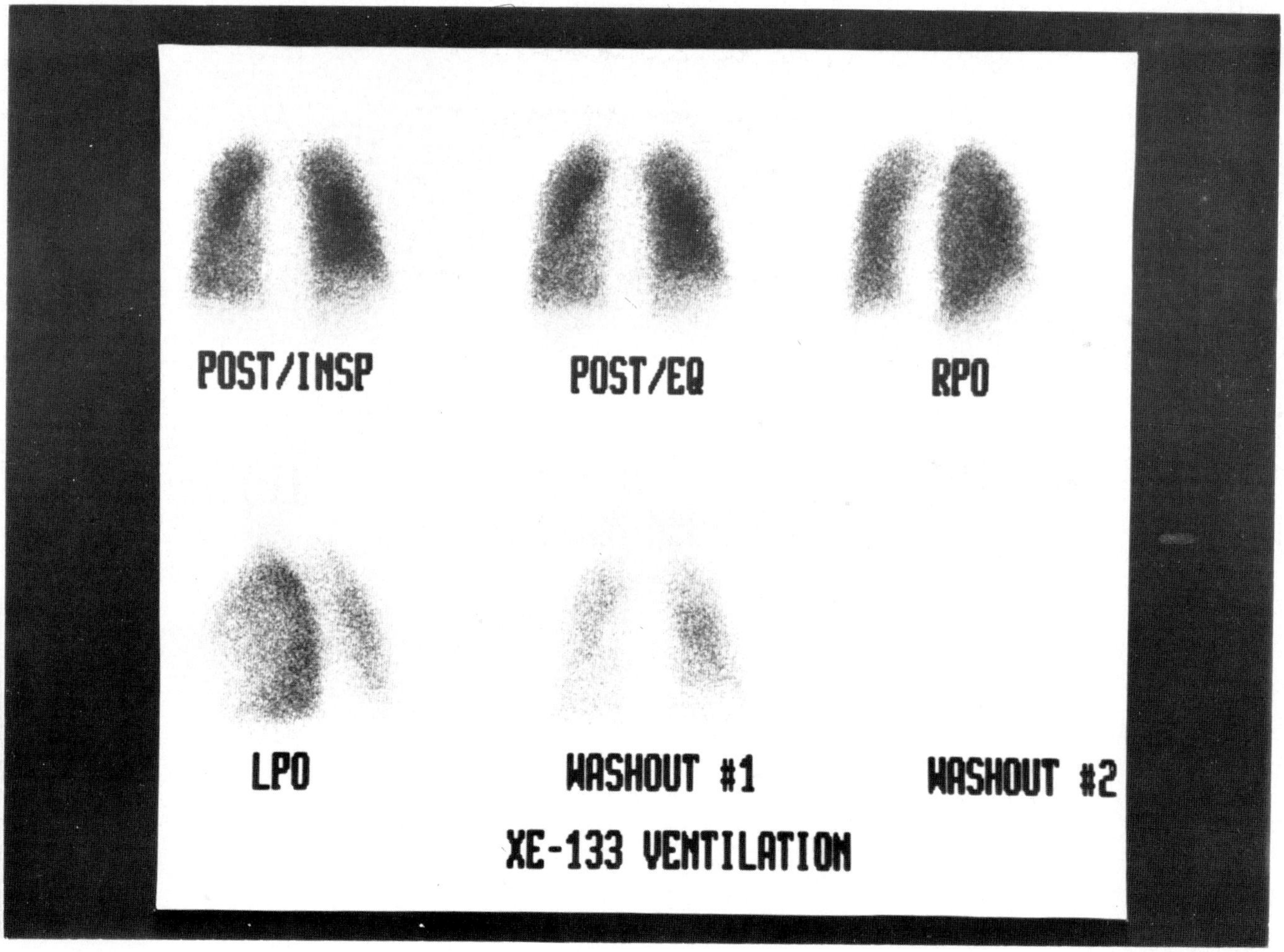

Figure 19

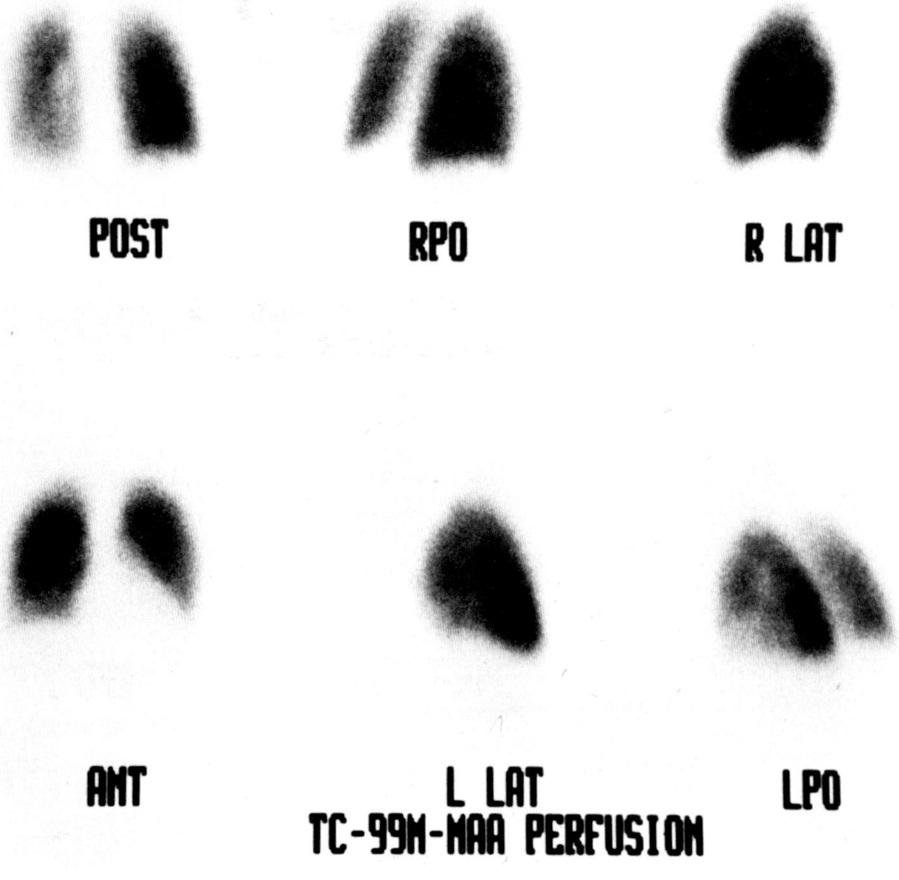

Figure 20

RADIOLOGY/IMAGING

ANSWERS

304-e	305-b	306-d	307-c	308-b	309-c	310-d	311-e
312-d	313-a	314-b	315-c	316-d	317-d		

ECHOCARDIOGRAPHY

RATIONALE 304-e

Most standard echographs use a crystal that emits a burst of sound at about 1-5 megaHertz (millions of cycles each sec) for extremely short periods.

Signal processing changes echoes into meaningful displays. Three standard modes are used. In A-mode, the amplitude of a spike rising from baseline indicates the intensity of the echo. B-mode means that the brightness of the image illustrates intensity of the echo. By introducing time in one direction (usually horizontal), an M-mode display shows motion. Much more complex and useful displays are available and, with multiple crystals, cross-sectional or if three-dimensional, views of structures are obtained.

Because echoes from the pericardium can be distinguished from other structures, small effusions, perhaps as small as 16 ml, can be detected. Motion of the left ventricular wall can be displayed with ease. A pseudocyst of the pancreas of 200 ml is detected as are vegetations on the heart valves (particularly Candida which often causes giant vegetations). Pneumothorax, however, cannot be detected easily because ultrasound does not travel well through air in the lungs or air in a pneumothorax.

REFERENCES

Feigenbaum H (Ed): Echocardiography. Fourth Edition. Philadelphia, Lea & Febiger, 1986, pp 548-578

Horowitz MS, Schultz CS, Stinson EB, et al: Sensitivity and specificity of echocardiographic diagnosis of pericardial effusion. Circulation 1974; 50:239

Johnson ML: Echocardiography. In: The Heart. Fourth Edition. Hurst JW, Logue RB, Schlant RC, et al (Eds). New York, McGraw-Hill Book Company, 1978, pp 434-445

Roy P, Tajik AJ, Giuliani ER, et al: Spectrum of echocardiographic findings in bacterial endocarditis. Circulation 1976; 53:474

RATIONALE 305-b

Echocardiogram "b" shows a significant posterior pericardial effusion (aa). Note the transition from the left ventricular chamber (bb) to the endocardium (cc), myocardium (dd), epicardium (ee), and pericardium (ff) which merges with the echogenic lung parenchyma (gg). Note that the pericardial effusion decreases in width during diastolic filling and becomes more prominent during systole. A small posterior pericardial effusion may not be significant but should not be visualized during diastole. Posterior prominence of the pericardial effusion is expected due to the supine position of the patient during the echocardiogram. Pericardial effusion and pericardial tamponade are not uncommon in critical care patients, particularly those with renal failure. The hallmark of temporizing therapy for pericardial tamponade is maintaining adequate preload. Diuretic usage and the resultant preload reduction can be disastrous. Echocardiogram "a" shows an enlarged left ventricle (hh). Echocardiogram "c" is normal; note the normal E to F slope (ii) of the mitral valve. Compare this with the reduced E to F slope (jj) shown in echocardiogram "d" which demonstrates classic mitral stenosis.

REFERENCES

Berger HJ, Matthay RA: Noninvasive radiographic assessment of cardiovascular function in acute and chronic respiratory failure. Am J Cardiol 1981; 47:950

Dane TEB, King EG: Fatal cardiac tamponade and other mechanical complications of central venous catheters. Br J Surg 1975; 62:6

Shabetai R: Changing concepts of cardiac tamponade. Modern Concepts of Cardiovascular Disease 1983; 52:19

EDITORIAL COMMENT

Ultrasonography is finding increased utilization in diagnosis of effects and complications of blunt abdominal trauma which include (1) splenic injuries such as subcapsular hematoma, laceration, or intraparenchymal hematomas; (2) pancreatic injuries resulting in edema or pseudocyst formation; and (3) fracture and rupture of the diaphragm.

The 2-D echo doppler is now being utilized to accurately quantitate both pulmonary and systemic blood flow and to calculate flow ratios noninvasively. In addition it has been utilized for intracardiac shunt quantitation and left ventricular stroke volume and offers much promise in accurate noninvasive flow measurements.

ADDITIONAL REFERENCES

Kuligowska E, Mueller PR, Simeone JF: Ultrasound: Is it useful in upper abdominal trauma? Modern Medicine 1985

Valdes-Cruz LM, Sahn DJ: Two-dimensional echo doppler for noninvasive quantitation of cardiac flow: A status report. Modern Concepts of Cardiovascular Disease, American Heart Association 1982, 51:123

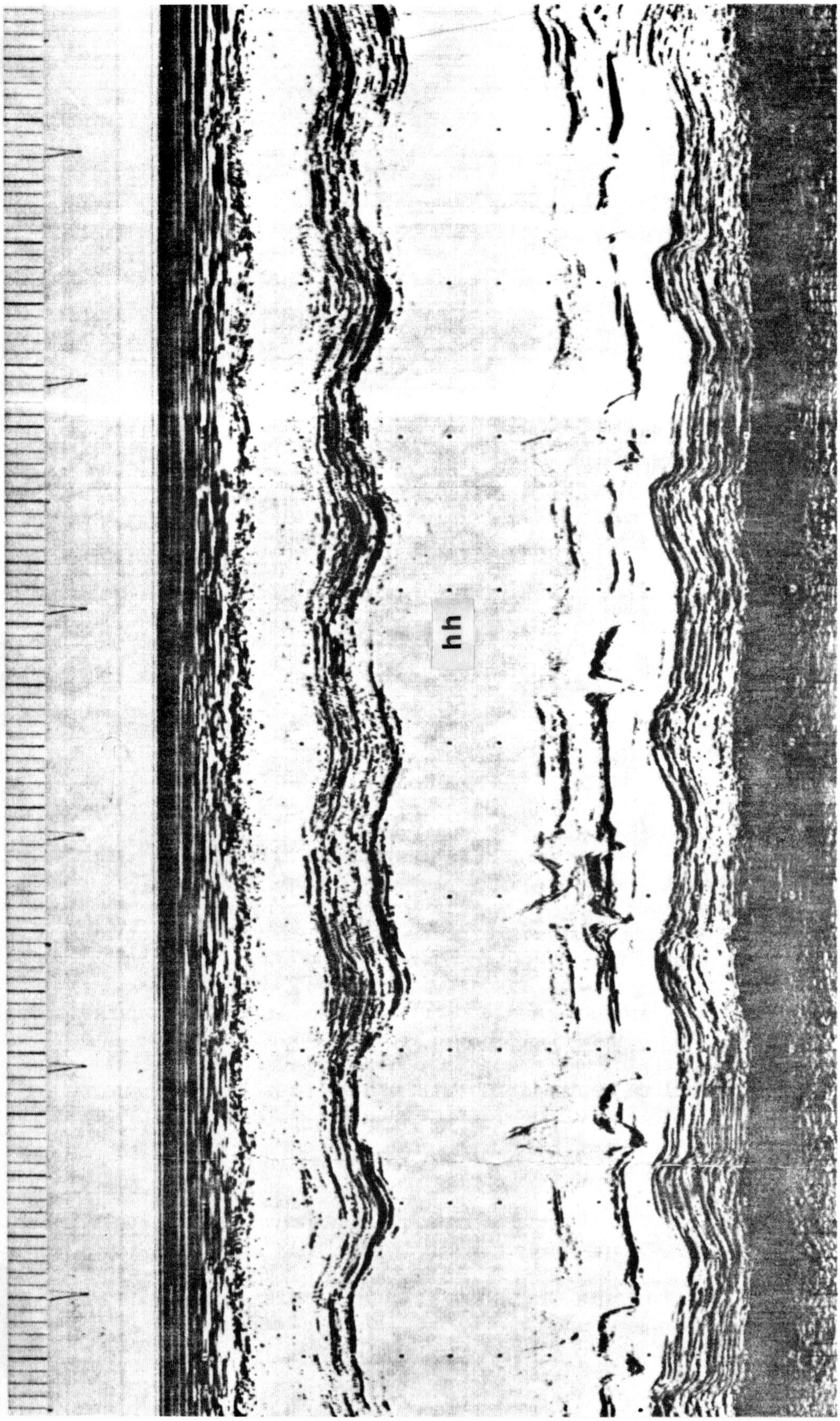

Echocardiogram - a

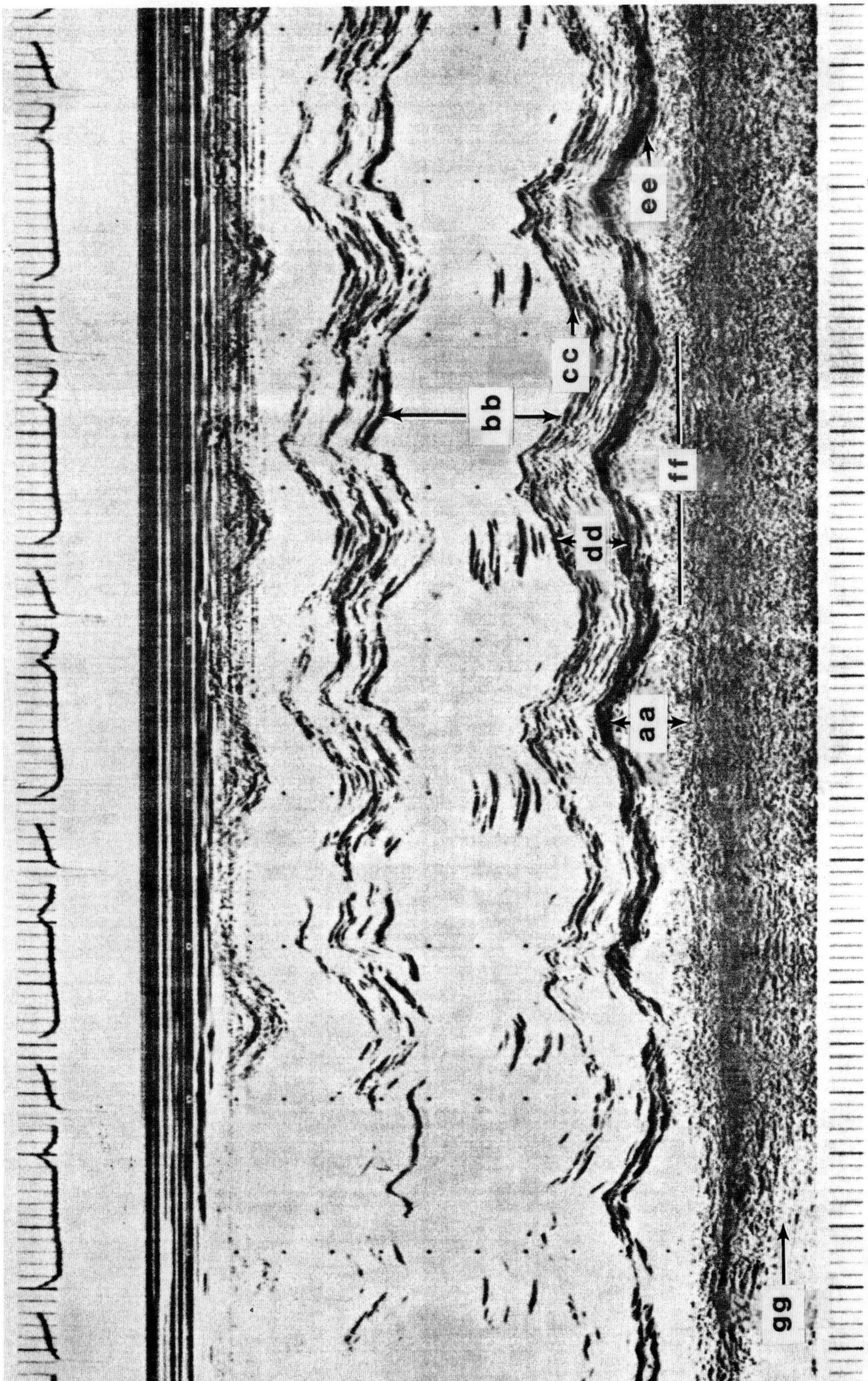

Echocardiogram - b

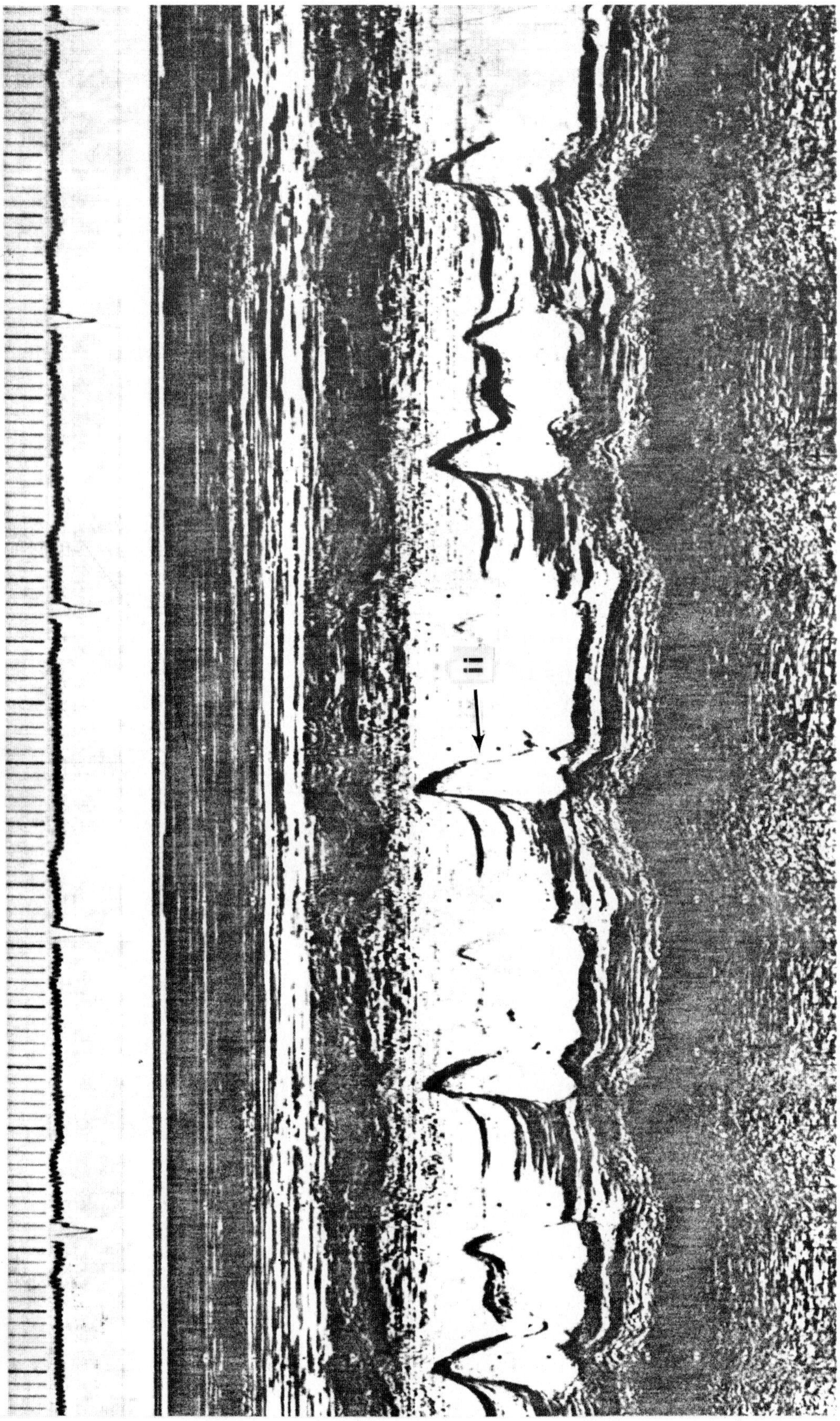

Echocardiogram - c

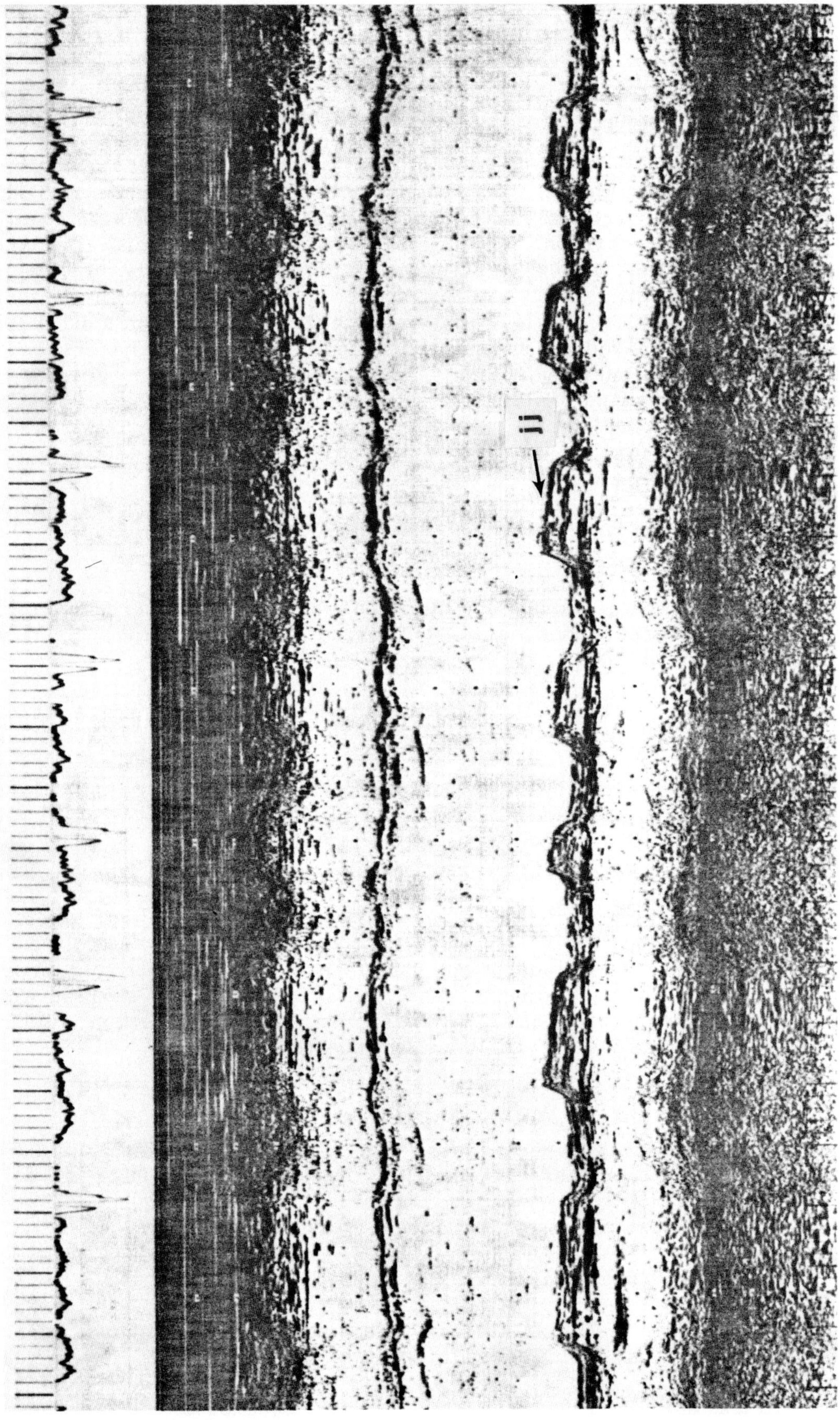

Echocardiogram - d

GENERAL

RATIONALE 306-d

The tip of the endotracheal tube in Figure 7 is in the right mainstem bronchus and clearly needs to be withdrawn. The pulmonary artery catheter and introducer never cross the midline from a left supraclavicular insertion site, and are therefore in an atypical position. The unusual catheter and introducer position suggests that the patient has a left-sided superior vena cava or that the catheter may not be within the vascular space through its proximal course. The catheter tip is probably in the right ventricular outflow tract or proximal main pulmonary artery. A wedged tracing obtained from this catheter position following balloon inflation is unlikely. Additionally, the introducer appears to be advanced to an excessive distance in this small adult.

REFERENCES

Caldwell SL, Sullivan KN: Artificial airways. In: Respiratory Care: A Guide to Clinical Practice. Second Edition. Burton GG, Hodgkin JE (Eds). Philadelphia, JB Lippincott Co., 1984, pp 493-521

Daily EK, Schoeder JS (Eds): Venous and pulmonary arterial pressure monitoring. In: Techniques in Bedside Hemodynamic Monitoring. Third Edition. St. Louis, CV Mosby Co., 1985, pp 55-100

Goodman LR, Putman CE: Intensive Care Radiology: Imaging of the Critically Ill. St. Louis, CV Mosby Co., 1978, pp 29-63

Sprung CL (Ed): The Pulmonary Artery Catheter: Methodology and Clinical Applications. Baltimore, University Park Press, 1983

RATIONALE 307-c

This patient has a tension pneumothorax which is a life-threatening process. The left lung is completely collapsed and the mediastinum is shifted to the right. Emergent decompression is essential. Acceptable treatment includes needle or catheter decompression, followed by tube thoracostomy.

REFERENCES

Kaye W: Invasive therapeutic techniques. In: Textbook of Advanced Cardiac Life Support. American Heart Association, 1981, pp 1-19

Putman CE, Goodman L: Imaging in the critically ill or injured. In: Critical Care: State of the Art. Vol 4. Shoemaker WC, Thompson WL (Eds). Fullerton, CA, Society of Critical Care Medicine, 1983, pp IV(A):1-63

Ross DS: Thoracentesis. In: Clinical Procedures in Emergency Medicine. Roberts JR, Hedges JR (Eds). Philadelphia, WB Saunders Co., 1985

Teplick SK, Clark RE: Various faces of tension pneumothorax. Postgrad Med 1974; 56:87

RATIONALE 308-b

The chest radiograph in Figure 9 demonstrates extensive subcutaneous and mediastinal emphysema, as well as free air under the right hemidiaphragm. In this patient, the findings were all caused by positive pressure ventilation and high level positive end-expiratory pressure.

Pulmonary barotrauma (PBT) is a common complication of ventilatory therapy. Investigators have demonstrated a relationship between PBT and the level of inspiratory airway pressure during positive pressure breathing.

Gas from ruptured alveoli may dissect into the pleural space causing pneumothorax or track proximally along pulmonary vascular sheaths causing pneumomediastinum. It may subsequently dissect tissue planes causing subcutaneous emphysema, pneumoretroperitoneum and pneumoperitoneum, and rarely pneumopericardium in the adult.

Presence of free air in the peritoneal cavity is worrisome as it may suggest a gastrointestinal perforation. In this case, the emphysematous changes resolved as the patient improved and was weaned from the ventilator and PEEP. A subsequent laparotomy (staging procedure for non-Hodgkins lymphoma) revealed no evidence of gastrointestinal pathology.

REFERENCES

Cullen DJ, Caldera DL: The incidence of ventilator-induced pulmonary barotrauma in critically ill patients. Anesthesiology 1979; 50:185

Leonidas JC, Hall RT, Rhodes PG, et al: Pneumoperitoneum in ventilated newborns. Am J Dis Child 1974; 128:677

Macklin CC: Transport of the air along sheaths of pulmonic blood vessels from alveoli to mediastinum: Clinical implications. Arch Intern Med 1939; 64:913

McLoud TC, Barash PG, Ravin CE, et al: Elevation of pulmonary artery pressure as a sign of pulmonary barotrauma (pneumothorax). Crit Care Med 1978; 6:61

Peterson GW, Baier H: Incidence of pulmonary barotrauma in a medical ICU. Crit Care Med 1983; 11:67

RATIONALE 309-c

When the chest radiograph in Figure 11 is compared to that in Figure 10, new opacification of the right hemithorax is noted. Unilateral opacification of a hemithorax is associated with a variety of conditions including lung collapse, pleural fluid, pneumonitis, thoracic bandages, rotation and others. The rapid occurrence of hemithoracic opacification following central line insertion and fluid infusion suggests an extravascular/intrapleural position of the catheter tip. A lateral decubitus or upright chest radiograph should demonstrate layering of the pleural fluid.

In this case, the pleural fluid was parenteral alimentation fluid infused through a malpositioned catheter. Radiographic conformation of vascular catheter position is critical. The medial displacement of the catheter tip in Figure 11 suggests an extravascular location.

The electrocardiogram is normal.

REFERENCES

Feliciano DV, Mattox KL, et al: Major complications of percutaneous subclavian vein catheters. Am J Surg 1979; 138:869

Weiner P, Sznajder I, et al: Unusual complications of subclavian vein catheterization. Crit Care Med 1984; 12:538

RATIONALE 310-d

Pericardial effusion commonly increases the size of the cardiopericardial silhouette. If the effusion is less than a few hundred milliliters, however, no apparent change may be present. Lung fields may be clear but often, especially with acute pericarditis, there is an associated left pleural effusion. Straightening of the left heart border and bulging of the right heart border are characteristic. As the patient's position is changed, the vascular pedical shadow size may vary. The left atrial appendage is sometimes seen as the most inferior of three "bumps" on the upper left heart border on posterior-anterior films. It is prominent when the left atrium is enlarged, as in mitral valve disease. Even were the left atrium enlarged, a pericardial effusion tends to obliterate this part of the left heart border shadow. See Figure 21.

REFERENCES

Felson B: Chest Roentgenology. Philadelphia, WB Saunders Co., 1973, p 395

Fowler NO: Cardiac Diagnosis and Treatment. Second Edition. Maryland, Harper and Row, 1976, pp 867-868

Fowler NO (Ed): The Pericardium in Health and Disease. New York, Futura Publishing Co., 1985, p 164

Meschan RM: Analysis of Roentgen Signs in General Radiology. Philadelphia, WB Saunders Co., 1973, pp 1139-1143

EDITORIAL COMMENT

Pulmonary barotrauma in mechanically ventilated patients continues to be a prominent occurrence in the intensive care unit. Positive end-expiratory pressure (PEEP) apparently influences barotrauma as it affects peak inspiration pressure (PIP). Theoretically, PEEP might decrease PIP by improving (increasing) compliance.

Pulmonary interstitial emphysema (PIE) was radiographically detected in 13 of 15 patients with adult respiratory distress syndrome (ARDS), 10 of whom also had pneumothorax. In 5 of these patients PIE was documented radiographically prior to and within 12 hours of development of the pneumothorax. Barotrauma correlated with peak inspiratory airway pressure of 40 cm of water or greater but not with mean airway pressure or positive end-inspiratory pressure alone. Time on the respirator at peak airway pressures above 40 cm of water along with clinical severity of ARDS and associated pulmonary pathology (such as COPD or concurrent bacterial pneumonia) increased probability of barotrauma.

The resolution time of pneumothorax (PTX) in neonates has recently been studied. After tube thoracotomy placement 28% resolved in 24 hours, 50% in 96 hours and 83% in 168 hours. All persistent leaks over 168 hours were in neonates requiring ventilatory assistance.

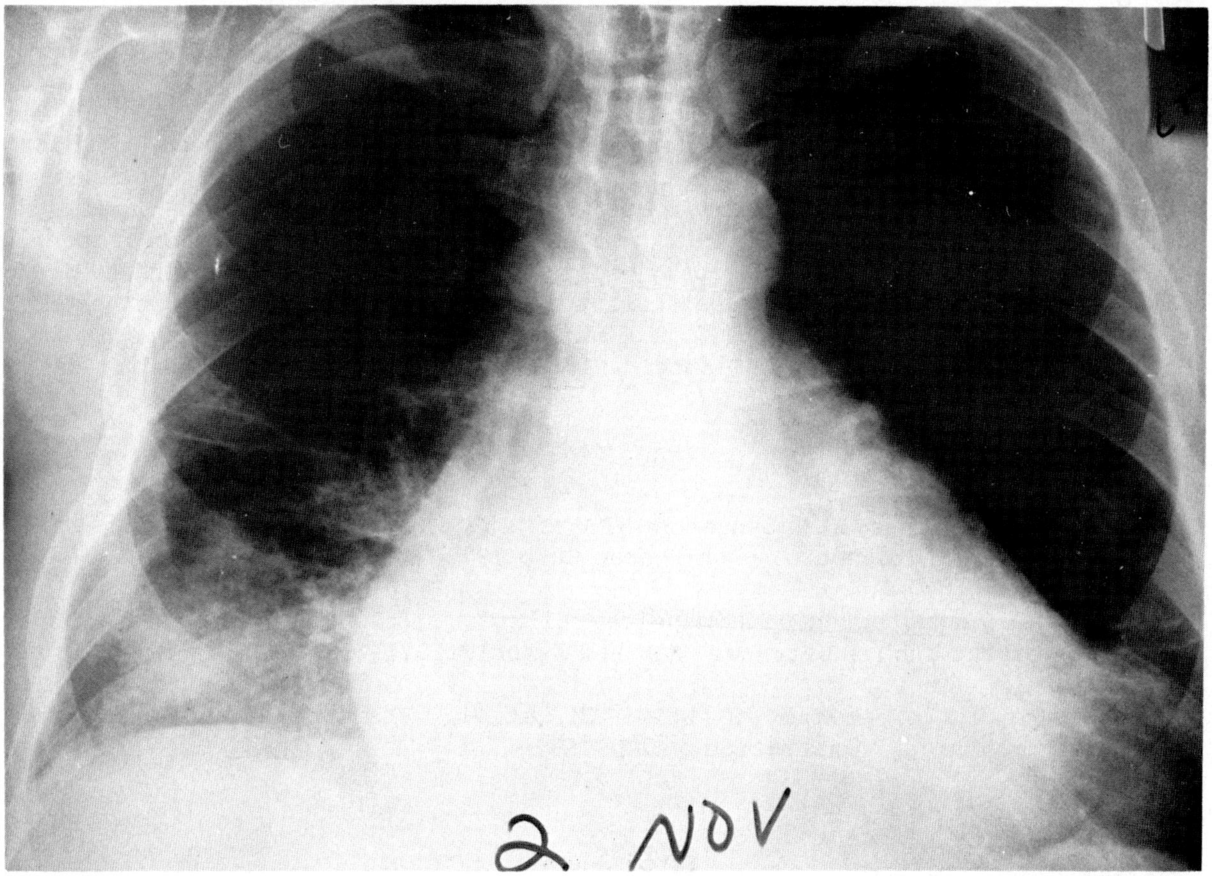

Figure 21

Case reports continue to demonstrate problems with PA catheter introducer sheath insertion complications particularly in smaller adult patients and in the left sided internal jugular approach. One should be leery of inserting the introducer sheath to its full length in most patients. Complications may be associated with trauma to the vein wall or exit of the introducer sheath from the vascular space.

ADDITIONAL REFERENCES

Bhatia J, Mathew OP: Resolution of pneumothorax in neonates. Crit Care Med 1985; 13:417

Woodring JH: Pulmonary interstitial emphysema in the adult respiratory distress syndrome. Crit Care Med 1985; 13:786

INTUBATION/MECHANICAL VENTILATION

RATIONALE 311-e

Overinflation of the alveoli leading to the development of interstitial pulmonary emphysema, mediastinal and subcutaneous emphysema, pneumoretroperitoneum, pneumothorax, and pneumoperitoneum was described first by Charles C. Macklin in 1937. Pneumoperitoneum as a complication of mechanical ventilation since then has been described in a few reports. Because of pneumoperitoneum, these patients may be erroneously subjected to a laparotomy for suspected hollow viscus perforation. Peak inspiratory pressure can be decreased by (1) decreasing tidal volume, (2) prolonging inspiratory time (decreasing flow rate), or (3) increasing compliance. (1) and (2) may not be practical due to patient pathology.

REFERENCES

Leininger BJ, Barker WL, Langston HT, et al: Tension pneumoperitoneum and pneumothorax in the newborn. Ann Thorac Surg 1970; 4:359

Macklin CC: Pneumothorax with massive collapse from experimental local over-inflation of the lung substance. Can Med Assoc J 1973; 36:414

Stringfield JT III, Graham JP, Watts CM, et al: Pneumoperitoneum: A complication of mechanical ventilation. JAMA 1976; 235:744

RATIONALE 312-d

Changes in distal endotracheal tube (ET) tip position on the chest radiograph may not always imply movement of the tube itself but, instead, changes in neck posturing and/or different phases of respiration. Flexion of the neck and decreased inspiration will both move the ET tube tip closer to the carina, and neck extension and increased inspiration will move tip further from carina.

It is therefore possible, even when the ET tube is noted to be at or above the carina on chest radiograph, that during expiration or neck flexion, the tube will be moved into an unsatisfactory position.

REFERENCES

Goodman LR, Putman CE: Intensive Care Radiology: Imaging of the Critically Ill. Philadelphia, WB Saunders Co., 1983, pp 18-20

Goodman LR, Putman CE: Radiological evaluation of patients receiving assisted ventilation. JAMA 1981; 245:858

Putman CE, Goodman L: Imaging in the critically ill or injured. In: Critical Care: State of the Art. Vol 4. Fullerton, CA, Society of Critical Care Medicine, 1983, pp IV(A):1-63

EDITORIAL COMMENT

The value of routine daily chest radiographs in a medical intensive care unit can be predicted. The incidence of unexpected radiographic changes increases with the number of catheters or intrathoracic tubes. The majority of the significant findings, however, are unrelated to the presence of the tube or catheter. The tube and catheter count therefore reflects the degree of clinical instability. Patients in a medical intensive care unit with uncomplicated cardiac disorders and nonpulmonary, noncardiac conditions do not benefit from routine daily chest radiographs.

Thermal dye indicator dilution technique determination of extravascular lung water has been used to ascertain the value of the portable chest radiograph to predict pulmonary edema. Results indicate a poor correlation. Only large changes in extravascular lung water can be accurately predicted based on radiographic scoring. This probably relates at least partially to the inability to obtain a fully upright inspiratory film due to patient illness and/or cooperation.

A malpositioned endotracheal tube is the most likely complication of intubation to be demonstrated by postintubation radiographs. Evaluation of tracheal tube tip position with a fiberoptic bronchoscope is more rapid than radiograph conformation of site of placement and is as reliable.

ADDITIONAL REFERENCES

Halperin BD, Feeley TW, Mihm FG, et al: Evaluation of the portable chest roentgenogram for quantitation extravascular lung water in critically ill adults. Chest 1985; 88:649

O'Brien D, Curran J, Conroy J, et al: Fibre-optic assessment of tracheal tube position. A comparison of tracheal tube position as estimated by fibre-optic bronchoscopy and by chest x-ray. Anaesthesia 1985; 40:73

Strain DS, Kinasewitz GT, Lowell VE, George RB: Value of routine daily chest x-rays in the medical intensive care unit. Crit Care Med 1985; 13:534

===

PEDIATRICS

===

RATIONALE 313-a

The chest radiographs in Figures 12 and 13 demonstrate ball-valve hyperinflation of the left lung secondary to left mainstem bronchus foreign body obstruction. This patient aspirated a pretzel. The expiratory film reveals marked air trapping in the left lung secondary to the ball-valve effect of the foreign body in the left mainstem bronchus. The left lung appears more radiolucent and the mediastinum has shifted to the right. None of the other options listed are associated with an inspiratory or expiratory mediastinal shift.

The child who has aspirated a foreign body may present with a persistent cough. Alternately, a history of the sudden onset and subsequent resolution of coughing, choking, vomiting and/or cyanosis may be obtained. Following the acute episode, the child may develop signs of airway obstruction and/or infection. Localized or diffuse wheezing may be heard.

Asymmetrical chest expansion may be detected on physical exam. A normal chest radiograph is not uncommon in this setting. Inspiratory and expiratory chest radiographs are extremely helpful but may be difficult to obtain in an uncooperative child.

The foreign body is most easily removed with rigid bronchoscopy. Although there has been some success reported with fiberoptic bronchoscopy in adults for removal of small foreign bodies, no data support this practice in small children.

REFERENCES

Blaser S, Naveh Y, Friedman A: Foreign body in the airway: A review of 200 cases. Am J Dis Child 1980; 134:68

Cohen SR, Lewis GB, Herbert WI, et al: Foreign bodies in the airway. Five-year retrospective study with special reference to management. Ann Otol 1980; 89:437

Cotton E, Yasuda K: Foreign body aspiration. Pediatr Clin North Am 1984; 4:937

Logvinoff M, Taussig LM: Foreign body aspiration in childhood. Ariz Med 1980; 27:77

EDITORIAL COMMENT

Signs and symptoms of upper airway obstruction may relate to the position of the foreign body in the trachea itself. If a tracheal foreign body leads to a partial obstruction and is outside the thoracic cavity (above the jugular notch) it produces predominantly inspiratory obstruction, and if inside the thoracic cavity produces predominantly expiratory obstruction. A fixed tracheal obstruction secondary to a foreign body causes pronounced inspiratory and expiratory obstruction regardless of location. Flow volume loops readily differentiate these two conditions and are valuable in cooperative patients.

In small children, however, this information is not usually attainable. The diagnostic triad of wheezing, coughing, and decreased breath sounds is more common in late diagnosis. This triad may be incomplete in greater than 50% of patients. The chest radiograph may be normal early after aspiration and show atelectasis or consolidation later.

ADDITIONAL REFERENCES

Cottong E, Yasuda K: Foreign body aspiration. Pediatr Clin North Am 1984; 31:937

Wiseman NE: The diagnosis of foreign body aspiration in childhood. J Pediatr Surg 1984; 19:531

POSTOPERATIVE

RATIONALE 314-b

The patient whose chest radiograph is shown in Figure 14 developed fever and progressive opacification of the right hemithorax two days following resection of an esophageal carcinoma. The meniscus extending across the right hemithorax is compatible with a significant pleural effusion. One should be alerted to the possibility of suture-line breakdown. This is especially true in a patient who appears to be getting worse and who has associated findings such as increased temperature and elevated white count. Thoracentesis in this patient revealed an amylase of greater than 13,000, a pH of 6.2 and a white count of 30,000 with PMN predominance. The LDH was 1100. A very low pH (often less than 6), a high amylase (which is salivary), and a high WBC count are classic findings in esophageal rupture or in a patient who has suture line breakdown following esophageal surgery. With such characteristic pleural fluid findings, a diagnostic thoracentesis is an extremely high-yield procedure for ruling in or out this diagnostic possibility. An indium-labeled WBC scan may be helpful in locating occult infection, and ultrasound and CT may be helpful in differentiating various pleural and chest parenchymal diagnostic possibilities; however, in this case the high yield, simple and straightforward procedure of choice is diagnostic thoracentesis.

REFERENCES

Bellman MH, Rajaratnam HN: Perforation of the esophagus with amylase-rich pleural effusion. Br J Dis Chest 1974; 68:18

Dye RA, Laforet EG: Esophageal rupture: Diagnosis of pleural fluid pH. Chest 1974; 66:454

Maulitz RM, et al: The pleuropulmonary consequences of esophageal rupture: An experimental model. Am Rev Respir Dis 1979; 120:363

Sherr HP, Light RW, Merson MH, et al: Origin of the pleural fluid amylase in esophageal rupture. Ann Intern Med 1972; 76:985

Skinner DB, Little AG, DeMeester TR: Management of esophageal perforation. Am J Surg 1980; 139:760

TRAUMA

RATIONALE 315-c

The chest radiograph shown in Figure 15 demonstrates a sternal fracture indicative of significant trauma. Blunt chest trauma is associated with an increased incidence of myocardial contusion.

The severity of myocardial contusion ranges from subclinical to findings of severe heart failure. Ventricular dysrhythmias may lead to sudden death. Recently, more sophisticated tests such as 2-D echocardiography and gated radionuclide angiography have been added to CK-MB measurement and electrocardiographic data, and have improved diagnostic capability in this disorder.

If myocardial contusion is suspected, the patient should be monitored for potential ventricular dysrhythmias, even when clinically stable. Electrocardiographic monitoring for at least 72 hours has been suggested in traumatized patients with documented myocardial contusions.

REFERENCES

Gay WC, McCabe JC: Trauma to the Chest. In: Principles of Trauma Care. Third Edition. Shires GT (Ed). New York, McGraw-Hill Book Company, 1985, pp 267-290

Jugdutt BI, Sussex BA, Sivaram CA, et al: Right ventricular infarction: Two-dimensional echocardiographic evaluation. Am Heart J 1984; 107:505

Kron IL, Cox PM Jr: Cardiac injury after chest trauma. Crit Care Med 1983; 11:524

Kumar SA, Puri VK, Mittal VK, et al: Myocardial contusion following nonfatal blunt chest trauma. J Trauma 1983; 23:327

Saunders CR, Doty DB: Myocardial contusion. Surg Gynecol Obstet 1977; 144:595

Snow N, Richardson JD, Flint LM: Myocardial contusion: Implications for patients with multiple traumatic injuries. Surgery 1982; 92:744

VENTILATION/PERFUSION LUNG SCANNING

RATIONALE 316-d

Pulmonary embolism is a common disease process in immobilized patients. Tachypnea, tachycardia, chest tightness and hypoxemia are consistent with this diagnosis. The ventilation-perfusion lung scintigram shown in Figures 16 and 17 demonstrates multiple unmatched segmental and subsegmental perfusion defects most consistent with multiple pulmonary emboli. The patient is also at risk for fat embolization. Although perfusion defects may be seen with fat embolization, they are rarely of this size on the $\dot{V}/\dot{Q}$ scan. Anticoagulation is indicated in this patient. Considering the magnitude of the perfusion defects and the cardiopulmonary arrest, streptokinase might be considered in this patient. Most would obtain angiographic documentation of pulmonary embolization prior to streptokinase therapy. Extensive trauma 4 days previously may, however, preclude its use.

REFERENCES

Bell W, et al: The clinical features of sub-massive and massive pulmonary emboli. Am J Med 1977; 62:355

Deykin D: Current status of anticoagulant therapy. Am J Med 1982; 72:659

Goodman LR, Putman CE: Intensive Care Radiology: Imaging of the Critically Ill. St. Louis, CV Mosby Co., 1978, pp 194-199

Marder J: The use of thrombolytic agents: Choice of patient, drug administration, laboratory monitoring. Ann Intern Med 1979; 90:802

Rosennow E, Osmundson P, Brown M: Pulmonary embolism. Mayo Clin Proc 1981; 56:161

Secker-Walker RH: The lung. In: Textbook of Nuclear Medicine: Clinical Applications. Rocha AFG, Harbert JC (Eds). Philadelphia, Lea & Febiger, 1979, pp 188-262

RATIONALE 317-d

The ventilation-perfusion ($\dot{V}/\dot{Q}$) lung scan shown in Figures 19 and 20 is normal. The central (less dense) areas on both ventilation and perfusion scans represent heart and hilum. The lungs are perfused uniformly. Ventilation is distributed normally and clears without delay.

A normal $\dot{V}/\dot{Q}$ lung scan excludes clinically significant pulmonary emboli (PE). A "high probability" $\dot{V}/\dot{Q}$ lung scan is helpful diagnostically and may preclude the need for pulmonary arteriography in a patient with significant risk factors for PE.

A "high probability" $\dot{V}/\dot{Q}$ lung scan is characterized by multiple segmental or larger perfusion defects with a normal ventilation scan (Figures 16 and 17).

Most clinicians feel, however, that even in the presence of a high probability $\dot{V}/\dot{Q}$ lung scan, an arteriogram is required if:

(1) The patient is young and without strong risk factors. (Oral contraceptives are not considered high risk.)

(2) Streptokinase therapy is anticipated.

(3) An inferior vena cava filter or plication is planned.

$\dot{V}/\dot{Q}$ lung scans that are neither normal nor "high probability" offer little help in the differential diagnosis of PE. A pulmonary arteriogram is usually warranted in this "indeterminant" setting.

REFERENCES

Hull RD, Hirsh J, Carter CJ, et al: Pulmonary angiography, ventilation lung scanning, and venography for clinically suspected pulmonary embolism with abnormal perfusion lung scan. Ann Intern Med 1983; 98:891

Robin ED: Overdiagnosis and overtreatment of pulmonary embolism: The emperor may have no clothes. Ann Intern Med 1977; 87:775

Sasahara AA, Sharma GVRK, Barsamian EM, et al: Pulmonary thromboembolism. JAMA 249:29

Viamonte M, Koolpe H, Janowitz W, et al: Pulmonary thromboembolism - Update. JAMA 1980; 243:2229

EDITORIAL COMMENT

Diagnostic and treatment dilemmas still remain for physicians involved in evaluation of patients suspected to have pulmonary embolism. The most helpful study is a normal perfusion scan which allows elimination of clinically significant pulmonary embolus from the differential diagnosis. Unfortunately, abnormal perfusion scans are nonspecific and often not very helpful in the differential diagnosis of pulmonary embolism. Multiple segmental or larger perfusion defects with normal ventilation scanning in radiographically normal areas are highly specific for pulmonary embolism and in most circumstances do not require angiographic documentation. Exceptions included the need for placement of a vena cava umbrella or streptokinase therapy. Documentation of proximal deep vein thrombosis by either venography or impedance/plethysmography (IPG) offers very useful data in this patient population as it necessitates anticoagulation therapy irrespective of results of ventilation-perfusion lung scanning. It also increases the predictive value of ventilation perfusion lung scanning. Angiography may still be required in those situations where perfusion scanning is neither normal nor high probability because of the short term and long term morbidity/mortality risks posed by heparin therapy or its alternatives.

Matched ventilation perfusion defects, although seen with pulmonary embolism, are also seen with multiple other acute and chronic pulmonary processes. If the ventilation defect is smaller than the perfusion defect, pulmonary embolism is more likely. If the perfusion defect is smaller than the ventilation defect a primary ventilatory process is more likely. These, however, are certainly not absolute criteria.

(Note: See additional questions and discussion of pulmonary embolism diagnosis in Section 15.)

ADDITIONAL REFERENCES

Goodman PC: Pulmonary angiography. Clin Chest Med 1984; 5:465

Hull RD, Hirsh J, Carter CJ, et al: Diagnostic value of ventilation-perfusion lung scanning in patients with suspected pulmonary embolism. Chest 1985; 77:819

Hull RD, Raskob GE, LeClere JR, et al: The diagnosis of clinically suspected venous thrombosis. Clin Chest Med 1984; 5:439

Polak JF, McNeil BJ: Pulmonary scintigraphy and the diagnosis of pulmonary embolism: A perspective. Clin Chest Med 1984; 5:457

Sors J, Safran D, Stern M, et al: An analysis of the diagnostic methods for acute pulmonary embolism. Intensive Care Med 1984; 10:81

Section 17

318. Decreased serum ionized calcium concentrations are observed LEAST often in:

   a. Patients given 10 units of ACD banked blood in 3 hours
   b. Patients with pseudohypoparathyroidism
   c. Acute central neurogenic hyperventilation
   d. Hypoalbuminemia
   e. Neonatal tetany

319. Which ONE of the following statements about calcium metabolism is NOT correct?

   a. Hypomagnesemia decreases release of and/or response to parathormone.
   b. Calcium chloride given intravenously may increase cardiac dysrhythmias in digitalis intoxication.
   c. Hypocalcemia is associated with a shortened QT interval on ECG.
   d. Calcium chloride given intravenously antagonizes adverse electrical effects of hyperkalemia.

320. A 36-year-old female with metastatic breast carcinoma is admitted to the ICU with a serum calcium of 18.4 mg/dl. Which of the following is the least acceptable method of treatment?

   a. Corticosteroids
   b. Mithramycin
   c. 0.9% NaCl
   d. Sodium polystyrene sulfonate

321. Causes of laboratory measured hypocalcemia (total and/or ionized) include all but which ONE of the following?

   a. Hypoalbuminemia
   b. Thyroid surgery
   c. Alkalosis
   d. Acute pancreatitis
   e. Hypermagnesemia

322. The colloid-crystalloid controversy continues. Certain principles, however, are clear. Which of the following is incorrect?

   a. Crystalloid resuscitation is much less expensive than colloid resuscitation.
   b. The therapeutic endpoint (maximum volume expansion) occurs more rapidly with crystalloid resuscitation.
   c. Isotonic crystalloid resuscitation requires much larger volumes than does colloid resuscitation.
   d. The risk of pulmonary edema is greater with crystalloid resuscitation.

323. Hemodialysis is performed most safely in which ONE of the following settings?

a. Bleeding due to decreased platelet adhesiveness
b. Intracranial hemorrhage
c. Acute gastrointestinal hemorrhage
d. Significant hypotension

324. Which ONE of the following represents the LEAST favorable setting for the use of therapeutic peritoneal dialysis?

a. Extensive abdominal trauma
b. Postoperative adhesions
c. Massive obesity
d. Presence of a colostomy
e. Ruptured diaphragm

325. A 56-year-old male developed a biliary fistula following a cholecystectomy. He is a known alcoholic. A nasogastric tube is in place. Profuse persistent diarrhea is present. His serum magnesium is 1.0 mg/dl (lower limit of normal is 1.5 mg/dl).

Which ONE of the following statements about this patient is MOST correct?

a. The primary reason for magnesium deficiency is most likely nasogastric suctioning.
b. Aminoglycoside therapy may worsen this disorder by altering proximal renal tubular magnesium reabsorption.
c. The intestinal mucosa is the primary regulatory organ of magnesium homeostasis.
d. Most body magnesium stores exist in the extracellular fluid.

326. A patient has a blood glucose of 1000 mg/dl, blood urea nitrogen of 100 mg/dl, serum sodium of 150 mEq/L, serum potassium of 3 mEq/L, serum chloride of 110 mEq/L, and serum carbon dioxide of 24 mEq/L. The total serum osmolality is:

a. 300 mOsm/kilogram plasma
b. 306 mOsm/kilogram plasma
c. 356 mOsm/kilogram plasma
d. 391 mOsm/kilogram plasma
e. 426 mOsm/kilogram plasma

327. Which ONE of the numbers below is closest to the calculated serum osmolality (mOsm/L) of a patient with a sodium of 120 mEq/L, glucose of 54 mg/dl and BUN of 6 mg/dl?

a. 245
b. 255
c. 265
d. 275
e. 285

328. Each of the following are causes of hypokalemia EXCEPT:

a. Secondary hyperaldosteronism associated with malignant hypertension
b. Magnesium deficiency
c. Nasogastric suctioning
d. Rhabdomyolysis associated with renal failure

329. Nonoliguric acute renal failure often causes which change in urine solute concentrations?

a. Decreased urine sodium and decreased urine creatinine
b. Decreased urine sodium and normal urine creatinine
c. Decreased urine sodium and increased urine creatinine
d. Increased urine sodium and decreased urine creatinine
e. Increased urine sodium and increased urine creatinine

330. A laboratory report of a urine sodium concentration of 2 mEq/L is most likely caused by:

a. Increased aldosterone effect
b. Inadequate sodium chloride in intravenous fluids
c. Nonoliguric acute renal failure
d. Inappropriate antidiuretic hormone secretion
e. Liver dysfunction

331. In a patient who is developing acute tubular necrosis, which ONE of the following observations is MOST likely to be correct?

a. Urine volume increases
b. Urine creatinine concentration increases
c. Urine sodium concentration increases
d. Diuretic response to furosemide increases
e. Diuretic response to dopamine increases

332. Which ONE of the following statements is MOST correct following an ischemic insult to the kidneys?

a. A urine osmolality of 380 mOsm/L and a urine sodium of 25 mEq/L make the diagnosis of acute renal failure unlikely.
b. If immediate use of furosemide results in increased urine output, prognosis may improve.
c. If hypovolemia is corrected, the use of either thiazides, furosemide, dopamine or nitroprusside will increase renal blood flow.
d. The development of nonoliguric renal failure is common but does not alter prognosis.

333. Postoperative oliguric renal failure in the adult:

a. Is associated with an overall mortality of 50% or more
b. Is usually due to direct injury to the kidneys at the time of operation
c. Is infrequently associated with sepsis in those patients who subsequently die
d. Is usually reversible through the use of essential amino acid infusion

334. Which ONE of the following has LEAST correlation with the hepatorenal syndrome?

a. Abnormal urine sediment
b. Ascites
c. Jaundice
d. Hepatic encephalopathy

335. Indications for dialysis in children with acute renal failure include all of the following EXCEPT:

a. Volume overload
b. To improve renal function
c. Hyperkalemia
d. Acidosis
e. To facilitate more aggressive nutritional support by controlling vascular volume

336. The fractional excretion of filtered sodium (FENa) is MOST reliable in predicting presence or absence of renal injury in which ONE of the following circumstances?

a. Acute renal failure induced by radiographic contrast medium
b. Acute renal failure following cardiac surgery
c. Myoglobin-induced acute renal failure
d. Severe volume depletion with azotemia

337. A previously healthy 17-year-old male has been involved in a high speed motorcycle accident. His injuries include multiple long bone fractures, multiple rib fractures, a left pneumothorax and a ruptured spleen. Following fluid resuscitation, chest tube insertion, exploratory laparotomy with splenectomy and orthopedic stabilization, he is admitted to the ICU. Twelve hours after injury, in spite of apparently adequate volume expansion, the patient's urine output drops to 5 cc/hr.

A urinalysis reveals:

Color	Brown	Microscopic
pH	5	
Specific gravity	1.015	WBC 0-2 per H.P.F.
Occult blood	4+	RBC 0-1 per H.P.F
Protein	1+	Epithelial cells 0
Bilirubin	0	Casts 1-2 per H.P.F.
Glucose	0	granular casts
Ketones	0	Bacteria 0

Which ONE of the following findings is LEAST likely to be associated with this condition?

a. Hypocalcemia
b. Elevated fibrin split products
c. Pink serum
d. Tall peaked T waves on EKG

338. A 69-year-old patient is admitted to the ICU lethargic but without focal neurologic signs. Examination is unremarkable except that the patient's mucous membranes are somewhat dry. Vital signs: pulse 100, BP 105/60, respiratory rate 18, temperature 36.6°C (98°F).

Laboratory data (on admission):

Hct	45
WBC	18,000
Na^+	105 mEq/L
Cl^-	79 mEq/L
K^+	2.8 mEq/L
HCO_3^-	28 mEq/L
Glucose	128 mg/dl
BUN	25 mg/dl

The most likely cause of the hyponatremia is:

a. IADH
b. Adrenal insufficiency
c. Diuretic use
d. CNS infection
e. Nephrotic syndrome

ANSWERS

318-d	319-c	320-d	321-e	322-d	323-a	324-e	325-b
326-d	327-a	328-d	329-d	330-e	331-c	332-d	333-a
334-a	335-b	336-d	337-c	338-c			

CALCIUM

RATIONALE 318-d

The concentration of ionized calcium in serum is reduced when citrate is given (as with multiple transfusions), in pseudohypoparathyroidism, hyperventilation and neonatal tetany. Calcium in serum is about half bound to proteins, especially albumin. In hypoalbuminemia the total calcium concentration may be reduced, because of lessened protein binding, but the concentration of ionized calcium is unchanged and tetany is uncommon.

REFERENCES

Raisz, LG: Calcium metabolism. Recent advances. DM 1972; 18:1

Yendt EL: Disorders of calcium, phosphorus, and magnesium metabolism. In: Clinical Disorders of Fluid and Electrolyte Metabolism. Maxwell MH, Kleeman CK (Eds). Second Edition. New York, McGraw-Hill Book Company, 1972, pp 401-404

RATIONALE 319-c

Hypercalcemia, not hypocalcemia, characteristically causes shortening of the QT interval. Hypercalcemia produces shortening of the PR interval, lengthening of the QRS complex duration, but shortening of the ST segment thereby shortening the QT interval. The short QT interval is one of the most reliable signs of severe hypercalcemia and, in this respect, hypercalcemia mimics digitalis. Because of the shorter refractory period and slowed conduction velocity in hypercalcemia, it may predispose to arrhythmias. In hypocalcemia there is QT prolongation due to ST prolongation with a normal T wave.

Hyperkalemic electrical effects on the heart are antagonized to a large extent by intravenous administration of calcium, but this occurs without any change in serum potassium concentrations.

Athough hypocalcemia, and especially a decrease in ionized calcium, is common in the critically ill patient, parathormone concentrations are actually increased. Hypomagnesemia, however, does decrease parathormone release, target organ response to parathormone, and also the response of bone calcium deposits to hypocalcemia. Calcium may increase digitalis intoxication arrhythmias, and reduction of calcium activity (with citrate or EDTA) has been employed to treat digitalis toxicity.

REFERENCES

Christy JH, Clements SD Jr: Endocrine and metabolic disorders. In: The Heart. Fourth Edition. Hurst JW, Logue RB, Schlant RC, et al (Eds). New York, McGraw-Hill Book Company, 1978, pp 1734-1755

Moe GK, Farah AE: Digitalis and allied cardiac glycosides. In: The Pharmacological Basis of Therapeutics. Fifth Edition. Goodman LS, Gilman A (Eds). New York, Macmillan Publishing Co. Inc., 1975, pp 653-682

Parfitt AM, Kleerekopes M: Clinical disorders of calcium, phosphorus, and magnesium metabolism. In: Clinical Disorders of Fluid and Electrolyte Metabolism. Third Edition. Maxwell MH, Kleeman CR (Eds). New York, McGraw-Hill Book Company, 1980, pp 947-1151

Underwood PS, Lamba A: Parathormone and ionized calcium in critically-ill patients with sepsis. Crit Care Med 1979; 7:136

RATIONALE 320-d

Hypercalcemia may be treated in a variety of ways including EDTA, furosemide, oral and/or intravenous phosphate, calcitonin, mithramycin, corticosteriods and dialysis.

Sodium polystyrene sulfonate is a cation exchange resin that exchanges sodium for potassium in the gut. It is useful in the treatment of hyperkalemia.

REFERENCES

Parfitt AM, Kleerekopes M: Clinical disorders of calcium, phosphorus, and magnesium metabolism. In: Clinical Disorders of Fluid and Electrolyte Metabolism. Third Edition. Maxwell MH, Kleeman CR (Eds). New York, McGraw-Hill Book Company, 1980, pp 949-1151

Shoemaker WC: Fluids and electrolytes in the adult. In: Critical Care: State of the Art. Vol 3. Shoemaker WC, Thompson WL (Eds). Fullerton, CA, Society of Critical Care Medicine, 1982, pp III(N):1-96

RATIONALE 321-e

Less than 1% of the body's calcium is in the blood and less than half of the total serum calcium exists as free ions (the physiology important state). The balance of calcium is bound to proteins and a very small part is complexed with phosphate or citrate. For every 1.0 gm/dl change in serum albumin, there is a 0.8 increment or decrement in total serum calcium. Body calcium homeostasis regulates ionized calcium only and is not binding-protein dependent. Therefore, measured serum calcium may fluctuate as protein concentration varies without a significant physiological effect as ionized protein may remain constant.

The binding of calcium to albumin and other proteins is pH dependent. An acid pH decreases binding producing a higher ionized calcium level. Alkalosis increases binding and can result in true clinical hypocalcemia with low ionized calcium.

Postoperative neck surgery, i.e., thyroidectomy, may result in removal, damage, or interruption of the vascular supply of the parathyroid glands with resultant hypoparathyroidism and hypocalcemia.

Acute pancreatitis may result in hypocalcemia. Postulated reasons include decreased albumin and glucagon-induced release of thyrocalcitonin.

Hypomagnesemia, not hypermagnesemia, is associated with hypocalcemia via impairment of parathyroid hormone response to hypocalcemia. The main mechanism is impairment of release of parathyroid hormone which is magnesium dependent. Magnesium is the cofactor involved in its release. There is experimental work showing the resistance of PTH action at the level of bone.

REFERENCES

Avioli LV, Haddad JG: Vitamin D. Current Concepts Metabolism 1973; 22:507

Chernow B: Hormonal and metabolic considerations in critical care medicine. In: Textbook of Critical Care. Shoemaker WC, Thompson WL, Holbrook PR (Eds). Philadelphia, WB Saunders Co., 1984, pp 646-664

John HT, Wills MR, Marcus RT: Changes in plasma-calcium concentration following subtotal thyroidectomy. Br J Surg 1966; 53:685

Krane SM: Calcium, phosphate and magnesium. In: The International Encyclopedia of Pharmacology and Therapeutics. Rasmussen H (Ed). London, Pergamon Press, 1970, pp 19-59

Robertson GM Jr, Moore EW, et al: Inadequate parathyroid response in acute pancreatitis. N Engl J Med 1976; 294:512

Rude RK, Oldham SB, Sharp CF Jr, et al: Parathyroid hormone secretion in magnesium deficiency. J Clin Endocrinol Metab 1978; 47:800

Taylor B, Sibbald WJ: Ionized hypocalcemia in critically ill patients with sepsis. Can J Surg 1978; 21:429

COLLOID/CRYSTALLOID

RATIONALE 322-d

Crystalloid resuscitation is fifty times less expensive than colloid resuscitation. The risk of pulmonary edema seems related more to the presence or absence of sepsis than to the type of resuscitation fluid employed. The subject is, however, controversial and papers can be found to support either side. There is a general consensus that the volume required in crystalloid resuscitation is approximately 1.5 - 3.0 times that needed during colloid resuscitation. The volume expansion that occurs with crystalloids is at a maximum immediately upon infusion and decreases thereafter. With colloids the maximum volume expansion occurs one-half to one hour after completion of the infusion.

REFERENCES

Hauser CJ, et al: Oxygen transport responses to colloids and crystalloids in critically ill surgical patients. Surg Gynecol Obstet 1980; 150:811

Poole G, et al: Comparison of colloids and crystalloids in resuscitation from hemorrhagic shock. Surg Gynecol Obstet 1982; 154:577

Shoemaker WC, et al: Fluid therapy in emergency resuscitation. Crit Care Med 1981; 9:367

Skillman JJ, et al: Randomized trial of albumin vs. electrolyte solutions during abdominal aortic operations. Surgery 1975; 78:291

Virgilio RW, et al: Crystalloid vs. colloid resuscitation: Is one better? Surgery 1979; 85:129

EDITORIAL COMMENT

Crystalloid vs. colloid resuscitation remains controversial. Several points can be reliably made concerning choices available. (1) Blood (preferably whole) should be available for acute hemorrhage in excess of 2 liters. For rapid blood volume increase, if blood is not immediately available or is inappropriate, colloids are the fluids of choice. Hydroxyethyl starch (a synthetic colloid) offers more rapid volume expansion than saline and maintains this beneficial effect for 24 to 36 hours. An alternative choice, albumin, is considerably more expensive. (2) Animal experimental work done in attempt to demonstrate colloid ability to reduce pulmonary edema has failed to demonstrate any benefit. (3) Since crystalloid is distributed across all body partitions it seems preferable to colloid in total body volume depletion. In cases, however, where there may be intravascular volume depletion without total body sodium depletion, such as in the selective postoperative patient, colloid may be a more reasonable choice. (4) Another potential use for colloid is in acute hypovolemic states when limited intravenous access is available. In these situations colloid infusion gives a more rapid increase in blood pressure.

Hypertonic saline and lactated Ringer's solution are equally effective in most situations. Hypertonic saline may, however, represent a potential alternative for treatment of low volume states when aggravation of intracranial hypertension is a consideration during resuscitation.

ADDITIONAL REFERENCES

MacIntyre E, Bullen C, Machin SJ: Fluid replacement in hypovolemia. Intensive Care Med 1985; 11:231

Prough DS, Johnson C, Poole GV, et al: Effects on intracranial pressure of resuscitation from hemorrhagic shock with hypertonic saline versus lactated Ringer's solution. Crit Care Med 1985; 13:407

Sturm JA, Wisner DH: Fluid resuscitation of hypovolemia. Intensive Care Med 1985; 11:227

Twigley AJ, Hillman KM: The end of the crystalloid era? Anaesthesia 1985; 40:860

DIALYSIS

RATIONALE 323-a

Symptomatic uremia, volume overload, hyperkalemia, and acidosis refractory to conservative measures are the major indications for hemodialysis. Uremia causes decreased platelet adhesiveness which may lead to significant bleeding. Dialysis may improve platelet function in the uremic patient and, therefore, decrease the bleeding tendency.

Hemodialysis is contraindicated in patients who are at high risk of bleeding during heparinization and in those who are hemodynamically unstable. Included among this group are patients with active gastrointestinal bleeding, intracranial hemorrhage, and subdural hematoma. Significant hypotension and evidence of pericardial tamponade are examples of hemodynamic contraindications.

REFERENCES

Fang LST: Hepatorenal syndrome. In: Manual of Intensive Care Medicine. Rippe JM, Csete ME (Eds). Boston, Little Brown and Co., 1983, pp 237-238

Manis T, Friedman EA: Dialytic therapy for irreversible uremia. N Engl J Med 1979; 301:1260,1321

RATIONALE 324-e

Peritoneal dialysis (PD) may be difficult in some or all of the situations listed. A ruptured diaphragm is the most unfavorable setting. Some would say that PD is absolutely contraindicated in this situation. Extensive abdominal trauma makes PD difficult due to leaking from drain sites or wounds. Peritoneal dialysis is not absolutely contraindicated in this setting but should be avoided if other options are available. Massive obesity makes catheter insertion difficult, but adequate clearances can be obtained once the catheter is correctly placed. Extensive adhesions may make catheter placement difficult as the risk of bowel perforation is greater than usual in this setting. Additionally, adhesions may decrease the surface area of dialysate/peritoneum contact resulting in an inadequate clearance. Presence of a colostomy is a relative but not absolute contraindication to PD.

Peritoneal dialysis is the oldest form of dialysis and remains an effective tool. This technique has many advantages over hemodialysis. It has less adverse hemodynamic effects, is more efficient in removing larger molecules (especially certain drugs) and can be performed with minimal equipment.

Peritoneal dialysis remains the treatment of choice for acute renal failure with hemodynamic compromise, secondary to rhabdomyolysis (unless the patient is extremely catabolic or hypervolemic) or complicated by acute hemorrhagic pancreatitis. It is a slower form of dialysis than hemodialysis and may not be adequate for the patient with a severe catabolic state or lactic acidosis. The clearance rate of PD is only 1/5 that of hemodialysis. Peritonitis remains the major complication of peritoneal dialysis.

FAVORABLE AND UNFAVORABLE SITUATIONS FOR PERITONEAL DIALYSIS*

	FAVORABLE		UNFAVORABLE
1.	Children	1.	Diseased peritoneal vasculature
2.	Blood access problems	2.	Traumatized or postoperative abdomen
3.	Fragile cardiovascular status	3.	Diaphragmatic defects or respiratory compromise
4.	Noncatabolic patient	4.	Intestinal adhesions
5.	Hemodialysis not available	5.	Need to remove small molecular weight substances rapidly
6.	Need to remove high molecular weight molecules		

*From: Nolph KD, Sorkin M: Peritoneal dialysis in acute renal failure. In: Acute Renal Failure. Brenner BM, Lazarus JM (Eds). Philadelphia, WB Saunders Co., 1983, pp 689-710

REFERENCES

Boen ST: Kinetics of peritoneal dialysis: Comparison with artificial kidney. Medicine 1961; 40:243

Cairns KB: Clinical and hemodynamic results of peritoneal dialysis for severe cardiac failure. Am Heart J 1968; 76:227

Chopra MP, et al: Peritoneal dialysis for pulmonary edema after acute myocardial infarction. Br Med J 1970; 3:7

Jones JH: Peritoneal dialysis. Br Med J 1971; 27:165

Nolph KD: New directions in peritoneal dialysis concepts and applications. Kidney Int 1980; 18:S111

Vaamonde CA: Peritoneal dialysis: Current status. Postgrad Med 1977; 62:148

EDITORIAL COMMENT

A bicarbonate bath may be more advantageous than acetate bath in the septic patient who is prone to hypotension during peritoneal dialysis. When the two baths were compared there was less of a hypotensive effect with the bicarbonate than with the acetate. No difference in peripheral vascular resistance was demonstrated between the groups. This was explained by increased myocardial contractility during the peritoneal dialysis with bicarbonate. It was postulated that this is due either to better cardiac contractility associated with less metabolic acidosis or to a diminution in extracellular potassium concentration, more pronounced with the bicarbonate bath. The bicarbonate bath should be considered in patients with significant metabolic acidosis, particularly in those patients with sepsis and decreased cardiac output.

Peritoneal dialysis should also be considered in the severely hypothermic patient who does not respond to passive external rewarming techniques. Passive external rewarming has been very successful in reversing the metabolic changes associated with severe hypothermia without producing hypotension which can be associated with active external rewarming. Possible complications with internal rewarming (peritoneal dialysis) are an increased incidence of ventricular fibrillation and a more rapid decrease in plasma potassium. It may be reasonable to initiate potassium supplements to the exchange or by intravenous route and to consider prophylactic bretylium therapy. Femoral-femoral arterial venous bypass with blood warming is the internal rewarming method of choice if available.

ADDITIONAL REFERENCES

Huyghebaert M, Dhainaut J, Monsallier JF, et al: Bicarbonate hemodialysis of patients with acute renal failure and severe sepsis. Crit Care Med 1985; 13:840

O'Connor JP: Use of peritoneal dialysis in severely hypothermic patients. Ann Emerg Med 1985; 15:104

MAGNESIUM

RATIONALE 325-b

Hypomagnesemia is a common and frequently overlooked problem in critical care patients. It results from a decreased intake or excessive loss of magnesium. Hypomagnesemia may occur during long periods of relative starvation and poor dietary intake of magnesium.

Magnesium deficiency develops in a wide variety of clinical conditions, including alcoholism, diarrhea, hypercalcemia, and hypophosphatemia. It has also been associated with diuretic and aminoglycoside therapy. Clinical signs include seizures, mental status changes, weakness, and cardiac dysrhythmias.

Magnesium is an essential intracellular cation, second only to potassium in intracellular concentration. The magnesium content of the extracellular fluid accounts for less than 1% of the body stores; the remainder is present either intracellularly (50%) or in the skeleton (50%).

Magnesium is absorbed in the small intestine. This absorption is, however, loosely controlled and the major regulator is the kidney. Excessive magnesium losses may occur via the GI tract with malabsorptive states, prolonged nasogastric suction, diarrhea, or biliary fistulae. Fluid from the lower GI tract is much richer in magnesium than is the fluid from the upper GI tract and, therefore, lower GI fluid loss is more likely to produce hypomagnesemia than is gastric fluid loss. The biliary fistula and profuse diarrhea in this patient are probably the major sites of magnesium loss.

A variety of renal disorders can impair magnesium reabsorption and cause hypomagnesemia. However, with advanced renal disease, hypermagnesemia occurs from impaired renal magnesium excretion.

Aminoglycosides are toxic to proximal tubules. Proximal tubular dysfunction, i.e., Fanconi Syndrome, may be seen in early aminoglycoside toxicity. This includes phosphaturia, uricosuria, aminoaciduria and glucosuria. This presumably is the mechanism for magnesium loss as the proximal tubule absorbs 30% of filtered magnesium. The thick ascending limb is the primary regulator of magnesium reabsorption however.

REFERENCES

Chernow B, Smith J, Rainey TG, et al: Hypomagnesemia: Implications for the critical care specialist. Crit Care Med 1982; 10:193

Chernow B, Zaloga GP: SCCM - Ions for society members: Sulfate, chloride, calcium, and magnesium. In: Critical Care: State of the Art. Vol 5. Shoemaker WC, Thompson WL (Eds). Fullerton, CA, Society of Critical Care Medicine, 1984, pp V(K):28-33

Cronin RE, Knochel JP: Magnesium deficiency. Adv Intern Med 1983; 28:509

Quamme GA, Dirks JH: Magnesium transport in the kidney. Am J Physiol 1980; 239:F393-F401

Ryzen E, Wagers PW, Singer FR, et al: Magnesium deficiency in a medical ICU population. Crit Care Med 1985; 13:19

EDITORIAL COMMENT

In a recent study, twenty percent of patients in a medical ICU had significant hypomagnesemia. There is no data available that predicts which subset of patients will have or become hypomagnesemic. Hypomagnesemia was the most common electrolyte disturbance identified in this study.

ADDITIONAL REFERENCE

Reinhart RA, Desbiens NA: Hypomagnesemia in patients entering the ICU. Crit Care Med 1985; 13:506

OSMOLALITY

RATIONALE 326-d 327-a

Osmolality is the total number of particles in an aqueous solution expressed as mOsm/L H_2O. Serum osmolality can be calculated using the following equation:

$$\text{Serum Osmolality} = 2 \times [Na^+] + BUN/2.8 + glucose/18$$

If the measured serum osmolality exceeds the calculated value by more than 5-10 mOsm/L H_2O, then either unidentified osmoles are present or pseudohyponatremia exists. Unidentified osmoles may be in the form of mannitol, glycerol, ethanol, or others. Pseudohyponatremia implies that the measured serum sodium is a falsely low estimate of the true serum sodium concentration. This occurs when a significant volume of plasma is made up of a non-aqueous component such as triglycerides or protein as in hyperlipoproteinemia or multiple myeloma.

REFERENCES

Gennari FJ: Serum osmolality: Uses and limitations. N Engl J Med 1984; 310:102

Goldberg M: Hyponatremia. In: Symposium on Body Fluid and Electrolyte Disorders. Bech LH (Ed). Med Clin North Am 1981; 65:251

Maffly RH: The body fluids: Volume, composition and physical chemistry. In: The Kidney. Second Edition. Brenner BM, Rector FC Jr (Eds). Philadelphia, WB Saunders Co., 1981, p 76

Skorecki KL, Brenner BM: Body fluid homeostasis in men: A contemporary overview. Am J Med 1981; 70:77

EDITORIAL COMMENT

The fractional excretion of sodium (FENa) is elevated in acute renal parenchymal disease and is utilized to predict acute renal failure vs. prerenal azotemia. In the absence of diuretic use a high value suggests that renal failure has developed. However, if there are osmotic agents present, the FENa may be high in the presence of prerenal azotemia. A new equation using the last two digits of the specific gravity has been utilized to identify osmotic agents without the independent measurement of osmolality. The presence of unidentified osmoles implies that the high FENa is secondary to the osmotic agent present and not due to renal failure. If the unidentified osmole measurement is negative then one should feel confident that the high FENa is not due to unmeasured osmoles.

ADDITIONAL REFERENCE

Goldsmith DI, Martinez AB, Schwartz GJ: Identification of osmotically active solutes in urine. Crit Care Med 1985; 13:468

POTASSIUM

RATIONALE 328-d

Rhabdomyolysis causes hyperkalemia, not hypokalemia. Hyperaldosterone states and nasogastric suctioning are well known causes of potassium deficiency. Magnesium deficiency causes hypokalemia by impairing normal functioning of the sodium potassium ATPase pump.

REFERENCES

Chernow B, Smith JA, Rainey TG, et al: Hypomagnesemia: Implications for the critical care specialist. Crit Care Med 1982; 10:193

Levinsky NG: Fluids and electrolytes. In: Harrison's: Principles of Internal Medicine. Tenth Edition. Petersdorf RG, et al (Eds). New York, McGraw-Hill Book Company, 1983, pp 220-230

Oh M, Carroll HJ: Electrolyte disorders. In: The Pharmacologic Approach to the Critically Ill Patient. Chernow B (Ed). Baltimore, Williams & Wilkins Co., 1983, pp 715-728

EDITORIAL COMMENT

McGovern recently suggested that anesthesia not be postponed secondary to decreased serum potassium between 2.5 - 3.5 mEq/L. Although this may be reasonable in patients with no known cardiac disease and who are not taking digitalis it is ill advised for patients at risk for serious arrhythmias.

Severe depression of serum potassium level can be associated with coma and seizures.

ADDITIONAL REFERENCES

McGovern B: Hypokalemia and cardiac arrhythmias. Anesthesiology 1985; 63:127

Phelan DM, Worthley LIG: Hypokalemic coma. Intensive Care Med 1985; 11:257

RENAL FAILURE

RATIONALE 329-d

Acute renal failure is characterized by a decreased glomerular filtration rate with a 20- to 100-fold reduction in the rate of excretion of creatinine. Concomitant tubular dysfunction limits reabsorption of water, salt and other solutes so that the small amount of creatinine filtered into the tubule appears in the urine together with a relatively large volume of salt and water, resulting in low concentrations in urine of creatinine. Sodium reabsorption is impaired in the damaged kidney and increased concentrations of sodium appear in urine. Although these changes in urine solutes are common in oliguric acute renal failure, they are not as reliable in nonoliguric renal failure.

REFERENCES

Brater DC, Their SO: Renal disorders. In: Clinical Pharmacology, Basic Principles in Therapeutics. Second Edition. Melmon KL, Morrelli HF (Eds). New York, Macmillan Publishing Co. Inc., 1978, pp 349-387

Harrington JT, Cohen JJ: Measurement of urinary electrolytes: Indications and limitations. N Engl J Med 1975; 293:1241

Levinsky NG, Alexander EA: Acute renal failure. In: The Kidney. Brenner BM, Rector FC Jr (Eds). Philadelphia, WB Saunders Co., 1976, pp 806-837

RATIONALE 330-e

Sodium reabsorption occurs partly in the distal tubule under the influence of aldosterone, but aldosterone effects would not reduce urine sodium concentrations less than 5 mEq/L even in severe salt loss. Sodium reabsorption also occurs in the proximal tubule, and this is enhanced in severe liver disease possibly by the "third factor" effect. Enhanced proximal tubular sodium reabsorption interferes with the countercurrent mechanism of the loop of Henle and makes it difficult for the patient to excrete either water or salt appropriately. Patients with severe liver disease often produce urine with very low concentrations of sodium.

REFERENCES

Reynolds TB: The hepatorenal syndrome. In: The Liver and its Diseases. Schaffner F, Sherlock S, Leevy CM (Eds). New York, Intercontinental Medical Book Corp, 1974, pp 307-313

Schiff L (Ed): Liver kidney interrelationships. In: Diseases of the Liver. Fourth Edition. Philadelphia, JB Lippincott Co., 1975, pp 445-465

RATIONALE 331-c

Acute tubular necrosis is the name that has been applied to a syndrome of acute renal failure due to intrinsic renal dysfunction produced by a diverse group of clinical insults. Hemodynamically mediated and nephrotoxic acute renal failure are the most common causes of this syndrome. There is great variation in both the duration and the severity of circulatory insufficiency that produces acute renal failure. Nephrotoxic agents that commonly cause acute renal failure are aminoglycoside antibiotics, heavy metals, organic solvents and methoxyflurane. After the initial insult, multiple factors including persistent renal vasoconstriction, tubular obstruction, back leakage of filtrate, and decreased glomerular capillary permeability work synergistically to perpetuate acute renal failure even after the primary insult has been removed.

As a result of the renal parenchymal damage, the kidney stops performing most of its functions. The urine volume often decreases and typically varies between 50-400 ml daily. The urine that is produced will have decreased concentrations of the substances normally filtered by the glomerulus, such as urea and creatinine. The substances normally reabsorbed by the tubules, such as sodium, will be found in the urine in increased amounts. The kidney in acute tubular necrosis is unable to concentrate or dilute, so the urine that is produced will be isotonic. The response to diuretic agents (e.g., furosemide, dopamine) will be diminished. The morphology of the urinary sediment is usually quite characteristic in acute tubular necrosis containing dirty brown granular casts, renal tubular cells, and renal tubular cell casts.

Reversible prerenal azotemia is likely if urine osmolality is greater than 500 mOsm/kg, the urinary sodium is less than 20 mEq/L, urine-to-plasma urea nitrogen concentration ratio is greater than 8, and the urine-to-plasma creatinine ratio is greater than 40. Acute tubular necrosis is suggested by urine osmolality less than 350-mOsm/kg, osmolar clearance less than 80 ml/hr, free water clearance close to zero (10 ml/hr), a urine-to-plasma urea nitrogen ratio less than 3, and a urine-to-plasma creatinine ratio less than 20.

Nonoliguric acute renal failure also occurs in the same clinical settings as oliguric tubular necrosis, although it seems to be more frequent in patients with nephrotoxicity. Recent studies suggest that nonoliguric acute renal failure may account for 20%-30% of all cases of acute renal failure. The mean daily urine volume in a recent series of 54 patients with this syndrome was 1280 ml. Urinary diagnostic indices in nonoliguric acute renal failure are often intermediate between those seen in prerenal azotemia and acute tubular necrosis. The morbidity and mortality of nonoliguric acute renal failure, although significant, is less than that of oliguric acute renal failure.

The role of diuretic agents, prophylactically or therapeutically, in acute renal failure is controversial. At present, no well-controlled clinical trials have been reported to answer this question, but many clinicians feel that patients with oliguric renal failure may sometimes respond to a trial of mannitol or furosemide with increased urine output. Because the outcome in patients with nonoliguric renal failure is considerably better than in patients with oliguric renal failure, increasing urine flow might be a valid goal even if other aspects of renal function are not altered.

Patients with fixed oliguric acute tubular necrosis will almost certainly not respond to diuretics and may suffer hearing loss if potent diuretics are given repeatedly in large doses, especially if injected rapidly intravenously. The only justification for a trial of diuretics is an attempt to convert oliguric to nonoliguric acute renal failure early in the course of the renal failure; although urine output may be increased, it is not clear that this alone will alter the ultimate outcome.

REFERENCES

Anderson RJ, Linas SL, Berns AS, et al: Nonoliguric acute renal failure. N Engl J Med 1977; 296:1134

Baek SM, Makabali GG, Brown RS, et al: Free water clearance patterns as predictors and therapeutic guides in acute renal failure. Surgery 1975; 77:632

Harrington JT, Cohen JJ: Acute oliguria. N Engl J Med 1975; 292:89

Levinsky NG, Alexander EA: Acute renal failure. In: The Kidney. Brenner BM, Rector FC Jr (Eds). Philadelphia, WB Saunders Co., 1976, p 807

Lucas CE, Zito JG, Carter KM, et al: Questionable value of furosemide in preventing renal failure. Surgery 1977; 82:314

Miller TR, Anderson RJ, Linas SL, et al: Urinary diagnostic indices in acute renal failure. A prospective study. Ann Intern Med 1978; 89:47

Patak RV, Lifschitz MD, Stein JH: Acute renal failure: Clinical aspects and pathophysiology. Cardiovasc Med 1979; 4:19

RATIONALE 332-d

Ischemic insults to the kidneys are a major cause of acute renal failure (ARF). Nonoliguric renal failure occurs more frequently than was previously recognized (30%-50%) and carries a better prognosis than oliguric renal failure. The prompt correction of hypovolemia with restoration of cardiac output is the most important single therapy for the postischemic injury. Furosemide, mannitol, dopamine and nitroprusside may all increase renal blood flow and thereby ameliorate renal damage. Furosemide, mannitol and dopamine increase solute clearance which may also have a beneficial effect. Thiazide diuretics increase renal vascular resistance and decrease renal blood flow. Assuming adequate intravascular volume is present, attempts to convert oliguric to nonoliguric renal failure with furosemide or mannitol may improve prognosis.

The analysis of urine electrolytes and osmolality is helpful in diagnosing ARF. However, recent studies have emphasized the limitation of these parameters. Urinary sodium concentrations between 10-40 mEq/L, osmolalities as high as 500 mOsm/L, and FENa between 1%-6% are non-definitive studies. In addition, variable values may occur in patients who develop renal dysfunction without complete renal failure after an ischemic insult.

REFERENCES

Anderson RT, et al: Nonoliguric renal failure. N Engl J Med 1977; 296:1134

Espinel CH: The FENa test. JAMA 1976; 236:579

Fink M: Are diuretics useful in treatment for prevention of acute renal failure? South Med J 1982; 75:329

Miller RT, et al: Urinary diagnostic indices in acute renal failure. Ann Intern Med 1978; 89:47

Oken D: On the differential diagnosis of acute renal failure. Am J Med 1981; 71:916

RATIONALE 333-a

Postoperative renal failure remains one of the most devastating of surgical complications. Overall mortality is greater than 50% in most series despite advances in dialytic and nutritional support. This is due, in part, to the seriousness of associated illness. The cause of acute renal failure (ARF) in the surgical patient is rarely direct damage at surgery. Rather, a combination of decreased cortical perfusion with tubular and capillary damage from ischemia and/or toxins is thought to be the most likely etiology. Sepsis is the most common associated factor in those patients who die of ARF following surgery, with gastrointestinal hemorrhage running second as an associated cause of death. There have been reports indicating that in some patients the course of ARF postsurgery can be improved by the judicious use of hyperalimentation with solutions of essential L-amino acids, but this is largely a supportive measure and has not reversed the high mortality rates associated with the complication.

REFERENCE

Manual of Surgical Intensive Care by the Committee on Pre and Postoperative Care of the American College of Surgeons. Philadelphia, WB Saunders Co., 1977, pp 287-298

RATIONALE 334-a

Hepatorenal syndrome occurs with severe liver disease in patients who typically have ascites, jaundice, and hepatic encephalopathy. It is accompanied by a progressive drop in urine output to less than 400 cc/day and the development of azotemia. Mortality, however, is usually related to other causes. Despite vigorous support, hepatorenal syndrome is accompanied by rapid and irreversible deterioration of renal function. The urine sediment remains benign even in the presence of progressive renal deterioration. The urinary sodium concentration in hepatorenal syndrome is usually less than 10 mEq/L. The fractional excretion of sodium is less than 1 and the urinary osmolality is usually only slightly greater than the serum osmolality.

REFERENCES

Conn HO: A rational approach to the hepatorenal syndrome. Gastroenterology 1973; 65:321

Fang LST: Hepatorenal syndrome. In: Manual of Intensive Care Medicine. Rippe JM, Csete ME (Eds). Boston, Little Brown & Co., 1983, pp 235-236

Papper S: Renal failure in cirrhosis. In: The Kidney in Liver Disease. Epstein M (Ed). New York (North Holland), Elsevier, 1978

Wong PY, et al: The hepatorenal syndrome. Gastroentereology 1979; 77:1326

RATIONALE 335-b

The indications for initiating dialysis in children with acute renal failure (ARF) remain controversial. The decision to begin dialysis requires an understanding of potential risks and benefits of the procedure, as well as the natural history of ARF in various clinical settings.

Generally accepted indications for dialysis include: (1) severe or persistent hyperkalemia; (2) intractable hypertension, heart failure or pulmonary edema from volume overload; (3) severe and persistent acidosis; and (4) uremic complications such as encephalopathy or pericarditis. Dialysis is rarely initiated on the basis of an elevated BUN alone unless the BUN is extremely elevated (> 160 mg/dl) or is rapidly rising (> 40 mg/dl/day).

Dialysis is an important adjunct in the nutritional support of patients with ARF. Although studies conflict regarding the benefit of parenteral nutrition in patients with ARF, it is generally accepted as useful. An additional indication for dialysis in patients with ARF may be to control vascular volume "to make room for" nutritional volume requirements.

Dialysis does NOT improve renal function.

REFERENCES

Anderson RI, Schrier RW: Nonoliguric acute renal failure. N Engl J Med 1977; 296:1134

Hakim RM, Lazarus JM: Hemodialysis in acute renal failure. In: Acute Renal Failure. Brenner BM, Lazarus JM (Eds). Philadelphia, WB Saunders Co., 1983

Leonard CD, Luke RG, Siegel RR: Parenteral essential amino acids in acute renal failure. Urology 1975; 6:154

Mauer SM, Lynch RE: Hemodialysis techniques for infants and children. Pediatr Clin North Am 1976; 23:843

Siegal NJ: Acute renal failure. In: Contemporary Issues in Nephrology: Pediatric Nephrology. Vol 12. Tune BM, Stanley AM, Brenner BM, et al (Eds). New York, Churchill Livingstone, 1984, pp 297-320

RATIONALE 336-d

A primary function of the kidney is volume preservation. The normal kidney efficiently reabsorbs > 99% of filtered Na in a volume depleted patient. Damaged renal tubules, however, are unable to conserve Na. The FENa is the percentage of Na filtered at the glomerulus that is eventually excreted. It is calculated by dividing the Na excreted by the Na filtered.

$FENa = (U_{Na} \times V) / (P_{Na} \times GFR)$

or

$FENa = (U_{Na} \times V) / (P_{Na} \times U_{Cr}/P_{Cr} \times V)$

Rearranging and cancelling volume

$FENa = (U/P)Na / (U/P)Cr \times 100$

Where:
V = Volume
U = Urine
P = Plasma
Cr = Creatinine
GFR = Glomerular Filtration Rate

This test is usually reliable in differentiating prerenal from renal azotemia. A FENa > 3% is usually predictive of renal damage although > 6% adds additional reliability. A value < 1% is usually predictive of prerenal or early postrenal (obstructive) azotemia.

Recent literature suggests that the FENa is not as sensitive or as specific a test as was previously thought. It is particularly unreliable or invalid in certain settings. Recent use of diuretics renders the test noninterpretable. Acute renal failure caused by radiographic contrast media or myoglobin, for unexplained reasons, have been associated with a low rather than a high FENa. Patients with acute renal failure following cardiac surgery may have a low FENa without oliguria. These patients are more likely to have a diminished arterial pressure, decreased renal plasma flow and higher filtration fractions than other patients with postoperative renal failure or prerenal azotemia.

REFERENCES

Bastl CP, Rudnik MD, Narins RG: Diagnostic approaches to acute renal failure. In: Contemporary Issues in Nephrology. Vol 6. New York, Churchill Livingstone Inc., 1980

Espinel CH: The FeNa test: Use in the differential diagnosis of acute renal failure. JAMA 1976; 236:579

Handa SP, Morrin PAF: Diagnostic indices in acute renal failure. Can Med Assoc J 1967; 96:78

Hibberman M, et al: Acute renal failure following cardiac surgery. J Thorac Cardiovasc Surg 1979; 77:880

Miller TJ, Schrier RW: Urinary diagnostic indices in acute renal failure: A prospective study. Ann Intern Med 1978; 89:47

Shrier RW, Conger JD: Acute renal failure: Pathogenesis, diagnosis, and management. In: Renal and Electrolyte Disorders. Second Editon. Schrier RW (Ed). Boston, Little, Brown & Co., 1980

Zarick S, et al: Fractional excretion of sodium. Arch Intern Med 1985; 145:108

RHABDOMYOLYSIS

RATIONALE 337-c

Rhabdomyolysis may be associated with multiple disorders including hypoxia, primary muscle injury (trauma), infectious diseases affecting muscle, and muscle injury by toxins.

Myoglobin is a red pigment found in skeletal muscle and myocardium. The function of myoglobin is to bind oxygen and facilitate its delivery to the site of oxidative metabolism in the muscle cell. When muscle is injured, myoglobin is released into the bloodstream. Myoglobin, unlike hemoglobin, does not cause pink discoloration of the serum. Because of relatively little protein binding and a low molecular weight (myoglobin 17,000; hemoglobin 68,000), myoglobin is easily filtered and rapidly excreted into the urine. Both hemoglobin and myoglobin are grossly visible in the urine when their respective concentration reaches 100/mg/dl. The orthotoluidine reaction (hemoccult) does not differentiate between hemoglobin and myoglobin. A well known and dreaded complication of rhabdomyolysis is acute renal failure. Hyperkalemia and hyperphosphatemia are common and are caused by release of these substances by injured muscle cells. Hypocalcemia may occur because of deposition of calcium salts in injured skeletal muscle and because of the decreased PTH activity and decreased vitamin D production associated with hyperphosphatemia. Disseminated intravascular coagulation is common in severe rhabdomyolysis.

REFERENCES

Knachel JP: Rhabdomyolysis and myoglobinuria. Annu Rev Med 1982; 33:435

Lach F, Felsenfeld AJ: Pathophysiology of altered calcium metabolism in rhabdomyolysis induced renal failure. N Engl J Med 1981; 305:117

SODIUM

RATIONALE 338-c

Hyponatremia below levels of 120 mEq/L may cause coma and seizures. The differential diagnosis is frequently divided into three major subgroups based on an evaluation of the patient's extracellular fluid content. Those with increased ECF and edema have heart failure, liver cirrhosis or nephrotic syndrome. Those without edema who appear euvolemic have either H_2O intoxication, nonoliguric renal failure, inappropriate ADH or factitious disease caused by hyperlipidemia or hypoproteinemia. Those who appear volume contracted have diuretic-induced disease, adrenal insufficiency, or salt wasting nephropathy.

This patient is volume contracted (dry mucous membrane, pulse 100, BP 105/60, BUN 25, Hct 45) and hyponatremic. Hyponatremia, hypochloremia and hypokalemia are consistent with diuretic-induced disease. These serum electrolyte levels may occur with conventional dosages of thiazide diuretics. If the patient has been replacing free water without salt, he may not be volume contracted. Urinary sodiums may be high or low. Serum potassium levels are uniformly low in contradistinction to the elevated levels expected in adrenal insufficiency.

REFERENCES

Fichman MP: Diuretic-induced hyponatremia. Ann Intern Med 1971; 75:853

Narins RG, et al: Diagnostic strategies in disorders of fluid electrolyte, and acid base disorders. Am J Med 1982; 72:498

EDITORIAL COMMENT

Pseudohyponatremia is a potential cause of measured hyponatremia. It can be caused by elevated concentrations of nonsodium containing elements of serum such as lipids or proteins. In this situation, when a dilutional method is used to measure sodium, the dilution occurs only in that area of plasma that is occupied by the sodium and not in that area that is occupied by the lipid or protein. Calculations assume that the fluid added prior to measurement has diluted the entire serum but in actuality has only diluted that portion which was occupied by sodium. This produces a falsely low calculated sodium. Measurement by direct potentiometry involves no sample dilution and, therefore, sodium measurements are uneffected by hyperlipidemia or hyperproteinemia. However, if measured by flame photometry or indirect potentiometry, the measurements will be falsely low.

ADDITIONAL REFERENCE

Mbbs TC, Kiechle FL: Pseudohyponatremia. Am J Emerg Med 1985; 3:236

Section 18

339. During cardiac arrest, each of the following drugs may be given via the intratracheal route (i.e., down the endotracheal tube) EXCEPT:

a. Epinephrine
b. Sodium bicarbonate
c. Atropine
d. Lidocaine

340. Which ONE of the following statements concerning the physiology of cardiopulmonary resuscitation (CPR) is FALSE?

a. An increase in carotid blood flow during CPR is NOT synonomous with increase in cerebral blood flow.
b. An increase in right atrial diastolic pressure as a single variable has a deleterious effect on myocardial blood flow.
c. Epinephrine's potent beta-adrenergic effect makes it an essential agent for most successful resuscitations.
d. Some studies have demonstrated the heart acts as a passive conduit during closed chest CPR.

341. In performing cardiopulmonary resuscitation in the infant, the greatest cardiac output can be achieved by which ONE of the following techniques?

a. Use two fingers to compress the upper half of the sternum.
b. Use two fingers to compress the lower half of the sternum.
c. Use the usual adult position of hands, but press gently.
d. Wrap both hands about the chest with thumbs compressing the sternum.
e. Use the heel of just one hand with a rocking motion up and down the sternum.

342. During cardiopulmonary resuscitation in a child, what energy level should be used in the first attempt at closed-chest defibrillation?

a. 2 watt-sec/kg body weight
b. 5 watt-sec/kg boby weight
c. 20 watt-sec/kg body weight
d. 50 watt-sec/kg body weight
e. 400 watt-sec/kg body weight

343. Which of the following is the most acceptable initial electrical dose for defibrillation of a 44-pound, 5-year-old child in ventricular fibrillation?

a. 200 watt/sec
b. 40 watt/sec
c. 250 joules
d. 5 joules
e. 150 watt/sec

344. A 17-month-old, 22-pound female is found cyanotic, apneic and pulseless after being submerged in fresh water for 10 minutes. A cardiac monitor shows ventricular fibrillation. In addition to ventilation and external cardiac compression, which of the following is appropriate initially?

a. Intravenous calcium chloride 10 cc of a 10% solution
b. Intravenous epinephrine 1.0 cc of a 1:1,000 solution
c. Synchronized cardioversion
d. Intravenous $NaHCO_3$ 10 mEq

RESUSCITATION

ANSWERS

339-b 340-c 341-d 342-a 343-b 344-d

RATIONALE 339-b

Epinephrine, atropine and xylocaine have each been successfully given via the endotracheal (ET) tube. Sodium bicarbonate causes alkali bronchial injury and should not be given via the ET tube.

REFERENCE

Silverberg RA, Weil MH: Cardiopulmonary pharmacology. In: The Pharmacologic Approach to the Critically Ill Patient. Chernow B (Ed). Baltimore, Williams & Wilkins Co., 1983, pp 140-159

RATIONALE 340-c

An increase in carotid blood flow does not necessarily mean improved cerebral blood flow since carotid blood flow is distributed between the extracerebral and cerebral vessels. In addition, cerebral blood flow during CPR correlates more directly with the difference between carotid artery pressure and intracranial pressure. Interventions that increase carotid blood flow do not uniformly improve cerebral blood flow, as these techniques may also increase intracranial pressure. Volume loading, for example, increases carotid blood flow but may decrease cerebral blood flow.

Coronary perfusion pressure during resuscitation equals the difference between aortic diastolic pressure and right atrial diastolic pressure. Some CPR techniques increase aortic diastolic pressure but also increase right atrial diastolic pressure and, therefore, do not improve myocardial blood flow. Volume loading increases cardiac output but may decrease myocardial blood flow. Continuous abdominal binding does not increase myocardial perfusion pressure although it increases arterial pressure and flow.

The major beneficial effect of epinephrine during CPR is its alpha or vasoconstrictive properties and not its beta-adrenergic effects. Dogs given the beta-adrenergic agonist isoproterenol alone could not be resuscitated. In contrast, animals treated with an alpha-adrenergic stimulating agent were resuscitated. Epinephrine or the alpha-adrenergic stimulating drugs result in an increase in the aortic diastolic pressure during external chest compression whereas isoproterenol does not. Defibrillation and resuscitation are successful in animal studies when epinephrine is given alone or in combination with a beta-adrenergic blocker, yet are unsuccessful when epinephrine is given in combination with an alpha-adrenergic blocking drug.

Although the heart may actually be squeezed in some arrest situations by CPR maneuvers, recent data suggest that closed-chest compression produces a generalized rise in intrathoracic pressure that is applied to the pulmonary vascular bed as well as the heart. Thus, the heart may act as a conduit for blood, rather than a pump during external cardiac massage.

REFERENCES

Ditchey RV, Lindenfeld J: Potential adverse effects of volume loading on perfusion of vital organs during closed-chest resuscitation. Circulation 1984; 69:181

Ewy GA: Current status of cardiopulmonary resuscitation. Modern Concepts of Cardiovascular Disease 1984; 53:43

Luce JM, Cary JM, Ross BK, et al: New developments in cardiopulmonary resuscitation. JAMA 1980; 244:1366

Michael JR, Guerci AD, Koehler RC, et al: Mechanisms by which epinephrine augments cerebral and myocardial perfusion during cardiopulmonary resuscitation in dogs. Circulation 1984; 69:822

Ralston SH, Voorhees WD, Babbs CF: Intrapulmonary epinephrine during prolonged cardiopulmonary resuscitation: Improved regional blood flow and resuscitation in dogs. Ann Emerg Med 1984; 13:79

Redding JS, Pearson JW: Evaluation of drugs for cardiac resuscitation. Anesthesiology 1963; 24:203

Yakaitis RW, Otto CW, Blitt CD: Relative importance of alpha- and beta-adrenergic receptors during resuscitation. Crit Care Med 1979; 7:293

EDITORIAL COMMENT

When epinephrine administered through an endotracheal tube during CPR is compared to intravenous injection, larger quantities are required to produce the same blood level and effect with endotracheal administration. However, if larger dosages of epinephrine are given endotracheally to compensate for this deficiency and a successful resuscitation results, there is a large overshoot in blood level secondary to increased absorption through the bronchial pulmonary tree after re-establishment of pulmonary circulation. Therefore, it is impractical to suggest that larger quantities of endotracheal epinephrine be given to compensate for decreased initial absorption.

Epinephrine, atropine, lidocaine, naloxone, bretylium, and diazepam have all shown potential utility for endotracheal administration. Any substance whose particle size is 0.1 - 6.0 µm or less can be rapidly absorbed into the pulmonary capillary network. Although there may be physicochemical advantages to administering drugs desolved in water, normal saline solution appears to be the diluent of choice as saline exerts a less detrimental effect on arterial oxygen tension. This is probably because water is more likely to disrupt surfactant protection.

Although drug absorption may occur at all levels of the respiratory tract from the trachea to the alveoli, the most efficient drug absorption takes place at the alveolar level. It is imperative, therefore, to maximize absorption that drugs be delivered as far distally as possible. Devices are currently available which will widely disperse medication in a spray form into the lower respiratory tract.

Not more than 5-10 cc of fluid should be administered. Volumes greater than this regardless of the diluent may have an adverse effect on surfactant and result in atelectasis and pulmonary damage. Following instillation, 5-10 rapid ventilations with a breathing bag are recommended to force the fluid distally.

When the central venous route of drug administration is compared to the peripheral venous route in the CPR setting, peak drug levels are attained more rapidly with the former. The disadvantage lies in the time delay necessary for placement of a central venous line as well as the logistic difficulty in placement while the patient undergoes closed chest compression. If a central venous line is already in place it is the best choice for drug administration.

Significant levels of lidocaine can be obtained by endotracheal lidocaine administration.

Dose response curves have been developed. It has been shown that although depth of installation of drugs administered by the endotracheal route may not be a major factor in determining levels, forced manual hyperventilation after administration assures optimal distal delivery of the endotracheally administered medication.

The predominant mechanism of blood flow during closed chest CPR remains unknown. Several published works suggest that forward flow during closed chest CPR is predominantly dependent upon changes in intrathoracic pressure and is not directly related to compression of the heart itself. Other investigators demonstrated mitral valve closure during compression systole and valve opening during compression diastole. This indicates a nonpassive component to blood flow during CPR.

The fact remains that closed chest CPR generates only a small percentage of the needed myocardial and cerebral blood flow.

ADDITIONAL REFERENCES

Bass E: Cardiopulmonary arrest - Pathophysiology and neurologic complications. Ann Intern Med 1985; 203(6 pt 1):920

Bircher N, Safar P: Cerebral preservation during cardiopulmonary resuscitation. Crit Care Med 1985; 13:185

Deshmukh HG, Weil MH, Rackow EC, et al: Echocardiographic observations during cardiopulmonary resuscitation: A preliminary report. Crit Care Med 1985; 13:904

Greenberg MI, Spivey WH: Comparison of deep and shallow endotracheal administration of dionosil in dogs and effect of manual hyperventilation. Ann Emerg Med 1985; 14:209

Hedges JR, Barsan WB, Doan LA, et al: Central versus peripheral intravenous routes in cardiopulmonary resuscitation. Am J Emerg Med 1984; 2:385

McDonald JL: Serum lidocaine levels during cardiopulmonary resuscitation after intravenous and endotracheal administration. Crit Care Med 1985; 13:914

Ralston SH, Tacker WA, Showen L, et al: Endotracheal versus intravenous epinephrine during electromechanical dissociation with CPR in dogs. Ann Emerg Med 1985; 14:1044

RATIONALE 341-d

The heart of the infant resides relatively higher in the chest than that of the adult. Thus, compression should be applied in the midsternal area. Good cardiac output can be achieved by positioning the fingertips of both hands in the spinal/paraspinal area and compressing the sternum with the thumbs of both hands. This method has been demonstrated to be superior to one- or two-finger compression on the sternum. Care must be taken, however, not to restrict chest expansion with the hands. Only the fingertips and thumbs should be in contact with the chest. This limits the usefulness of this technique to the infant.

Other factors to be remembered in the resuscitation of the child include: the airway is more flexible and hyperextension of the neck may lead to collapse of airway; it arises higher in the neck than in the adult and intubation is, thus, somewhat different; the airway is narrower and produces a greater resistance to flow in the nonintubated patient; ventilatory and cardiac compression rates are higher; the tidal volume is smaller in the child (7 ml/kg body weight); depth of compression is less than in an adult (a depth of one-fourth to one-third of the thickness of the child is sufficient); etiology of the cardiac arrest in children is almost never due to coronary artery disease; similarly, the frequency of dysrhythmias is less than in an adult resuscitation and when they occur they are frequently self-limited. Finally, the outcome of pediatric resuscitation is better than that of adults. In one study, in-hospital noncritical care unit children who arrested were resuscitated 78% of the time with 47% subsequently leaving the ICU in satisfactory condition.

REFERENCES

Ehrlich R, Emmett SM, Rodriquez-Torres R: Pediatric cardiac resuscitation team: A 6-year study. J Pediatr 1974; 84:152

Greenburg MI: The use of endotracheal medication in cardiac emergencies. Resuscitation 1984; 12:155

Thaler MM, Stobie GH: An improved technic of external cardiac compression in infants and young children. N Engl J Med 1963; 269:606

Todres ID, Rogers MD: Methods of external cardiac massage in the newborn infant. J Pediatr 1974; 86:781

RATIONALE 342-a

Data by Tacker et al. suggest that the optimal defibrillation dose for children is 2 watt-seconds (joules)/kg body weight. This dose should be reduced in children suspected of being digitalis toxic. Dosage should be increased if lower amounts fail.

Although the ideal electrode position is anterio-posterior on the chest, this is usually impractical in resuscitation situations. An acceptable alternative is to position the electrodes on the right parasternal area (2nd rib) and left midclavicular to axillary region at the xiphoid level.

REFERENCES

Chameides L, Brown GE, Rage JR, et al: Guidlines for defibrillation in infants and children. Report of the American Heart Association Target Activity Group: Cardiopulmonary resuscitation in the young. Circulation 1977; 56(Suppl):502A

Gutgesel NP, Tacker WA, et al: Energy dose for ventricular defibrillation of children. Presented at Society for Pediatric Research, 1974

Tacker WA Jr, Galioto FM, Giulliani I, et al: Energy dosage for human trans-chest electrical ventricular defibrillation. N Engl J Med 1974; 290:214

EDITORIAL COMMENT

Caputo and associates demonstrated the sequence of events in a pediatric canine model of anoxic cardiopulmonary arrest. Hypertension occurred first followed by hypotension and finally asystole. Asystole occurred follwoing 4-5 minutes of total oxygen deprivation. Asystole occurring during a pediatric arrest may be associated with neurologic recovery if the anoxic insult is less than 15 minutes duration.

Forward flow during CPR in the infant may be more dependent on cardiac compression (vs. changes in intrathoracic pressure) when compared to the adult.

A prospective evaluation of pediatric cardiopulmonary resuscitation revealed four hospital discharges out of 26 arrests. Asystole was the rhythm present at time of initial treatment in 24 of the 26 patients.

ADDITIONAL REFERENCES

Caputo G, Delgado-Pareses C, Swedlow D, et al: Anoxic cardiopulmonary arrest in a pediatric animal model: Clinical and laboratory correlates of duration. Ped Emerg Care 1985; 1:57

Rosenberg NR: Pediatric cardiopulmonary arrest in the emergency department. Am J Emerg Med 1984; 2:497

RATIONALE 343-b

The electrical dose that will defibrillate most children without causing myocardial damage has not been firmly established. The available data suggest an initial dose of 2 watt/sec (joules) per kg. The energy dose should be doubled if the initial defibrillation attempt proves unsuccessful.

REFERENCE

Chameides L, Brown GE, Rage JR, et al: Guidlines for defibrillation in infants and children. Report of the American Heart Association Target Activity Group: Cardiopulmonary resuscitation in the young. Circulation 1977; 56(Suppl):502A

RATIONALE 344-d

Intravenous epinephrine is indicated in the treatment of ventricular fibrillation. The dose is 0.1 ml/kg of a 1:10,000 solution (.01 mg/kg). In a 10 kg child the initial dose would therefore be 0.1 mg. The dose of epinephrine given in choice a is ten times that amount and is therefore incorrect. When indicated, 25 mg/kg of calcium chloride is given intravenously. In a 10 kg child 10 cc of 10% $CaCl_2$ is equivalent to 100 mg/kg. Most modern defibrillators are available with the capacity for synchronized cardioversion. When the synchronizer circuit is activated, a QRS complex must be detected before countershock will be delivered. Countershock of ventricular fibrillation cannot be accomplished if the synchronizer circuit is activated.

The recommended dose of $NaHCO_3$ in cardiac arrest is 1 mEq/kg. In a 10 kg child this is equivalent to 10 mEq.

REFERENCES

Killip T: Synchronized DC precordial shock for arrhythmias. Safe new technique to establish normal rhythm may be utilized on an elective or emergency basis. JAMA 1963; 186:1

Standards and guidelines for cardiopulmonary resuscitation (CPR) and emergency cardiac care (ECC). JAMA 1980; 244(Suppl):453

EDITORIAL COMMENT

Studies continue to show the benefits of epinephrine in combination with defibrillation to convert ischemic ventricular fibrillation in the adult. Outcome is improved not by a greater success of countershock during resuscitation from ventricular fibrillation, but rather by an increase in the incidence of successful return of spontaneous circulation after defibrillation is successful.

The success of very low defibrillation currents in open chest defibrillation has been demonstrated with 31% of one joule shocks and 58% of 2.5 joule shocks successfully defibrillating 150 adult cardiac surgical patients evaluated prospectively.

A retrospective evaluation of high energy vs. low energy defibrillation supported the use of 360-400 joules energy as the choice for initial defibrillatory current in the adult. AHA ACLS recommendations remain 200 joules for initial countershock. As a high percentage of patients who were initially defibrillated reverted again to ventricular fibrillation, increased attention should be directed to use of antidysrhythmic drugs and correction of metabolic abnormalities in an attempt to improve survival in successfully defibrillated patients.

Early defibrillation is associated with improved neurologic recovery and survival. Incorporation of defibrillation as part of basic life-support could significantly reduce mortality and morbidity from cardiac arrest.

Evidence now exists that calcium chloride is ineffective in the resuscitation of refractory asystole in the prehospital cardiac arrest setting. There remains controversy over the effectiveness of calcium chloride in refractory electromechanical association. There may be a subset of patients who would benefit from calcium utilization in this circumstance although successful resuscitation and hospital discharge is extremely dismal in this group of patients.

Noninvasive external pacing is a viable alternative to other forms of temporary pacing and may be used as a temporizing measure while a transvenous pacer is inserted. Its primary utilization is in patients who acutely develop high degree heart block not reversed by atropine or isoproterenol. It has proven ineffective in patients presenting in asystole after prolonged CPR.

ADDITIONAL REFERENCES

Falk RH, Zoll PM, Zoll RH: Safety and efficacy of noninvasive cardiac pacing. N Engl J Med 1983; 19:1166

Lake CL, Duncan S, Nolan SP, et al: Low-energy defibrillation: Safe and effective. Am J Emerg Med 1985; 3:104

Morgan JP, Hearne SF, Raizes GS, et al: High-energy vs. low-energy defibrillation: Experience in patients (excluding those in the intensive care units) at Mayo Clinic-affiliated hospitals. Mayo Clin Proc 1984; 59:829

Otto CW, Yakaitis RW, Ewy GA: Effect of epinephrine on defibrillation in ischemic ventricular fibrillation. Am J Emerg Med 1985; 3:285

Stueven HA, Thompson B, Aprahamian C, et al: Lack of effectiveness of calcium chloride in refractory asystole. Ann Emerg Med 1985; 14:630

Stueven HA, Thompson B, Aprahamian C, et al: The effectiveness of calcium chloride in refractory electromechanical dissociation. Ann Emerg Med 1985; 14:626

Weaver WD, Copass MK, Bufi D, et al: Improved neurologic recovery and survival after early defibrillation. Circulation 1984; 69:943

Zoll PM, Zoll RH, Falk RH, et al: Enteral noninvasive temporary cardiac pacing: Clinical trials. Circulation 1985; 71:937

Section 19

345. A 62-year-old man underwent a left pneumonectomy and had an uneventful first postoperative week. On the eighth day after surgery, he began to have massive hemoptysis.

Which ONE of the options listed below represents the most appropriate immediate step in the management of this patient?

a. Obtaining a high quality chest radiograph in the radiology department
b. Placement of a chest tube in the operating room under sterile conditions
c. Placement of the patient in the left lateral decubitus position
d. Tracheal intubation
e. Bronchoscopy

346. A 37-year-old male who underwent an uncomplicated appendectomy 24 hours previously has the rapid onset of mid-abdominal pain, vomiting and abdominal distension. The abdominal exam reveals signs of peritoneal irritation. A plain film of the abdomen and subsequently a barium enema are obtained. A radiograph taken during the barium enema is shown in Figure 22.

Which ONE of the following is the most likely diagnosis?

a. Perforated viscus
b. Adynamic ileus
c. Cecal volvulus
d. Retained appendiceal stump
e. Sigmoid volvulus

347. A 63-year-old patient who underwent curative sigmoid colectomy three years ago for adenocarcinoma of the colon had an elective resection of an abdominal aortic aneurysm. On the first postoperative day, the patient passed a maroon colored diarrheal stool which was hemoccult positive.

Which ONE of the following statements is MOST appropriate regarding this patient?

a. Careful observation for further signs of bleeding
b. Flexible sigmoidoscopy should be performed
c. An emergency aortogram should be performed
d. A barium enema should be performed

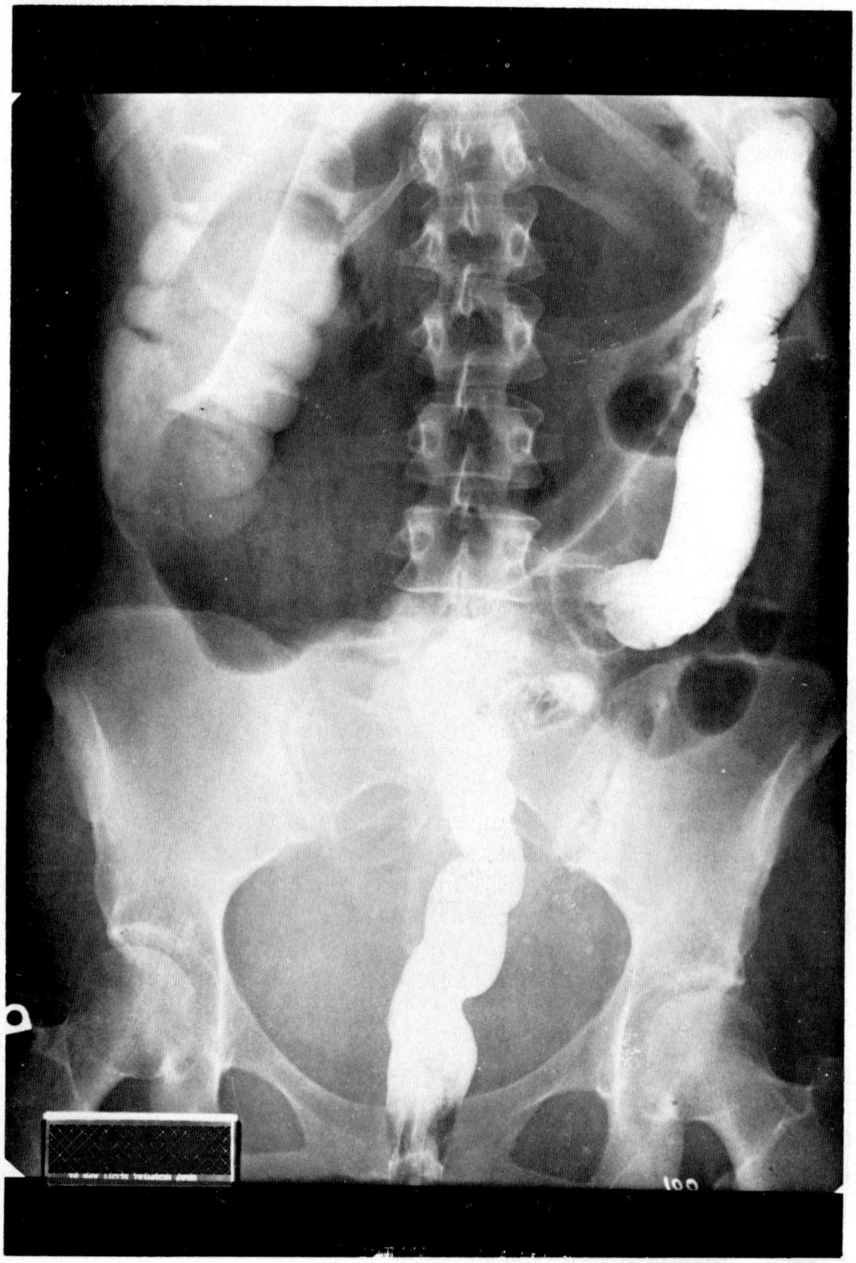

Figure 22

348. A 46-year-old male with a history of chronic pancreatitis had a median sternotomy and coronary artery bypass graft three days ago. He now develops chest pain and the new onset of serous drainage from his sternotomy incision. A previous chest radiograph obtained 24 hours earlier is unremarkable except for expected postoperative changes. A new radiograph is obtained and shown in Figure 23.

Which ONE of the following is the MOST likely diagnosis?

a. Mediastinal pancreatic pseudocyst
b. Clostridia perfringens wound infection
c. Pneumomediastinum
d. Sternal dehiscence
e. Pneumopericardium

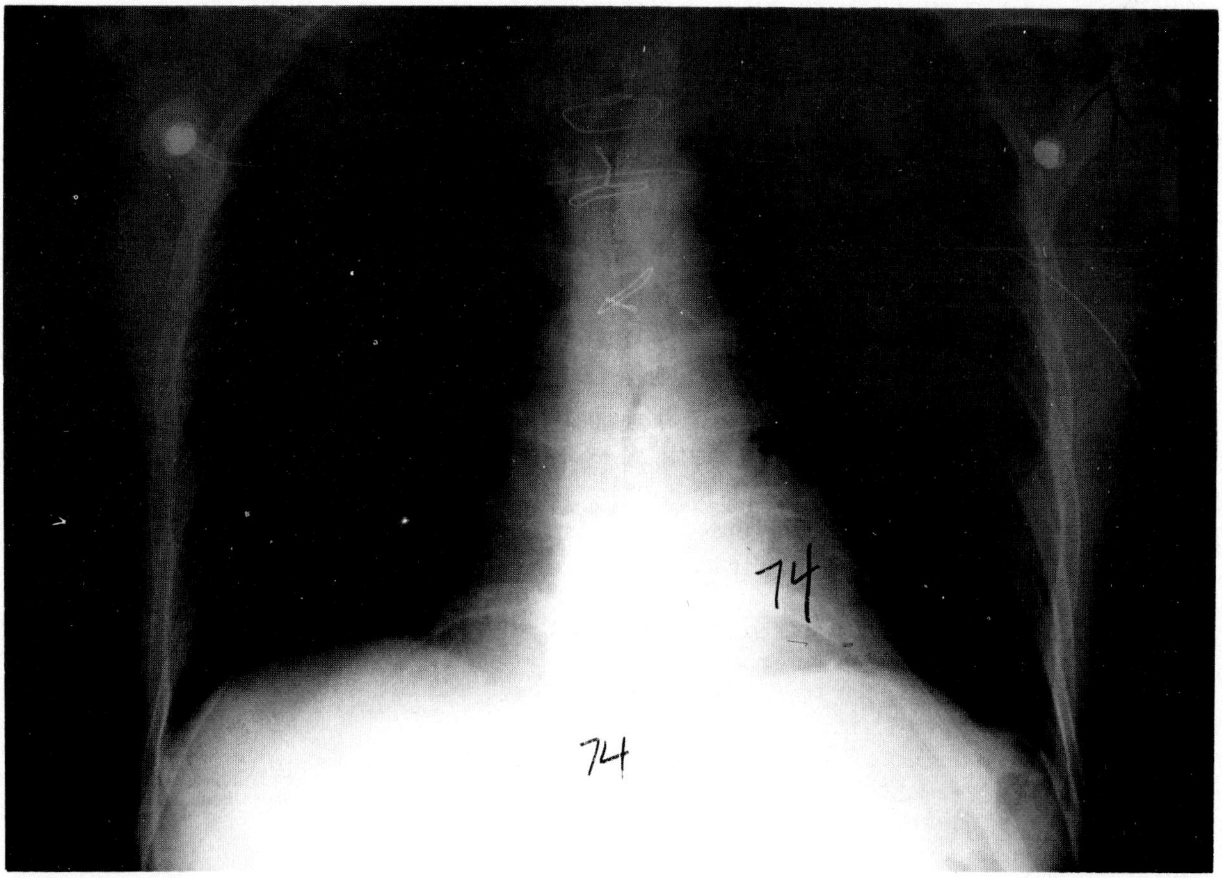

Figure 23

349. Postoperative fever (rectal temperature above 39°C):

a. Is safely dismissed as a result of atelectasis if it occurs within the first 24 hours of surgery
b. Is seen with similar frequencies following lower abdominal or lower extremity operations done under spinal vs. general anesthesia
c. If seen within the first 24 hours of surgery is not caused by a wound infection
d. Is a cause of increased metabolic demands by the patient

Questions 350-351 refer to the following case history: A 63-year-old male, 50 pack-year smoker is 18 hours post thoracotomy for repair of a thoracic aortic aneurysm. He has been extubated for 3 hours. The physician on call is notified that the patient has developed fever and a cough.

Physical Exam: T - 101°F, P - 100, BP - 120/80, R - 22

Lungs	- bilateral crackles
CV	- regular rate, no murmurs or gallops
Abdomen	- normal exam
Extremities	- no cyanosis, edema, or tenderness

Preop. ABG (Room Air):	pH 7.4	$PaCO_2$ 40 mm Hg	PaO_2 80 mm Hg
12 hrs. Postoperative ABG: (2 L/min nasal cannula)	pH 7.4	$PaCO_2$ 35 mm Hg	PaO_2 60 mm Hg

350. Which ONE of the following represents the MOST likely diagnosis?

a. Postoperative atelectasis
b. Pulmonary embolism
c. Aspiration pneumonia
d. Dressler's syndrome
e. Urinary tract infection

351. Which ONE of the following would NOT be an expected change in pulmonary function after thoracotomy?

a. Decreased vital capacity
b. Decreased functional residual capacity
c. $\dot{V}/\dot{Q}$ mismatching
d. Increased expiratory reserve volume

352. A 57-year-old male had an esophageal resection six days ago. Jejunostomy feeding began on the second postoperative day. A large unilateral pleural effusion is noted. Contrast studies reveal the suture line to be intact. The patient is afebrile and in no significant distress. A thoracentesis reveals thick, milky fluid.

Which ONE of the following statements about this case is FALSE?

a. An iatrogenic injury most likely occurred in the right hemithorax.
b. The cholesterol/triglyceride ratio is usually less than 1.
c. Selection of an enteral feeding formula relative to this patient's diagnosis may be beneficial.
d. A silver-methenamine stain of pleural fluid is usually diagnostic in this condition.

353. Which of the following statements regarding deep venous thrombosis (DVT) associated with elective abdominal surgery is true?

a. When utilized for prophylaxis against postoperative DVT, subcutaneous heparin (5000 units SQ, Q 12°) is best started after the operative procedure has been completed.
b. Venous doppler and impedance plethysmographic studies of the lower extremities are both noninvasive means of assessing the patency of deep veins of the lower extremity but are insensitive in the detection of DVT of thigh veins when compared to venography.
c. DVT of the calf veins frequently leads to clinically significant pulmonary embolism.
d. None of the above

354. A 38-week, 2000 gm infant was delivered without difficulty after having a normal pre-natal course. The infant did well until the first feeding, when she began coughing, choking, and became cyanotic. A diagnosis of tracheoesophageal fistula was made by passing a soft rubber catheter down the esophagus to the blind esophageal pouch. The diagnosis was confirmed radiographically. The infant was then taken to the operating room where fistula repair was accomplished without difficulty. In the ICU, she did well until the second postoperative day, when she became hypotensive and had a subsequent cardiac arrest from which she was not successfully resuscitated.

Which of the following is the MOST pertinent in this case?

a. No correlation exists between the type of tracheoesophageal fistula (TEF) and the incidence of other associated anomalies.
b. Cardiovascular anomalies are frequently associated with TEF.
c. The association of TEF with multiple congenital anomalies is extremely rare.
d. If cardiovascular anomalies are present, atrial septal defect and pulmonary stenosis are the cardiovascular anomalies most commonly associated with TEF.

355. A 2500 gm male infant is noted to have a scaphoid abdomen, and absence of breath sounds in the left chest at birth. Chest radiography confirms the diagnosis of congenital diaphragmatic hernia (CDH). He is taken to the operating room where a successful repair is performed. He is then transferred to the ICU.

Which ONE of the following statements about CDH and the management of this infant is CORRECT?

a. Pulmonary hypoplasia usually occurs contralateral to the side of the hernia.
b. Vigorous attempts should be made to expand the left lung immediately after a left-sided hernia repair since it is usually severely atelectatic.
c. The mortality rate for congenital diaphragmatic hernia has significantly decreased in the past two decades.
d. Increased right to left intracardiac shunting due to pulmonary artery vasoconstriction, especially in the hypoplastic lung, but also in the opposite lung, usually appears in the postoperative period.

356. Shortly after birth, a newborn child develops bilious vomiting. The infant's abdominal radiograph is shown in Figure 24.

Which ONE of the following statements is MOST correct regarding this case?

a. The esophagus is abnormal in most newborns with this disorder.
b. Web formation is the most likely etiology of this infant's problem.
c. The abdominal radiograph supports congenital duodenal obstruction.
d. Immediate surgery is imperative.

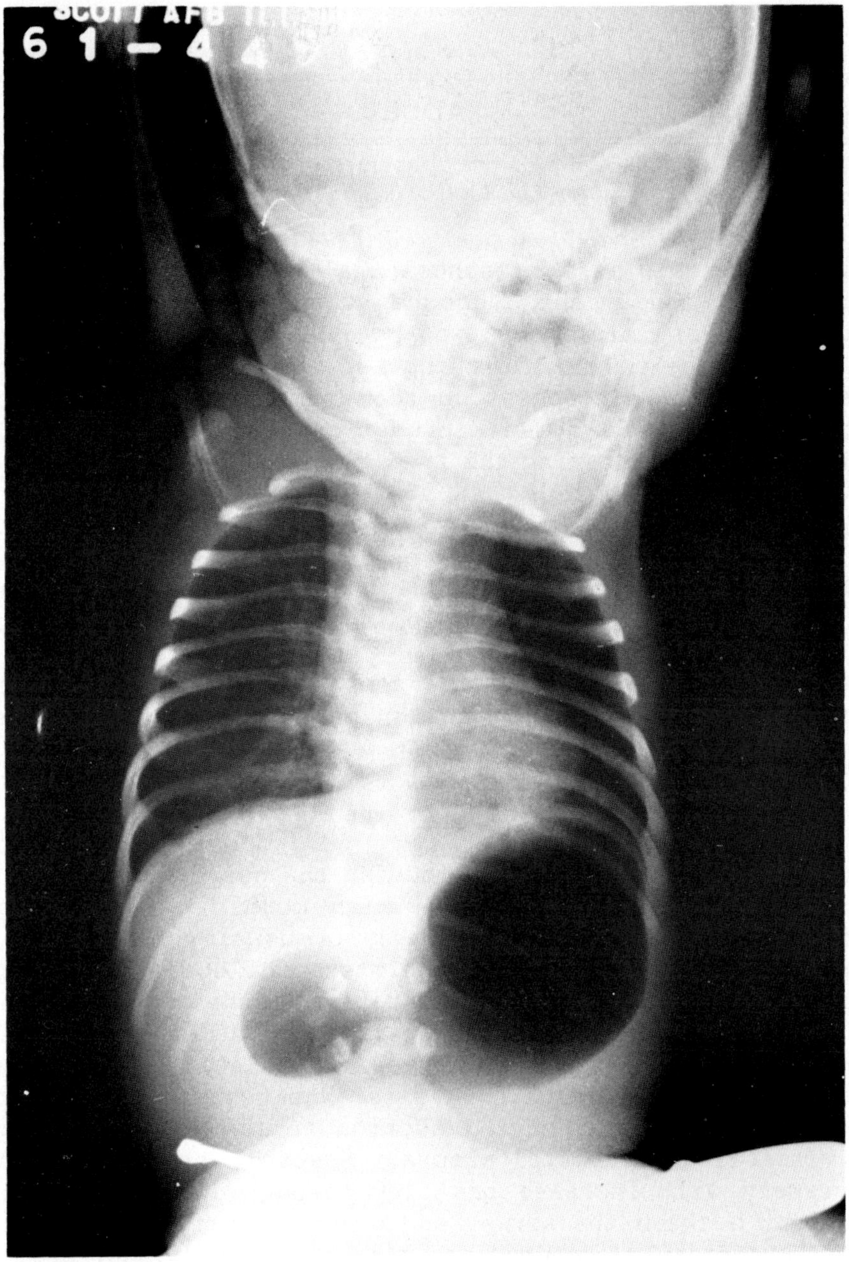

Figure 24

ANSWERS

345-c	346-c	347-b	348-d	349-d	350-a	351-d	352-d
353-d	354-b	355-d	356-c				

ADULT

RATIONALE 345-c

The most likely diagnosis is a bronchopleural fistula. The immediate risk is aspiration of fluid into right lung and subsequent asphyxiation. Therefore, the immediate treatment is placement of patient in the left lateral decubitus position (operated side down). Delaying this initial therapy to obtain a high quality chest radiograph or operating room time increases the patient's risk of aspiration and death. Tracheal intubation does not prevent fluid from the operated hemithorax from entering the tracheobronchial tree.

REFERENCES

DeMeester TR, LaFontaine E: The pleura. In: Gibbon's Surgery of the Chest. Sabiston DC, Spencer FC (Eds). Philadelphia, WB Saunders Co., 1983, pp 388-389

Pairolero PC, Payne WS: Postoperative complications in the thoracic surgical patient. In: Thoracic and Cardiovascular Surgery. Glenn WWL (Ed). Norwalk, Appleton-Century-Crofts, 1983, p 349

EDITORIAL COMMENT

Bronchopleural (BP) fistula occurring during the postoperative period following pulmonary resection is associated with high morbidity and mortality. After pneumonectomy the magnitude of the leak is usually large with significant associated respiratory insufficiency and risk of flooding and contamination of the contralateral lung. The most imperative issue is the establishment of adequate dependant drainage. Bronchopleural fistulas associated with penetrating or blunt chest trauma or mechanical ventilation-induced barotrauma are usually smaller and may not require surgical intervention. The latter fistulas may sometimes be closed by applying suction to a thoracotomy tube to promote adhesion of visceral and parietal pleura. However, one cannot predict if the suction conversely will increase gas flow through a fistula by increasing the pressure gradient between the airway and pleural space. In the case of post-pneumonectomy BP fistula, operative closure usually is preferable. High frequency jet ventilation may also facilitate closure of BP fistula. Endobronchial intubation may be beneficial emergently to isolate the intact bronchus in acute post-pneumonectomy BP fistula.

ADDITIONAL REFERENCES

Baldwin JC, Mark JBD: Treatment of bronchopleural fistula after pneumonectomy. J Thorac Cardiovasc Surg 1985; 90:813

Powner DJ, Cline CD, Rodman GH: Effect of chest tube suction on gas flow through a bronchopleural fistula. Crit Care Med 1985; 13:99

Sjostrand UH, Smith RB, Hoff BH, et al: Conventional and high-frequency ventilation in dogs with bronchopleural fistula. Crit Care Med 1985; 13:191

RATIONALE 346-c

Figure 22 demonstrates a cecal volvulus. A massively dilated cecum and dilated loops of small bowel are present. The column of barium stops at the site of obstruction.

Cecal volvulus may occur at any age but is most common in patients from 25-35 years of age. This disorder is characterized by nausea, vomiting, severe mid-abdominal colicky pain and moderate abdominal distension. Hyperresonance may be noted in the right lower quadrant. Severe abdominal pain with rebound tenderness indicate that strangulation may be present.

A plain abdominal radiograph is often diagnostic but on occasion may be difficult to interpret. Lack of lateral fixation allows the mobile cecum to be seen anywhere in the abdomen. A large mid-abdominal, gas-filled ovoid segment with distended small bowel loops and a relatively empty large bowel is characteristic of this disorder.

A barium enema may help localize the obstruction, but is infrequently necessary. Prompt surgical relief of the obstruction is the treatment of choice. Nonoperative measures are generally unsuccessful and the risk of strangulation in the closed-loop obstruction is high.

An adynamic ileus presents radiographically with multiple distended loops of small bowel and air fluid levels. The large mid-abdominal gas collection shown in Figure 22 is highly atypical of an adynamic ileus.

REFERENCES

O'Mara CS, Wilson TH Jr: Cecal volvulus: Analysis of 50 patients with long-term follow-up. Ann Surg 1979; 189:724

Schwartz SI, Shires GT, Spencer FC, et al: Colon, rectum and anus. In: Principles of Surgery. Fourth Edition. New York, McGraw-Hill Book Company, 1984, pp 1211-1214

Todd GJ, Forde KA: Volvulus on the cecum: Choice of operation. Am J Surg 1979; 138:632

RATIONALE 347-b

All patients undergoing abdominal aortic surgery with ligation of the inferior mesenteric artery (IMA) are at risk for colonic ischemia. Risk is higher for patients who have had prior colonic surgery. This diagnosis needs to be excluded if heme-positive stool develops postoperatively. The most appropriately diagnostic maneuver is examination of rectal mucosa by sigmoidoscopy. If only mucosal ischemia is present, careful observation is necessary. If, however, any signs of transmural necrosis are present or develop, re-exploration and resection of ischemic bowel is necessary before perforation occurs.

REFERENCES

Beebe HG (Ed): Complications in Vascular Surgery. Philadelphia, JB Lippincott Co., 1973, pp 60-63

Gomes MN, Schelinger D: Abdominal aortic aneurysms: A clinicopathological study. Ann Thorac Surg 1979; 27:479

Leonard JC, Hasleton PS: Dissecting aortic aneurysms: Diagnostic review and new technique. J Med 1979; 48:55

RATIONALE 348-d

Figure 23 demonstrates a radiolucent midsternal stripe not present on the previous chest radiograph. Development of this radiographic abnormality in association with chest pain and serous wound drainage is virtually diagnostic of sternal dehiscence. A midsternal stripe may be seen after median sternotomy without dehiscence, but the development of such a stripe several days postoperatively is highly suggestive of that diagnosis. Sternal dehiscence can, however, be seen in the absence of this radiographic finding.

Sternal dehiscence may be associated with pain, fever, or both. The presence of serous fluid drainage from the wound is compatible with the separation of the deepest wound layer. The most reliable sign of sternal dehiscence is palpable sternal separation with cough.

REFERENCES

Adams GW, Raven CE: Midline lucency following median sternotomy. Chest 1983; 83:793

Escovitz ES, Okulski TA, Lapayowker MS: The midsternal stripe: A sign of dehiscence following median sternotomy. Radiology 1976; 121:521

Stoney WS, Alford WC Jr, Burrus GR, et al: Median sternotomy dehiscence. Ann Thorac Surg 1978; 26:421

RATIONALE 349-d

Fever in the postoperative period is perhaps the most common of all postop complications. While a moderate temperature elevation occurring within the first 48 hours following general anesthesia is most likely due to atelectasis, fever cannot be safely dismissed. Both clostridial and streptococcal wound infections have been noted to occur within 24 hours of surgery, occasionally within a few hours of the procedure. General anesthesia and intubation alter the normal pulmonary physiology and predispose to atelectasis, which is not as common following spinal anesthesia. Metabolic demands are increased by fever at a rate of about 10% increase in metabolic requirement for each 1°C of elevation of body temperature.

REFERENCES

Goldman DR, Brown FH, Levy WK, et al: Medical Care of the Surgical Patient. Philadelphia, JB Lippincott Co., 1982, pp 482-506

Sabiston DC Jr (Ed): Textbook of Surgery. Philadelphia, WB Saunders Co., 1981, pp 180-184

RATIONALE 350-a 351-d

A "pulmonary complication" of surgery is defined as a postoperative temperature elevation with new physical findings on chest examination or the new appearance of radiographic findings with productive cough, purulent sputum, dyspnea or persistent fever. Postoperative complications are not restricted to patients with pre-existing lung disease but also occur in normal patients. Lung volume, pattern of breathing, gas exchange, and defense mechanisms are each affected, particularly in patients who have had thoracic or upper abdominal surgery, and in patients with pre-existing cardiopulmonary disease. Decreased functional residual capacity, vital capacity, tidal volume, expiratory reserve volume and weakened respiratory musculature contribute to alveolar collapse, ventilation-perfusion mismatching and hypoxemia. The decrease in functional residual capacity is caused by a breathing pattern of shallow tidal breaths without periodic maximal inflation, i.e., sighs.

Early ambulation, minimizing sedation, and incentive spirometry are efficacious in minimizing the risk of postoperative pulmonary complications.

REFERENCES

Bartlett RH: Pulmonary pathophysiology in surgical patients. Surg Clin North Am 1980; 60:1323

Iverson L, Ecker RR, Fox HE, et al: A comparative study of IPPB, the incentive spirometer, and blow bottles: The prevention of atelectasis following cardiac surgery. Ann Thorac Surg 1978; 25:197

Luce JM: Preoperative evaluation and perioperative management of patients with pulmonary disease. Postgrad Med 1980; 67:301

Tisi GM: Preoperative evaluation of pulmonary function. Am Rev Respir Dis 1979; 119:293

Van De Water JM: Preoperative and postoperative techniques in the prevention of pulmonary complications. Surg Clin North Am 1980; 60:1339

RATIONALE 352-d

Chylothorax is an important although infrequent cause of pleural effusion. The diagnosis is often complicated by superimposition of both a thoracic duct leak and other etiologies of pleural effusion, such as heart failure. Unless chylothorax is recognized and appropriate treatment rendered, severe nutritional depletion can result from continuous chyle leakage. Nonoperative management is usually successful. A very low fat diet causes a marked reduction of fistula flow and is conducive to spontaneous fistula closure. Use of a fat-poor enteral diet and placement of a chest tube for complete drainage of the effusion and re-expansion of the lung usually assists in reducing the chylous drainage significantly. Commercially available enteral formulas with a fat content no greater than 1 gram per liter, or a low fat diet supplemented with medium-chain triglycerides is beneficial in these patients. Chylous effusion is most commonly left-sided, but may be bilateral. Injury to the thoracic duct has been reported during operations involving the heart, aorta, esophagus, and left subclavian vessels. At the level of the fifth to seventh thoracic vertebra, the thoracic duct crosses from the right to the left side of the mediastinum and ascends extrapleurally along the left side of the esophagus. It crosses behind the aortic arch and the left subclavian artery. This anatomic relationship explains thoracic duct injury in trauma or operation in these areas. Thoracic duct damage below the level of the fifth or sixth thoracic vertebra results in a right-sided chylothorax. If the injury is above this level, the effusion is usually left-sided. In patients not receiving enteral feeding and in whom gastric suction is employed, delay in diagnosis is more likely. Likewise, the probability of chylothorax is increased if the infusion increases concomitantly with enteral feeding resumption, especially when the feeding is rich in fat. Analysis of the fluid reveals a high triglyceride and cholesterol/triglyceride ratio is usually less than 1. The fluid is lymphocyte predominant and the Sudan III stain, not Silver-Methenamine stain, may be positive in staining for fat globules.

REFERENCES

Cevese PG, Vecchioni R, D'Amico DF, et al: Postoperative chylothorax. J Thorac Cardiovasc Surg 1975; 69:966

Hughes RL, Mintzer RA, Hidvegi DF, et al: The management of chylothorax. Chest 1979; 76:212

Lam KH, Lim STK, Wong J, Ong GB: Chylothorax following resection of the esophagus. Br J Surg 1979; 66:105

Ramzy AI, Rodriguez A, Cowley RA: Pitfalls in the management of traumatic chylothorax. J Trauma 1982; 22:513

Teba L, Dedhia HV, Bowen R, et al: Chylothorax review. Crit Care Med 1985; 13:49

EDITORIAL COMMENT

Pleural effusions greater than one centimeter measured on a lateral decubitus chest radiograph when associated with a known or suspected bacterial pneumonia require thoracentesis to rule out an infected pleural space. If the pleural effusion is less than one centimeter then it can be followed and tapped if it reaches one centimeter or greater.

Chyliform pleural effusions are lipid pleural effusions that are not chylous. Instead of triglycerides, chyliform pleural effusions contain cholesterol as the major lipid component. These probably represent breakdown products of blood cells. Most of these are seen in patients with longstanding pleural thickening resulting from a previous therapeutic pneumothorax. The effusions are usually sterile and tend to recur. Patients with chronic symptoms associated with a recurrent chyliform pleural effusion may benefit from decortication.

ADDITIONAL REFERENCES

Hillerdal G: Chyliform (cholesterol) pleural effusion. Chest 1985; 88:426

Light RW: Parapneumonic effusions and empyema. Clin Chest Med 1985; 6:55

Mulders AV, Lacquet LM, Meighem WV, et al: Chylothorax complicating pneumonectomy. Thorax 1984; 39:954

RATIONALE 353-d

Subcutaneous heparin is an effective prophylactic agent in the management of deep venous thrombosis (DVT) occurring after elective thoracoabdominal surgery. Fifty percent of patients that develop DVT postoperatively have done so by the time the surgical procedure is completed. Therefore, it has been suggested that it is best to begin prophylactic heparin two hours before the surgery. The heparin should be continued postoperatively until the patient is fully ambulatory. Venous doppler and impedance plethysmographic studies have both been shown to be sensitive tests for the detection of DVT above the knee. An isolated thrombosis of soleal or tibial veins has been associated with perfusion defects on lung scans but these are usually clinically silent.

REFERENCES

Browse NL, et al: Fibrinogen-detectable thrombosis in the legs and pulmonary embolism. Br Med J 1974; 1:602

Clagert GP, Salzman EW: Prevention of venous thrombosis in surgical patients. N Engl J Med 1974; 290:93

Kakkar VV: The ^{125}I-labelled fibrinogen test and phlebography in the diagnosis of deep vein thrombosis. Milbank Mem Fund Q 1972; 50:206

Kakker VV, et al: Low doses of heparin in prevention of deep vein thrombosis. Lancet 1971; 2:669

Strandners DE, Thiele BL (Eds): Selected Topics in Venous Disorders. New York, Futura Publishing Co., 1981, pp 79-157

PEDIATRIC

RATIONALE 354-b

Tracheoesophageal fistula most commonly presents with proximal esophageal atresia and a tracheoesophageal fistula in the distal segment of the esophagus. This is the Kluth Type III presentation and comprises approximately 85% of all TEF. The incidence of associated cardiovascular anomalies is 14%-28%. Ventricular septal defect and patent ductus arteriosus are the most common defect. Multiple anomalies in other organ systems are found in 30%-55% of patients with esophageal atresia. Survivability seems to be closely correlated with birth weight. Infants with birth weights above 2.5 kg do much better than infants below this weight.

In the case cited above, post-mortem examination showed the presence of a preductal tight coarctation of the aorta. As the infant stabilized, her duct began to close, leaving her with essentially no flow to the aorta beyond the arch. The case stresses the importance of preoperative cardiovascular assessment and postoperative ICU monitoring of what is now a surgically correctable lesion in 70%-80% of cases.

REFERENCES

Calverley RK, Johnston AE: The anaesthetic management of tracheoesophageal fistula: A review of ten years' experience. Can Anaesth Soc J 1972; 19:270

German JC, Mahour GH, Woolley MM: Esophageal atresia and associated anomalies. J Pediatr Surg 1976; 11:299

Greenwood RD, Rosenthal A: Cardiovascular malformations associated with tracheoesophageal fistula and esophageal atresia. Pediatrics 1976; 57:87

Kluth D: Atlas of esophageal atresia. J Pediatr Surg 1976; 11:901

Koop CE, Schnaufer L, Broennle AM: Esophageal atresia and tracheoesophageal fistula: Supportive measures that affect survival. Pediatrics 1974; 54:558

EDITORIAL COMMENT

Patients with esophageal atresia and tracheoesophageal fistula who have severe respiratory distress and who require positive-pressure ventilation preoperatively represent a high risk group. Sudden loss of intragastric pressure may result in acute loss of effective ventilation pressure in those patients with high pulmonary resistance. This may occur during placement of a gastrostomy tube.

Resuscitation is not possible in certain patients until leakage from the esophagus is controlled by ligation of the fistula or transabdominal occlusion of the distal esophagus. Early thoracotomy and fistula ligation in these patients with respiratory distress syndrome is recommended.

Congenital diaphragmatic hernia presenting within the first 6 hours of life is associated with a 50% or greater mortality rate. Pulmonary vascular abnormalities coexist with pulmonary hypoplasia, a fact that has led to trials with pulmonary vasodilators. Although initial reports documented an improvement in ductal shunting with tolazoline, larger series still show a mortality rate of 45% or greater in patients who receive vasodilator therapy.

M-mode echocardiography has been used to measure ventricular ejection periods for correlation with the degree of pulmonary hypertension. This offers a method of following pulmonary vascular resistance. Evidence of decreasing resistance can then be used as an indication to attempt aggressive weaning.

ADDITIONAL REFERENCES

Hansen J, James S, Burrington J, et al: The decreasing incidence of pneumothorax and improving survival of infants with congenital diaphragmatic hernia. J Ped Surg 1984; 19:385

Reynolds M, Luck SR, Lappen R: The "critical" neonate with diaphragmatic hernia: A 21-year perspective. J Pediatr Surg 1984; 19:364

Templeton JM, Templeton JJ, Schnaufer L, et al: Management of esophageal atresia and tracheoesophageal fistula in the neonate with severe respiratory distress syndrome. J Pediatr Surg 1985; 20:394

RATIONALE 355-d

Congenital diaphragmatic hernia (CDH) with associated pulmonary hypoplasia occurs in approximately 1:2,000 live births and occurs most commonly on the left in a posterolateral defect (Foramen of Bochdalek). Pulmonary hypoplasia usually, but not always, occurs on the same side as the hernia. Surgical repair is usually accomplished within 24 hours of birth. The lung on the affected side is not merely atelectatic but truly hypoplastic, and vigorous attempts to expand that lung after surgical repair of the hernia often result in a tension pneumothorax in the opposite hemithorax. Indeed, this is the most common postsurgical cause of death in these infants. Increased right to left intracardiac shunting occurs secondary to pulmonary arterial vasoconstriction not only in the hypoplastic lung, but also many times in the "normal" lung.

This produces shunting through the foramen ovale and ductus arteriosus, often leading the patient into a vicious cycle of persistent fetal circulation. Extracorporeal membrane oxygenation (ECMO) and several pharmacologic agents such as tolazoline, morphine sulfate, prostaglandins, chlorpromazine and bradykinin have all been used with some, but not consistent, success. Despite significant advances in surgical, anesthetic, and intensive care techniques in the past 20 years, mortality from this congenital lesion is still 30%-50% overall and 50%-70% in those requiring surgical repair in the first 24 hours of life.

REFERENCES

Bloss RS, Aranda JV, Beardmore HE: Congenital diaphragmatic hernia: Pathophysiology and pharmacologic support. Surgery 1981; 89:518

Bray RJ: Congenital diaphragmatic hernia. Anesthesia 1979; 34:567

Wiener ES: Congenital posterolateral diaphragmatic hernia: New dimensions in management. Surgery 1982; 92:670

RATIONALE 356-c

Figure 24 demonstrates the "double bubble" sign of congenital duodenal obstruction. The "double bubble" represents air in the stomach and distended duodenum. This radiograph is compatible with complete obstruction because bowel gas is absent distal to the duodenum. Although a duodenal web may present in this manner, by far the most common etiology is duodenal atresia.

Vomiting usually begins within 24 hours of birth. The vomitus is bile-stained except in those rare individuals in whom the obstruction is proximal to the ampulla of Vater.

In most cases, immediate surgery is neither necessary nor desirable. One-third of infants with duodenal atresia have Trisomy-21. A thorough search for other anomalies and chromosomal karyotyping are warranted. The duodenum can be adequately decompressed with a nasogastric tube during this evaluation. Surgery should not be deferred, however, in cases of duodenal obstruction secondary to malrotation.

REFERENCES

Altman RP, Randolph JG, Anderson KD: Pediatric surgery. In: Principles of Surgery. Fourth Edition. Schwartz SI, Shires GT, Spencer FC, et al (Eds). New York, McGraw-Hill Book Company, 1984; pp 1649-1652

Leape LL, Holder TM: Pediatric surgery. In: Textbook of Surgery: The Biological Basis of Modern Surgical Practice. Twelfth Edition. Philadelphia, WB Saunders Co., 1981, pp 1372-1373

Shandling B: Congential and perinatal anomalies of the gastrointestinal tract and intestinal obstruction. In: Textbook of Pediatrics. Twelfth Edition. Behrman RE, Vaughn VC (Eds). Philadelphia, WB Saunders Co., 1983, pp 907-908

Section 20

Questions 357-358 refer to the same patient:

357. A 25-year-old man is involved in a motorcycle accident. Upon reaching the emergency room at 10 p.m., he is mildly confused but otherwise stable. Initial evaluation by the emergency room physician reveals no evidence of serious visceral injury other than the closed head injury. He is transferred to the ICU for observation.

Which of the following is LEAST likely to suggest the possibility of a traumatic thoracic aortic dissection?

a. History of a violent sudden deceleration injury
b. Findings of upper extremity hypertension or asymmetrical brachial artery blood pressures
c. Presence of a severe petechial reaction over the head and neck along with facial edema, chemosis, and subconjunctival hemorrhage
d. Findings of a paraplegia on physical exam
e. Evidence of a widening mediastinum or loss of aortic knob prominence on a chest radiograph

358. You see the patient at midnight. He has developed substernal and upper mid-back discomfort and a harsh precordial systolic murmur. Review of the chest radiograph is highly suggestive of the presence of a traumatic dissection of the thoracic aorta. All of the following are indicated EXCEPT:

a. Type and crossmatch for 8 units of blood.
b. Schedule aortography for the following morning.
c. Obtain an EKG if none was done in the emergency room.
d. Promptly notify the appropriate surgical service of the possible aortic injury.
e. Assess the patient for the possibility of concomitant injuries.

359. Which ONE of the following factors would have the MOST influence on survival of a patient with third-degree burns covering one-half of the body?

a. Sex
b. Race
c. Age
d. Trunk vs. extremity burn
e. Anterior vs. posterior location

Questions 360-365: Match each of the following questions or statements with the most appropriate of the lettered responses that follow. Each letter may be selected once, more than once, or not at all.

360. No penetration of eschar

361. Inhibition of carbonic anhydrase

362. Bone marrow suppression with neutropenia

363. Resistance of many Enterobacter cloacae species

364. Painful for 20-30 minutes after application to second degree burns

365. Which topical antimicrobial agent best penetrates the entire thickness of the burn eschar?

 a. Silver nitrate
 b. Silver sulfadiazine (Silvadene)
 c. Mafenide acetate (Sulfamylon)

Questions 366-368: Use the following information to answer the questions:

A previously healthy 40-year-old woman was involved in an auto accident at 4 p.m. She was the driver of the car and hit an embankment at 35 mph. Initial evaluation in the emergency room revealed an alert patient with a blood pressure of 120/80 and a pulse rate of 88. Examination of the chest is normal. Jugular venous distention is absent. A displaced fracture of the left humerus with distal ischemia is noted. There is tenderness over the left side of the abdomen in the area of an abrasion. A peritoneal lavage is performed, the results showed 10,000 RBC/mm^3. Admission labs include a hemoglobin/hematocrit of 12/39 respectively, clear urine, a normal chest radiograph and a normal EKG. Following satisfactory reduction of the left arm fracture, the patient is admitted to the ICU for overnight observation. In the early morning hours, her blood pressure drifts down to 70/40 with an increase in pulse rate to 130. The patient is mildly confused, but in no apparent distress. The fracture site is stable. Her physical examination is unchanged. The resident covering the ICU supports her pressure with a dopamine drip. The patient becomes lucid and her pressure is raised to 100/60. You see the patient on rounds at 9 a.m.

366. The most likely cause for the patient's clinical condition when you see her is:

 a. Myocardial contusion
 b. Loss of blood into fracture site
 c. Pulmonary contusion
 d. Ruptured spleen
 e. Cerebral contusion

367. All of the diagnostic and therapeutic measures outlined in the case were appropriate EXCEPT:

a. Dopamine infusion
b. Fracture reduction
c. Peritoneal lavage
d. Chest radiography
e. EKG

368. Which ONE of the following alternatives is most appropriate in the management of this patient?

a. Serial EKG and MB-CPK monitoring
b. Serial CBC checks
c. Blood gas analysis and serial chest films
d. Preparation for exploratory laparotomy
e. Echocardiography

369. A 25-year-old male is involved in a motor vehicle accident resulting in bilateral femoral and right tibial-fibial fractures. The fractures are treated with closed reduction and external traction. No other significant injury was evident during a thorough initial evaluation. Approximately 48 hours after the accident, he develops tachypnea and dyspnea. His arterial blood gases on room air are PaO_2 68 mm Hg, $PaCO_2$ 28 mm Hg, pH 7.52. Mental status changes are noted to have developed.

Which ONE of the following statements is most likely TRUE concerning this patient?

a. A ventilation/perfusion scan is usually diagnostic.
b. Thrombocytosis is an expected finding.
c. This clinical syndrome will usually resolve with supportive therapy only.
d. This syndrome is most often seen with rib fractures.

370. A 35-year-old previously healthy man is admitted to your service with multiple trauma secondary to an automobile accident. He is stabilized and breathing spontaneously. He develops increasing dyspnea and is noted to cough bloody sputum. Chest roentgenography shows no change in the fractured 1st and 2nd ribs on the right, but there is extensive mediastinal emphysema and a large pneumothorax.

Which ONE of the following conditions is the MOST likely to be present?

a. Lung contusion
b. Bronchial adenoma
c. Aspiration pneumonia
d. Bronchial rupture
e. Emphysematous bleb

371. A 36-year-old male suffered blunt abdominal and chest trauma in an automobile accident. An upright portable chest radiograph was obtained prior to ICU admission and is shown in Figure 25.

Which ONE of the following statements regarding this case is MOST correct?

a. A thoracostomy tube should be placed.
b. This injury is most common on the right.
c. A thoracentesis should be performed.
d. An operation will be required following stabilization.
e. Injury to visceral organs is unlikely in this patient.

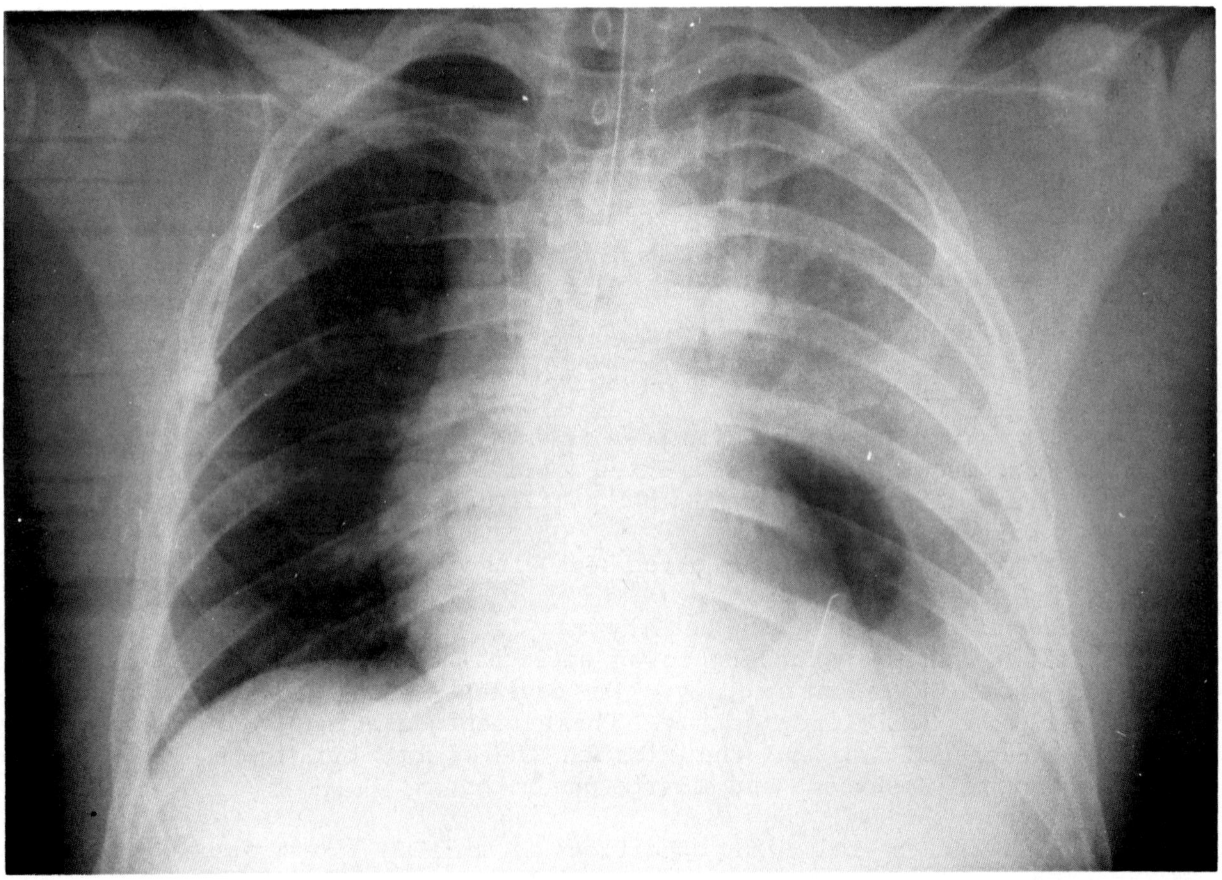

Figure 25

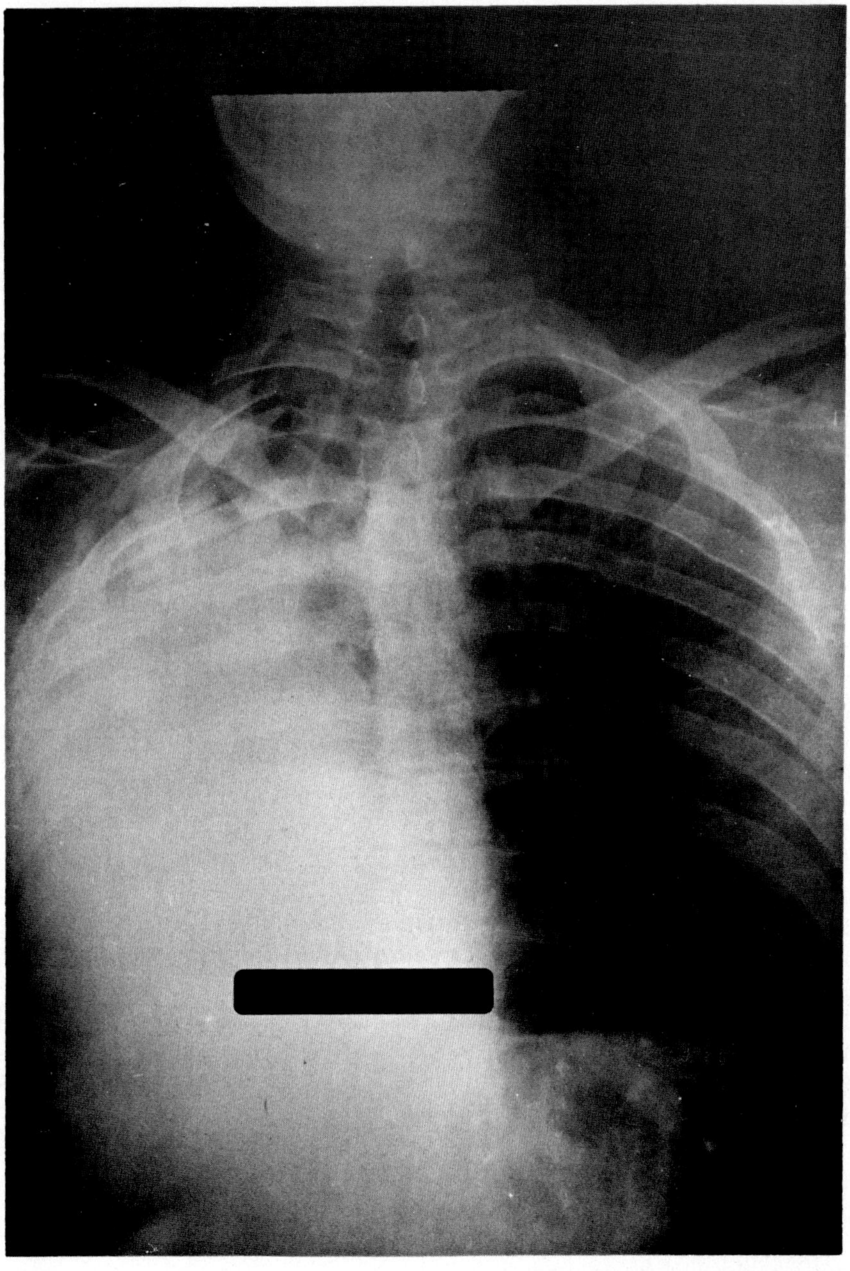

Figure 26

372. A 32-year-old male suffered massive chest trauma in a motor vehicle accident. Physical examination demonstrated subcutaneous emphysema over the right hemithorax. Based on the history above and the chest radiograph shown in Figure 26, which ONE of the following is the MOST likely diagnosis?

a. Fractured right bronchus
b. Ruptured right diaphragm
c. Massive right hemothorax
d. Right tension pneumothorax

373. The head injured patient commonly:

a. Hypoventilates
b. Is hypoxemic
c. Develops hypotension
d. Develops diabetes insipidus
e. None of the above

374. The prospect for recovery is improved in the head injured patient in all of the following EXCEPT:

a. Hypotension is quickly reversed.
b. The patient is under 20 years of age.
c. An intracranial hematoma is rapidly removed.
d. A mass lesion (as opposed to a diffuse lesion) is present.

375. Which ONE of the following statements is FALSE with reference to patients who sustain severe closed head injury?

a. Maintenance of airway and avoidance of hypotension in the pre-hospital phase of management will improve the eventual hospital outcome.
b. Early evacuation of intracranial hematomas in patients with neurologic symptoms decreases secondary insult to the brain and will improve hospital outcome.
c. Isoenzymes of creatine kinase may be found in the blood of head injured patients.
d. Controlled studies have proven that dexamethasone in adequate doses improves outcome in closed head injuries.

376. Which ONE of the following diagnoses is MOST compatible with the unenhanced CT scan of the head shown in Figure 27?

a. Subarachnoid hemorrhage
b. Epidural hematoma
c. Acute subdural hematoma
d. Hemorrhagic contusion

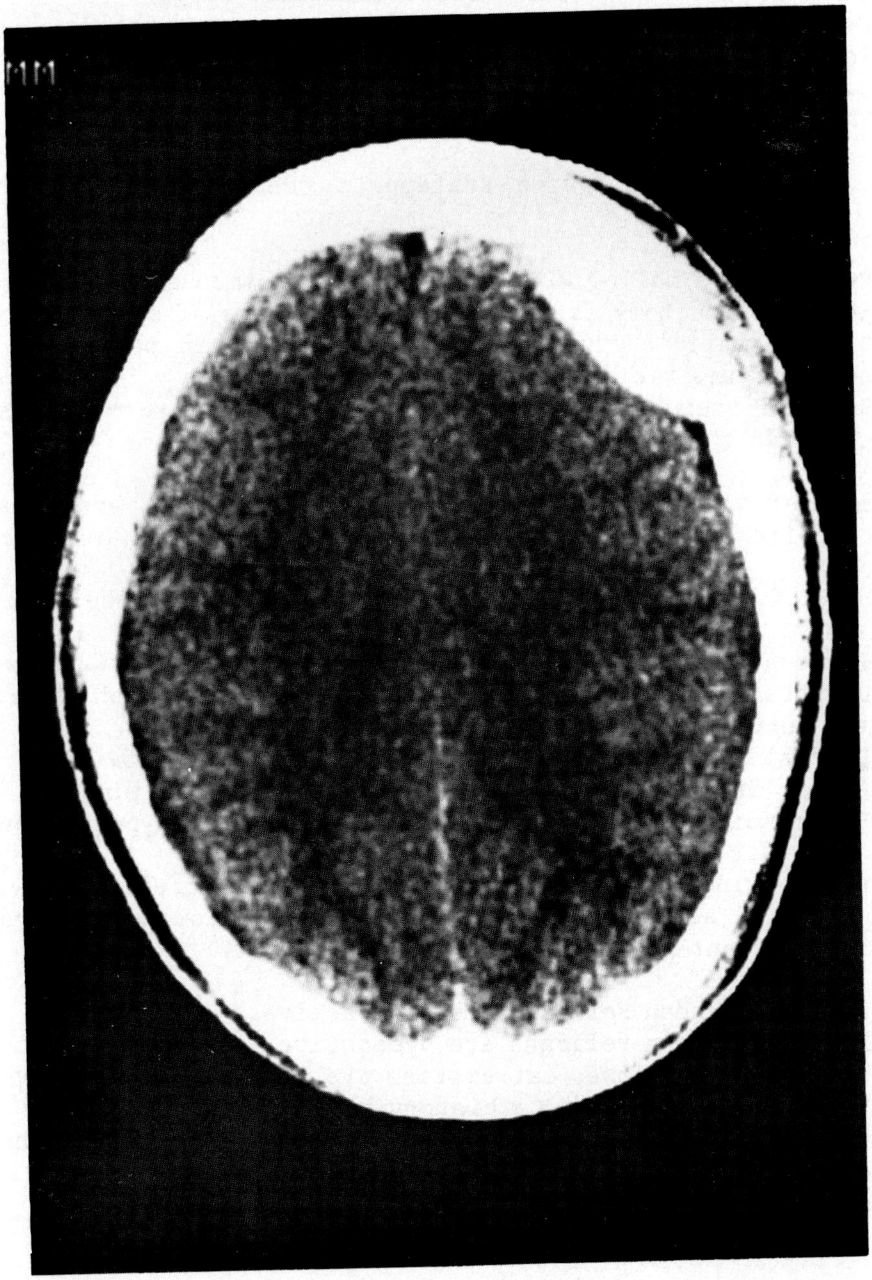

Figure 27

377. The metabolic response to severe injury includes all of the following EXCEPT:

a. Elevated plasma levels of catecholamines and glucocorticoids
b. Insulin resistance at the skeletal muscle level
c. Fat mobilization due to elevated catecholamine levels
d. Increased levels of branched-chain amino acids in the peripheral circulation
e. Increased plasma levels of glucagon

378. Which ONE of the following statements concerning pediatric trauma is TRUE?

a. Rupture of a hollow viscus is the most common abdominal injury.
b. Early splenectomy is indicated in all cases of splenic injury.
c. Diaphragmatic rupture is much more common in pediatric rather than adult trauma victims.
d. Rib and sternal fractures, and flail chest are much less common in children than in adults.

379. A three-year-old child suffered blunt chest and upper abdominal trauma in an automobile accident. His chest radiograph is shown in Figure 28.

Which ONE of the following statements concerning this child is INCORRECT?

a. Pulmonary contusion may cause his respiratory status to worsen.
b. Diaphragmatic rupture is less likely to be seen on the right than on the left.
c. Lateral decubitus chest radiographs should be obtained.
d. Aortic disruption is more likely than if this injury was in an adult.
e. Pericardial tamponade should be considered if hypotension develops.

380. You are managing a young athlete whose head perforated the windshield in an automobile accident. Which ONE of the following observations would be MOST important in determining his management?

a. All deep tendon reflexes are hyperactive.
b. All deep tendon reflexes are hypoactive.
c. Left upper and lower extremities are weaker than the right ones.
d. Two hours after giving a history he becomes somnolent.
e. On admission the left pupil is 1 mm larger than the right but equally reactive.

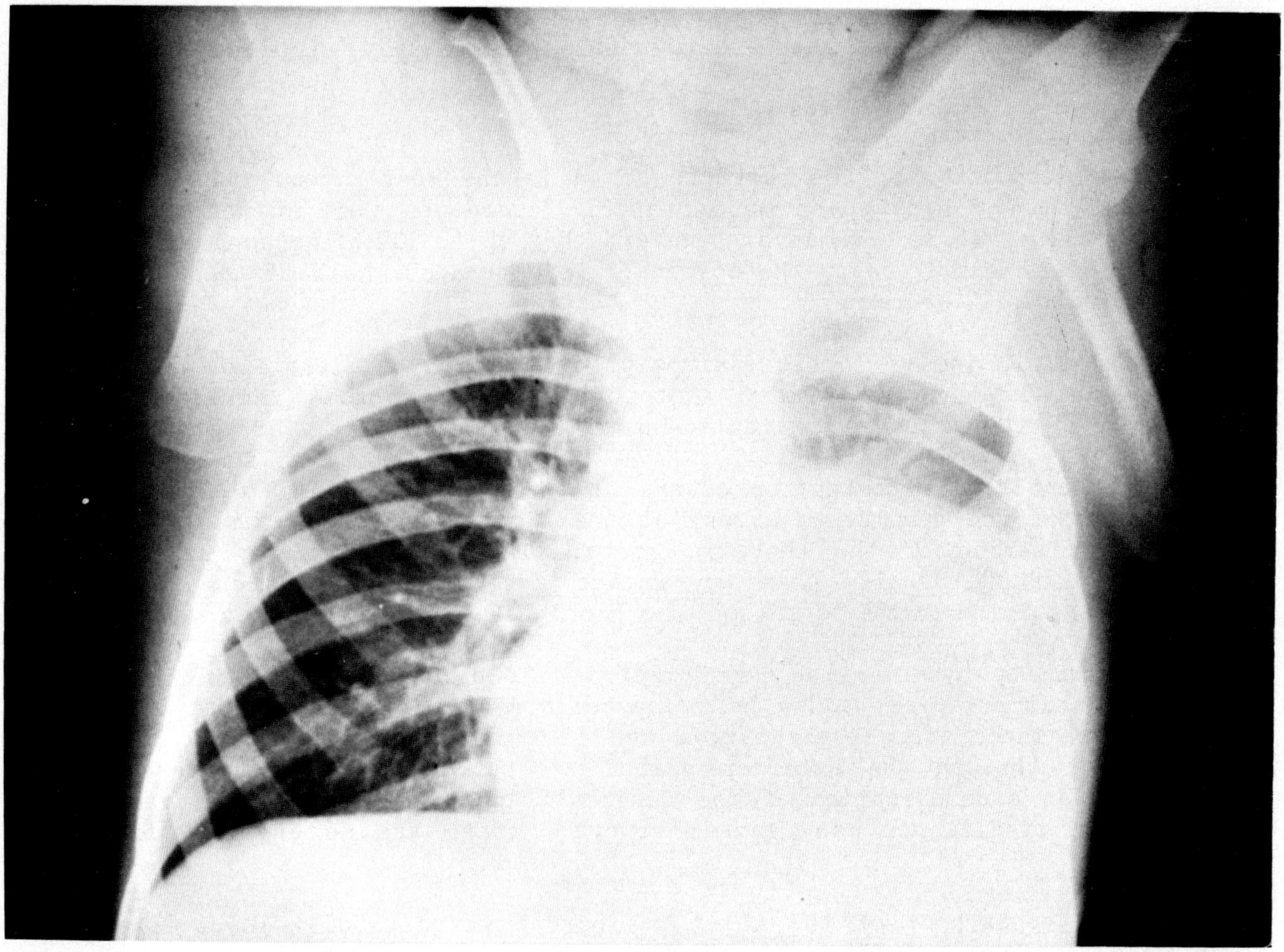

Figure 28

ANSWERS

357-c	358-b	359-c	360-a	361-c	362-b	363-b	364-c
365-c	366-d	367-a	368-d	369-c	370-d	371-d	372-a
373-b	374-d	375-d	376-b	377-d	378-d	379-d	380-d

AORTA

RATIONALE 357-c 358-b

Traumatic disruption of the thoracic aorta is the most common cause of death among victims of high speed motor vehicle accidents who do not reach the hospital alive. It is estimated, however, that up to 20% of persons who sustain such an injury live to reach the hospital. If untreated, half of these patients will die within 12 hours.

The usual mechanism of aortic disruption is a rapid deceleration, regardless of external evidence of injury. Noteworthy is a two-fold increase in the incidence of this injury in patients who are ejected from the vehicle.

Most frequently, the disruption occurs at the aortic isthmus, just distal to the origin of the subclavian artery at the ligamentum arteriosum, a point of relative fixation of the thoracic aorta. Those patients who survive the immediate injury usually have an intact adventitia and external elastic lamella, resulting in the formation of a highly dangerous false aneurysm.

Upper extremity hypertension, dyssymmetric blood pressures in the right vs. left brachial arteries, and a harsh systolic murmur can all result from the injury. An interesting presentation can be paraplegia, due to reduction in blood flow through the anterior spinal artery. Paraplegia is more often discussed as a complication of the surgical repair, but it can be primary to the injury itself. In many cases, however, there are no physical findings present.

It is the appearance of the chest radiograph which usually leads to aortography. A widening of the mediastinum and/or straightening of the left heart border are the common tipoffs to the possibility of injury. Less frequently noted are depression of the left mainstem bronchus and deviation of the trachea to the right. A bloody pleural effusion, usually on the left, will also suggest the possibility of aortic dissection.

The diagnosis ultimately rests upon the demonstration of the site of injury by aortography. In a minority of cases where exsanguinating hemorrhage into the chest is occurring, immediate thoracotomy is necessary. The majority of patients are temporarily stable and aortography, without delay, is the procedure of choice. As digital subtraction becomes more available, this may replace standard aortography. A high index of suspicion and rapid diagnostic and therapeutic intervention are important in preventing the high likelihood of a fatal outcome if the injury were to remain untreated.

In question 357, choice c lists findings suggestive of acute superior vena caval obstruction, seen with thoracic compression injuries and not associated with traumatic aortic dissection per se. Choice c is, therefore, the correct response.

In question 358, the correct response is b. While aortography is the procedure of choice, it should be undertaken with dispatch and not deferred for the several hours suggested by the answer. The remaining choices are all part of preparation for the anticipated surgery.

REFERENCES

Ayella RJ, Hankins JR, Turney SZ, et al: Ruptured thoracic aorta due to blunt trauma. J Trauma 1977; 17:199

Gayzaniga AB, Khuri EI, Mir-Sepasi HM, et al: Rupture of the thoracic aorta following blunt trauma. Arch Surg 1975; 110:1119

Marsh DG, Strum JT: Traumatic aortic rupture: Roentgenographic indications for angiography. Ann Thorac Surg 1976; 21:337

Symbas PN: Great vessel injury. Am Heart J 1977; 93:518

Wolfe WG: Traumatic aneurysms of the aorta. In: Textbook of Surgery. Thirteenth Edition. Sabiston DC (Ed). Philadelphia, WB Saunders Co., 1986, pp 1810-1815

EDITORIAL COMMENT

Most mediastinal enlargement after blunt chest trauma is not due to aortic rupture but rather to bleeding of smaller vessels. It is paramount, however, that traumatic rupture of the aorta be ruled out. This is done utilizing an unenhanced and enhanced thoracic CT scan or an aortogram. A mediastinal width on chest radiograph greater than 7.5 - 8 cm should be considered suspicious in the setting of chest trauma, but absolute measurements have not been as satisfactory as simple overall evaluation of the chest film. An upright PA inspiratory chest radiograph is optimum for this type of evaluation.

Following emergent cardiorrhaphy for penetrating blunt cardiac injuries, a significant percentage of delayed sequelae and complications occur in 4% to 56% of survivors. These sequelae frequently require secondary surgical corrections. Two-D echocardiography is useful in identifying myocardial damage, thrombi, pericardial effusion and valve disruption in these postoperative patients. In addition, pulsed-doppler echocardiography is useful in diagnosing shunts and valvular abnormalities.

ADDITIONAL REFERENCE

Mattox KL, Limacher MC, Feliciano DV, et al: Cardiac evaluation following heart injury. J Trauma 1985; 25:758

BURNS

RATIONALE 359-c

Age and percentage of surface area of burns have significant prognostic importance. Sex and race are not prognostic indices. There are currently no data to support a relationship between trunk or extremity burns and ultimate outcome, although on theoretical grounds there may be a difference. Whether anterior or posterior burns affect prognosis is also debatable, but one thing is clear; anterior trunk burns have a higher incidence of respiratory involvement and, thus, have the potential for greater lethality. As a general rule, burns of the same depth and extent (i.e., surface areas) are at greater risk for mortality in the very young (2 years) and the older (60 years) patient. Overall, survival from a 50% surface, full thickness burn is poor. Less than one-third of these patients will survive. Associated injuries and pre-existing diseases further influence outcome. Great strides have been made in the management of the burn patient in the past few years that are worthy of consideration. These fall into two major areas: resuscitation and burn wound management. We are just now beginning to unravel the complexities of metabolic changes in thermal injury. When this is more firm, then the third critical area, nutritional support, will further expand our therapeutic capabilities for these high risk, seriously ill patients.

Volume replacement with only electrolyte-containing fluids is currently favored for the first 24 hours. Whether this relates to documented local or distant (from burn site) capillary permeability is not entirely clear. However, some capillary leak is present, and it is not a good idea to infuse colloids with the possibility they may leak into the perivascular space and later draw out more fluids and further increase intravascular fluid requirements. Resuscitation in the first 24 hours with electrolyte solutions is effective and should be routinely employed. The "Parkland" formula is reasonable giving 4 ml lactated Ringer's per kilogram per percent burn in the first 24 hours. Resuscitation with hypertonic saline remains a debatable issue.

The question of nutritional support is real, and it is now believed that early and aggressive administration of calories is essential if one is to prevent late complications associated with the burn. Efforts directed at adequate replacement of maintenance calories as well as substrate for repair seems crucial if one is to avoid late complications. Energy expenditure in burns is great, and replacement must match expenditures lest vital functions, such as immunological competence, become compromised. Prompt and early attention to nutritional support in the burned patient, preferably by the enteral route, is a major requirement in burn patient management.

REFERENCES

Arturson MG: Metabolic changes following thermal injury. World J Surg 1978; 2:203

Curreri PW: Nutritional support of burn patients. World J Surg 1978; 2:215

Feller I, Crane KH: National burn information exchange. Surg Clin North Am 1970; 50:1425

Pruitt BA Jr: Advances in fluid therapy and the early care of the burn patient. World J Surg 1978; 2:139

Shea CM, Caulfield JB, Burke JB: Microvascular ultrastructure in thermal injury: A reconsideration of the role of mediators. Microvasc Res 1973; 5:87

RATIONALE 360-a 361-c 362-b 363-b 364-c 365-c

Mafenide acetate cream (Sulfamylon burn cream), 0.5% silver nitrate solution and 1% silver sulfadiazine (Silvadene) are commonly used topical antimicrobial burn wound agents. Each has its limitations.

Mafenide acetate cream may cause pain for about 20-30 minutes after application to second degree burns. It penetrates the entire eschar thickness and delivers adequate antimicrobial concentrations into the underlying tissues. This substance may also inhibit carbonic anhydrase and produce frank metabolic acidosis. Silver nitrate solution precipitates on contact and therefore does not penetrate the eschar. Silver sulfadiazine cream has been reported to cause bone marrow suppression with neutropenia. It is often ineffective against Enterobacter cloacae and may be ineffective against certain strains of Pseudomonas.

REFERENCES

Moncrief JA, Lindberg RB, Switzer WE: Use of topical antibacterial therapy in the treatment of the burn wound. Arch Surg 1966; 92:558

Pruitt BA: The Burn Patient: II. Later care and complications of thermal injury. Curr Probl Surg 1979; 16:5

EDITORIAL COMMENT

Routine administration of prophylactic low-dose penicillin in acutely burned, hospitalized patients offers neither protection against cellulitis and burn wound sepsis nor promotes selection of antibiotic-resistant bacteria.

Extensive dermal burns produce dysfunction of myocardial contractile mechanisms manifested by decreased contractility, slower isovolumic relaxation, and decreased diastolic compliance of the left ventricle in a guinea pig model.

A retrospective study suggested a decreased therapeutic efficacy of cimetidine when it was compared to antacid therapy in pediatric burn patients. The rapid clearance of cimetidine in the pediatric burn patient is offered as a possible explanation for this decreased efficiacy.

ADDITIONAL REFERENCES

Adams HR, Baxter CR, Izenberg SD: Decreased contractility and compliance of the left ventricle as complications of thermal trauma. Am Heart J 1984; 108:1477

Durtschi MB, Orgain C, Counts GW, et al: A prospective study of prophylactic penicillin in acutely burned hospitalized patients. J Trauma 1982; 22:11

Goodwin CW: Current burn treatment. In: Advances in Surgery. Vol 18. Shires GT (Ed). Chicago, Year Book Medical Publishers, 1984, pp 145-176

Martyn JAJ: Cimetidine and/or antacid for the control of gastric acidity in pediatric burn patients. Crit Care Med 1985; 13:1

DIFFERENTIAL DIAGNOSIS

RATIONALE 366-d 367-a 368-d

Shock in association with abdominal trauma is due to abdominal injury until proven otherwise. The spleen is the organ most often injured in blunt abdominal trauma, and delay in diagnosis is a major contributor to the mortality associated with splenic injuries. The presence of a normal EKG and chest film lend support to the abdomen as the likely cause of hypotension. Although significant occult blood loss can occur in a fracture site in the lower extremity and pelvis, the arm is less likely to be a cause for such a large occult volume loss. This patient's confusion is most likely secondary to hypotension.

A fracture in association with distal ischemia must be reduced. A chest radiograph and EKG are part of the complete evaluation of the multiple trauma patient.

Peritoneal lavage has increased significantly the reliability of determination of serious intraperitoneal injury in blunt trauma. It is a test properly reserved for use in equivocal cases of the need to explore the abdomen as it was in this patient on her initial presentation. There is a false negative rate of up to 5% associated with the use of peritoneal lavage. Thus, while a positive lavage is an absolute indication for laparotomy, a negative result does not discount the possibility of serious visceral injury. The negative abdominal lavage should have no bearing on the subsequent evaluation of the clinical course of the patient.

Shock following trauma is usually due to hemorrhage, and fluid resuscitation, not pressors, is the appropriate treatment. Therefore, dopamine infusion is incorrect.

In this patient, delay in treatment of the presumed hemorrhagic shock is her greatest threat. While peritoneal lavage is useful in questionable cases of the need for laparotomy and was appropriate when this patient was initially seen, there is nothing equivocal about shock. Shock in the presence of abdominal trauma requires laparotomy. While one might not be faulted for repeating a peritoneal lavage while awaiting arrival of the surgeon, this patient needs to be explored even if the repeat lavage is negative.

REFERENCES

Early Care of the Injured Patient by the Committee on Trauma of the American College of Surgeons. Third Edition. Alexander J (Ed). Philadelphia, WB Saunders Co., 1982, pp 142-148

Naylor R, Cohn D, Shires GT: Morbidity and mortality from injuries to the spleen. J Trauma 1974; 14:775

Zuidema G, Rutherford R, Ballinger W: The Management of Trauma. Third Edition. Philadelphia, WB Saunders Co., 1979, pp 457-461

EDITORIAL COMMENT

Goldstein and associates compared peritoneal lavage, intravenous pyelography, and computerized tomography in the evaluation of 103 patients with blunt abdominal trauma. They concluded that CT is the diagnostic modality of choice in the hemodynamically stable patient with nonpenetrating trauma when evaluating potential intra-abdominal injury or hematuria.

ADDITIONAL REFERENCE

Goldstein AL, Sclafani S, Kupperstein NH: The diagnostic superiority of computerized tomography. J Trauma 1984; 25:938

RATIONALE 369-c

This patient presents with the classic predisposing injuries, time course, and symptom development of fat embolism syndrome (FES). Supportive treatment is the primary mode of therapy and is usually successful. Positive end-expiratory pressure may be necessary in some cases. Steroids may be of value if instituted early, and recent data indicates their potential value as a prophylactic agent. Heparin therapy is not indicated and may actually increase the fatty acid levels. Radionuclide ventilation/perfusion scans are usually nonspecific in this setting and data do not support their usefulness in the FES. Although rib fractures have been reported with FES, long bone fractures are the hallmark of predisposition. Rib fractures would correlate best with lung contusion as the etiology of post-traumatic hypoxemia. Clinical FES classically develops in a small percentage of trauma victims with long bone fractures after 1-2 days. The three hallmarks of this syndrome are:

a. Hypoxemia (with hypocapnia)
b. Mental status changes
c. Petechiae

The chest film usually shows scattered infiltrates. A radiographic pattern consistent with ARDS may develop. Petechiae are usually, but not always, present. They are commonly found in the conjunctiva and in the axillary area.

Hypoxemia, petechiae, and mental status changes are due to intravascular lipid macroglobules. The lipid is embolized bone marrow from fracture sites. An additional source of lipid may be the intravascular formation of fatty complexes. These may be induced by chemical changes produced in the bloodstream by the trauma. The hypoxemia in FES develops later than that which would be expected from a lung contusion and earlier than with pulmonary emboli. Fat embolization syndrome occurs in approximately 2%-4% of lower extremity long bone fractures and increases with the number of fractures. Thrombocytopenia, neutrophilic leukocytosis, and low grade fever are variable findings. Thrombocytosis is not seen. Fat globules in the urine, although usually present, are a nonspecific finding and may be seen in the absence of the clinical syndrome.

REFERENCES

Moore PG, James OF: Pulmonary fat embolism. Semin Resp Med 1982; 3:275

Schonfeld SA: Fat embolism prophylaxis with corticosteroids: A prospective study in high-risk patients. Ann Intern Med 1983; 99:438

Wilson RF: Trauma. In: Textbook of Critical Care. Shoemaker WC, Thompson WL, Holbrook PR (Eds). Philadelphia, WB Saunders Co., 1984, pp 907-908

RATIONALE 370-d

In many patients with thoracic trauma in automobile accidents, there is no immediate, simple way to separate the rare patient whose bronchus has been ruptured from the usual who has no bronchial injury. The problem is even more complex because pneumothorax or other injury accompanying the bronchial rupture may satisfactorily respond to treatment at first in the same way as would be expected in a patient without bronchial injury. Signs of potential bronchial rupture are: (1) pneumothorax, (2) fracture of upper ribs, (3) subcutaneous emphysema, and (4) dyspnea. These are present in less than one-half of the total group of patients with bronchial injury. Presence of serious hemoptysis and fractured ribs should alert one to the possibility of an underlying airway injury. Bronchoscopy, followed by repair of the tracheobronchial injury, would be best. Normal blood gases are unlikely to be associated with serious lung contusion. Expectant management by measurement of hemoptysis, etc., does not appear to be warranted in a 35-year-old patient after an automobile accident. The results of pulmonary and bronchial arteriography are unlikely to be rewarding in this patient.

REFERENCES

Burke JF: Early diagnosis of traumatic rupture of the bronchus. JAMA 1962; 181:682

Munnell ER: Fracture of major airways. Am J Surg 1963; 105:511

RATIONALE 371-d

The radiograph in Figure 25 demonstrates the nasogastric tube and associated stomach gas in an apparent left hemithoracic location. Figure 29 was obtained after barium administration through the NG tube and confirms the diagnosis of diaphragmatic rupture.

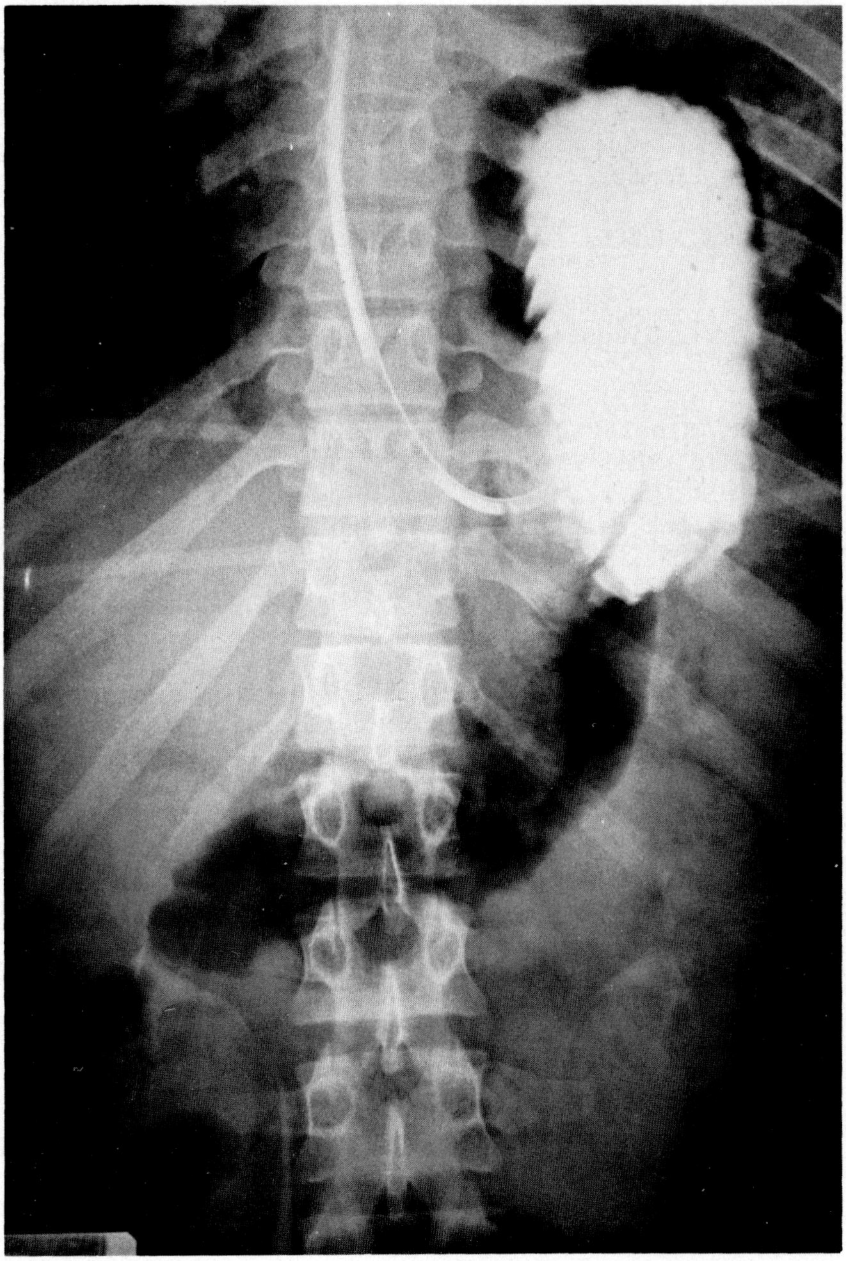

Figure 29

Diaphragmatic rupture is usually the result of severe thoracic or abdominal trauma. This condition is less likely following penetrating trauma. Although most common on the left where the liver does not offer protection, it may also develop on the right side. Variable amounts of consolidation and density may be present in the chest. Bowel air may or may not be noted. A mediastinal shift toward the side of rupture, however, is highly atypical. Because of the severity of trauma, associated injury to abdominal viscera is common. Emergency operation and repair of the defect is indicated.

REFERENCES

Cowley RA, Dunham CM: Shock Trauma/Critical Care Manual. Baltimore, University Park Press 1982, pp 130-131

Ebert PA, Gaertner RA, Zuidema GD: Traumatic diaphragmatic hernias. Surg Gynecol Obstet 1967; 129:59

Estrera AS, Platt MR, Mills LJ: Traumatic injuries of the diaphragm. Chest 1979; 75:306

Gourin AF, Garzon AA: Diagnostic problems in traumatic diaphragmatic hernia. J Trauma 1974; 14:19

Hagman J, Iguchi R, Kinsley J, et al: Diaphragmatic rupture following blunt trauma. Ann Emerg Med 1984; 13:49

Hill LD: Injuries of the diaphragm following blunt trauma. Surg Clin North Am 1972; 62:611

RATIONALE 372-a

Noted on the chest radiograph is a shift of the mediastinum to the right displayed most prominently by the tracheal air column. A massive right hemothorax generally causes a shift of the mediastinum and trachea to the left.

This patient had a fractured right bronchus. Fractures of the tracheobronchial tree most often result from blunt trauma to the anterior chest in vehicular accidents. They are uncommon and usually present with a persistent pneumothorax even after chest tube insertion. Pneumothorax may be absent in 30% of cases. They are often associated with pulmonary contusion which should also be considered as a primary diagnosis in this case. Pulmonary contusions may present as a massive patchy consolidation which progresses to uniform consolidation.

A right tension pneumothorax is associated with mediastinal shift to the left, NOT the right side. A ruptured right diaphragm should not shift trachea to that side.

REFERENCES

Bugge-Asperheim B, Svennevig JL, Birkeland S: Haemodynamic and metabolic consequences of lung contusion following blunt chest trauma. Scand J Thorac Cardiovasc Surg 1980; 14:295

Fraser RG, Pare JAP: Effects on the lungs of nonpenetrating trauma. In: Diagnosis of Diseases of the Chest. Fraser RG, Pare JAP (Eds). Philadelphia, WB Saunders Co., 1979, pp 1577-1588

Lynn RB, Iyengar K: Traumatic rupture of the bronchus. Chest 1972; 61:81

Richardson JD, Adams L, Flint LM: Selective management of flail chest and pulmonary contusion. Ann Surg 1982; 196:481

EDITORIAL COMMENT

Rupture of the trachea or bronchus occurs as a result of thoracic compression while the glottis is closed or as a result of direct penetrating tracheal trauma. Although tracheal and bronchial injuries are usually the cause of massive air leaks, esophagoscopy may also be indicated to ascertain any unsuspected esophageal injury. Traumatic bronchial injuries necessitate immediate operative intervention and repair of the defect. Surprisingly, hemoptysis is seen in only slightly less than one-half of the cases.

Since the diaphragm rises high into the chest during expiration, any wound below the 4th intercostal space anteriorly, the 8th interspace posteriorly, and the 6th interspace laterally may have penetrated the diaphragm. Diaphragmatic injury and injury to intra-abdominal organs should be suspected in this setting.

Peritoneal lavage in combination with chest radiography is reliable in identifying a ruptured diaphragm secondary to blunt trauma. Peritoneal lavage was positive in 89% of patients without other sources of intraabdominal hemorrhage. Chest radiography alone identified 41% of the diaphragm injuries. If the peritoneal lavage is negative, the radiograph is not diagnostic, and significant suspicion of diaphragm injury remains, water-soluble contrast material can be instilled through the lavage catheter into the peritoneal cavity in hopes of demonstrating the defect.

Diaphragmatic rupture is seen in both penetrating and blunt traumatic injuries to the chest or upper abdomen. If present, associated injuries may be as high as 50%-90%. The most commonly injured organs in penetrating trauma are the liver and stomach.

Recognition of traumatic diaphragm rupture requires awareness of the three phases of symptomatology: (1) the acute phase with symptoms of shock, respiratory distress and symptoms relating to injuries of other organs; (2) a latent phase, usually without symptoms; and (3) a late phase which may be as long as 35 years after injury, when the patient presents with symptoms of obstruction, strangulation, and hemorrhage. There is no reliable finding on the chest radiograph in the acute phase that documents a ruptured diaphragm unless there is herniation of intra-abdominal contents. This occurs only in a small percentage of patients.

Conservative management of isolated solid organ rupture, especially the spleen, is being increasingly utilized in selected cases, especially children. Diagnosis is made by an abdominal CT scan or by radionuclide scintigraphy. Hemodynamically stable patients should be vigilantly observed in the ICU and serial vital signs and hematocrits obtained. Need for transfusion is not an absolute indication for surgery.

ADDITIONAL REFERENCES

Ordog GJ, Wasserberger J, Balasubramaniam S: Tension gastrothorax complicating post-traumatic rupture of the diaphragm. Am J Emerg Med 1984; 2:219

Troop B, Myers RM, Agarwal NN: Early recognition of diaphragmatic injuries from blunt trauma. Ann Emerg Med 1985; 14:97

Webb WR, Moustoukas NM: Noncardiac thoracic trauma. Pulmonary Clinical Update - American College of Chest Physician 1985; 1:1

Webster VJ: Abdominal trauma: Preoperative assessment and postoperative problems in intensive care. Anaesth Intensive Care 1985; 13:258

HEAD TRAUMA

RATIONALE 373-b

As long as the airway remains unobstructed, head injured patients usually hyperventilate rather than hypoventilate. Apnea occurs during the late stages of herniation and brain stem compression. Hypotension should always alert the examiner to look for systemic sites of blood loss. Diabetes insipidus, although possible, is uncommon after head injury. Hypoxemia, on the other hand, has been documented in 40%-60% of all head injured patients presenting to the hospital. This disturbance in oxygenation may occur in the absence of obvious injury to the chest. Because hypoxia is an easily reversible cause of secondary brain injury, all head injured patients should be placed on supplemental oxygen.

REFERENCES

Safar P: Resuscitation after brain ischemia. In: Brain Failure & Resuscitation. Clinics in Critical Care Medicine. Grenvik A, Safar P (Eds). New York, Churchill Livingstone, 1981, pp 159-160

Frost EAM: Respiratory problems associated with head trauma. Neurosurgery 1979; 50:768

Jennett B, Teasdale G: Management of head injuries. Contemporary Neurology Series 20, 1981

Katsurado K, et al: Respiratory insufficiency in patients with severe head injury. Surgery 1973; 73:191

Rose MW: Avoidable factors contributing to death after head injury. Br Med J 1977; 2:615

RATIONALE 374-d

Hypotension and hypoxia are major reversible causes of secondary brain damage. In general, patients with diffuse brain injury have a better prognosis than do those with mass lesions. However, in those patients with mass lesions and brain compression, rapid removal of the lesion reduces secondary damage and improves outcome. The pediatric brain tolerates injury of any kind much better than does the adult brain.

REFERENCES

Jennett B: Scope and magnitude of the problem. In: Brain Failure & Resuscitation. Clinics in Critical Care Medicine. Grenvik A, Safar P (Eds). New York, Churchill Livingstone, 1981, pp 7-8

Jennett B, Teasdale G: Management of head injuries. Contemporary Neurology Series 20, 1981

RATIONALE 375-d

Immediately following the primary traumatic insult, the potential for secondary insult to the brain begins. The most serious errors found in the early treatment of head injuries are failure to maintain an adequate airway and failure to support the patient's blood pressure. Unfortunately, these errors were made in a significant percentage of patients in the large multinational studies of Jennett. If patients have expanding intracranial hematomas, the sooner they are removed, the smaller will be the secondary insult. Isoenzymes of creatine kinase are present in several types of neurologic disorders but are most common in traumatic head injuries. These include BB for the so-called brain specific isoenzyme as well as MB creatine kinase ("myocardium-specific"). Controlled studies have shown dexamethasone does not improve outcome in closed head injuries.

REFERENCES

Bakay RAE, Ward AA: Enzymatic changes in serum and cerebrospinal fluid in neurological injury. J Neurosurg 1983; 57:27

Braakman R, Schouten HJA: Megadose steroids in severe head injury - Results of a prospective double-blind clinical trial. J Neurosurg 1983; 58:326

Cooper PR, et al: Dexamethasone and severe head injury. J Neurosurg 1979; 51:307

Gudeman SK, Miller D: Failure of high-dose steroid therapy to influence intracranial pressure in patients with severe head injury. J Neurosurg 1979; 51:301

Hackenberry LE, Miner ME, Rea GL, et al: Biochemical evidence of myocardial injury after severe head trauma. Crit Care Med 1982; 10:641

Jennett B, Teasdale G: Management of Head Injuries. Philadelphia, FA Davis Co., 1981

Kaste M, et al: Creatine kinase isoenzymes in acute brain injury. J Neurosurg 1981; 54:511

RATIONALE 376-b

Epidural hematomas are classically seen on head CT scans as localized biconvex (lens shaped) high-density areas immediately adjacent to the cranial vault (Figure 27). They are commonly located in the area of the middle meningeal artery and are usually limited by suture lines. Acute subdural hematomas are usually concavoconvex spreading over the surface of the cerebral hemisphere. Hemorrhagic contusions appear as mass lesions of mixed high and low density within the substance of the brain tissue. Subarachnoid hemorrhage may be associated with a variety of CT abnormalities including subarachnoid, intracerebral or intraventricular blood.

REFERENCES

Becker DP, Miller JD, Young HF, et al: Diagnosis and treatment of head injury in adults. In: Neurological Surgery. Youmans IR (Ed). Philadelphia, WB Saunders Co., 1982, pp 1938-2083

New PF, Scott WR: Computed Tomography of the Brain and Orbit. Second Edition. Baltimore, William & Wilkins Co., 1975

Sutton D (Ed): A Textbook of Radiology and Imaging. Third Edition. Edinburgh, Churchill Livingstone, 1980, pp 1252-1265

EDITORIAL COMMENT

Acute brain edema occurs rapidly following fatal head injury. This likely occurs following disruption of the vasomotor centers in the hypothalamus and brainstem. Vasomotor paralysis then causes a sudden increase in cerebral blood flow and volume. This leads to sudden brain swelling which produces increased intracranial pressure, a decrease in cerebral perfusion pressure, and obstruction of venous outflow mechanisms. The resultant brain ischemia produces rapid acute brain edema. A vicious circle of further brain ischemia and brain edema ensues.

Steroid use in CNS injuries remains controversial. Although some experimental evidence supports the use of "high dose" steroids in treatment of CNS trauma, numerous clinical studies demonstrated no significant therapeutic effect. Critics of studies demonstrating no benefit argue that "high doses" were not used.

Steroid advocates recommend iv administration of at least 6 mg/kg of dexamethasone or 30 mg/kg of methylprednisolone for treatment of CNS trauma.

Most agree that if any benefit is to be gained, the steroid should be given as soon as possible following trauma.

ADDITIONAL REFERENCES

Braughler JM, Hall ED: Current application of "high-dose" steroid therapy for CNS injury. J Neurosurg 1985; 62:802

Yoshino E, Yamaki T, Higuchi T, et al: Acute brain edema in fatal head injury: Analysis by dynamic CT scanning. J Neurosurg 1985; 63:830

METABOLIC RESPONSE

RATIONALE 377-d

The hormonal response to severe injury includes elevated levels of catecholamines, glucagon, and glucocorticoids. Insulin levels relative to glucagon levels are markedly reduced. Insulin resistance has been shown to occur at the skeletal muscle level in severely traumatized patients. Protein, therefore, becomes a dominant caloric source available to the skeletal muscle. These factors result in the severe protein catabolism commonly seen in the traumatized patient. In addition, skeletal muscle catabolizes the branched-chain amino acids in this setting, resulting in decreased rather than increased levels of branched-chain amino acids in the peripheral circulation.

REFERENCES

Cerra FB, Mazuski J, Teasley K, et al: Nitrogen retention in critically ill patients is proportional to the branched-chain amino acid load. Crit Care Med 1983; 11:775

O'Donnell TF, Clowes GHA, Blackburn GL, et al: Proteolysis associated with a deficit of peripheral energy substrates. Surgery 1976; 80:192

Snelling CF, Woolf LI, Groves AL, et al: Amino acid metabolism in patients with severe burns. Surgery 1982; 91:474

Wilmore DW, Aulick LH: Metabolic changes in burned patients. Surg Clin North Am 1978; 58:1173

EDITORIAL COMMENT

Severely burned patients have an impairment in ability to metabolize sulfur-containing amino acids to inorganic sulfate. If high amounts of methionine-containing amino acids are given to burn patients they may develop signs of impaired trans-sulfurative degradation. The amount of methionine amino acids given to severely burned patients should, therefore, probably be monitored.

Patients with trauma sepsis have an accelerated synthetic rate of proteins essential for the maintenance of immunocompetence, preservation of organ function, and promotion of wound healing. This occurs in the liver and other visceral organs by the release of amino acids at rates at least 3-4 times normal through degradation of muscle protein. Although certain stress hormones play a role in this process, the principal stimuli to both muscle breakdown and hepatic acute phase protein synthesis are interleukin-1 and proteolysis-inducing factor elaborated by activated macrophages.

Savino studied 20 ventilator-dependent polytrauma patients and demonstrated that when measured energy expenditure (using indirect calorimetry) was compared between an intermittent mandatory ventilation (IMV) mode and an assist mode ventilation, the assist mode ventilation resulted in less work of breathing and less energy expenditure. Intermittent mandatory ventilation, although potentially useful in weaning, may not be appropriate in a catabolic trauma patient who is not ready to wean, particularly if the patient's spontaneous work of breathing is significant.

ADDITIONAL REFERENCES

Martensson J, Larsson J, Schildt B: Metabolic effects of amino acids solutions in severely burned patients: With emphasis on sulfur amino acids metabolism and positive breakdown. J Trauma 1985; 25:427

Pearl RH, Clowes GHA, Hirsch EF: Prognosis and survival as determined by visceral amino acid clearance in severe trauma. J Trauma 1985; 25:777

Savino JA, Dawson JA, Agarwar N: Metabolic cost of breathing in critical surgical patients. J Trauma 1985; 25:1126

PEDIATRIC TRAUMA

RATIONALE 378-d

Injury to solid organs predominates in pediatric abdominal trauma. The child's less developed abdominal musculature and flexible rib cage are attributable. Recent reports indicate that a large number of splenic injuries may be safely treated by careful observation or splenic repair and may resolve without the need for splenectomy. Because of the high incidence and severity of post-splenectomy sepsis and because of the important immunologic properties of the spleen, preservation of the spleen must be emphasized whenever possible. In these patients hepatic injury is diagnosed by ultrasonography, radionuclide scintigraphy, or computed tomography. Patients are maintained on restricted activity and vital signs followed if nonoperative management is planned. The receipt of blood transfusion is not an absolute contraindication to non-operative therapy as long as the patient remains hemodynamically stable. If there is significant nonhepatic injury requiring surgery or if the patient is deteriorating with hepatic trauma, operative intervention is necessary.

Diaphragmatic rupture appears less commonly in pediatric trauma victims than in adults but, when present, may be more subtle in its presentation. These ruptures are usually radial tears and most often located on the left side.

Because of the elasticity of the developing pediatric chest, rib and sternal fractures and flail chest are much less common in children than in adults. In fact, severe parenchymal thoracic injuries may be present with minimal or no signs of external trauma and with a normal initial chest radiograph.

REFERENCES

Berlatzky Y, Shiloni E, Krausz MM: Acute blunt traumatic rupture of the diaphragm in a child. Injury 1979; 11:62

Hood JM, Smythe BT: Nonpenetrating intra-abdominal injuries in children. J Pediatr Surg 1974; 9:69

Othersen HB Jr: Cardiothoracic injuries. In: Pediatric Trauma. Touloukian RJ (Ed). New York, John Wiley & Sons Inc., 1978, pp 305-368

Rowe MI, Marchildon MB: Pediatric trauma. In: Critical Care: State of the Art. Vol 2. Shoemaker WC, Thompson WL (Eds). Fullerton, CA, Society of Critical Care Medicine, 1981, pp II(K):13-15

RATIONALE 379-d

The chest radiograph shown in Figure 28 demonstrates left hemithoracic opacification and a fracture of the right scapula. The presence of a fractured scapula implies that significant trauma has occurred.

Diaphragmatic rupture appears less commonly in pediatric trauma victims and most often on the left side. They may be associated with thoracic opacification with or without presence of a bowel gas pattern with the thoracic cavity.

This child has suffered a significant chest trauma and has probably sustained some degree of pulmonary contusion. Worsening of his respiratory status over time is a distinct possibility.

Intercostal artery disruption may lead to hemothorax and opacification. A lateral decubitus radiograph of the chest is likely to identify blood or other fluid in the pleural space. Although diagnostic thoracentesis or chest tube insertion may be indicated in the critically injured patient, one must be wary of these procedures if diaphragmatic rupture is being strongly considered to avoid damage to abdominal organs.

A ruptured aorta is a rare occurrence in children because of the elasticity of the great vessels. Large arterial tears are more likely to occur in those arteries supplying heavy organs such as liver, spleen and kidneys. Mediastinal widening is most commonly secondary to small vessel hemorrhage. Pericardial tamponade must be strongly considered in any child with blunt chest trauma and hypotension.

REFERENCES

Berlatzky Y, Shiloni E, Krausz MM: Acute blunt traumatic rupture of the diaphragm in a child. Injury 1979; 11:62

Mustard WT, Trusler GA, Williams WG: Cardiovascular injuries. In: Care for the Injured Child. Salter RB (Ed). Baltimore, Williams & Wilkins Co., 1975, pp 143-149

Othersen HB Jr: Cardiothoracic injuries. In: Pediatric Trauma. Touloukian RJ (Ed). New York, John Wiley & Sons Inc., 1978, pp 305-368

Rowe MI, Marchildon MB: Pediatric trauma. In: Critical Care: State of the Art. Vol 2. Shoemaker WC, Thompson WL (Eds). Fullerton, CA, Society of Critical Care Medicine, 1981, pp II(K):13-15

EDITORIAL COMMENT

After the first few months of life, trauma to child passengers in motor vehicle accidents is the leading cause of death to children. Most states now have mandatory child restraining laws.

In the hemodynamically stable pediatric patient with no other abdominal trauma other than spleen or liver, most traumatologists favor diagnosis by radionuclide scintigraphy or computerized tomography followed in the stable patient by expectant observation with close monitoring of vital signs.

ADDITIONAL REFERENCES

Harris BH: Management of multiple trauma. Pediatr Clin North Am 1985; 32:175

Robertson LS: Motor vehicles. Pediatr Clin North Am 1985; 32:87

SPINAL CORD

RATIONALE 380-d

Hyperactive reflexes in the presence of downgoing toes are usually normal. Hypoactive (or absent) deep tendon reflexes could represent spinal cord trauma, and might persist for as long as 1-2 weeks after compressive damage to the spinal cord. Continued immobilization of the vertebral column (sandbags, neckbrace) is required until radiologic evaluation is complete. Dominance of one side (the same as the patient is "handed") is common. Cerebral or cord injury is still possible, of course. Depression of level of consciousness suggests compromise of both cerebral hemispheres, or of the brain stem; and progressive depression of wakefulness suggests a significantly enlarging mass lesion. Anisocoria is present in a small percentage of otherwise neurologically healthy individuals. More significance would be ascribed to a difference in reactivity, or to change in relative size.

REFERENCES

DeMyer W: Technique of the Neurologic Examination: A Programmed Text. Second Edition. New York, McGraw-Hill Book Company, 1974, pp 354-369

Plum F, Posner JB (Eds): The pathophysiology of signs and symptoms of coma. In: The Diagnosis of Stupor in Coma. Second Edition. Philadelphia, FA Davis Co., 1972, pp 6-8

EDITORIAL COMMENT

Complete spinal cord lesions block reflexes and eliminate caudal sensory and motor function. The following are well-established incomplete syndromes: (1) the central cord syndrome characterized by impairment of upper motor function rather than lower, with bladder dysfunction and variable sensory loss below the level of the lesion; (2) the Brown-Sequard syndrome resulting in ipsilateral paralysis and loss of touch and vibration sense, proprioception, and contralateral loss of temperature and pain sensation; 3) the anterior cord syndrome involving paralysis and hyperesthesia below the lesion level with proprioception preserved as well as touch and vibration; 4) the posterior cord syndrome with all motor and sensory functions preserved except touch and temperature.

ADDITIONAL REFERENCE

Luce JM: Medical management of spinal cord injury. Crit Care Med 1985; 13:126